Advances in
Disease Vector Research

Advances in Disease Vector Research

Edited by

Kerry F. Harris
Virus Vector Laboratory, Department of Entomology, Texas A&M University, College Station, Texas 77843, USA

Advances in Disease Vector Research

Volume 8

Edited by Kerry F. Harris

With Contributions by
T.V. Barrett D.T. Brown T.R. Burkot
C.R. Davies R.C. Gergerich R. Gothe
L.D. Jones M.L. Miller M. Mogi A.W.H. Neitz
P.A. Nuttall H.A. Scott T. Sota R.A. Wirtz

Springer-Verlag
New York Berlin Heidelberg London
Paris Tokyo Hong Kong Barcelona

Kerry F. Harris
Virus Vector Laboratory
Department of Entomology
Texas A&M University
College Station, TX 77843, USA

Volumes 1 and 2 of *Current Topics in Vector Research* were published by Praeger Publishers, New York, NY.

ISSN: 0934-6112

Printed on acid-free paper.

Typeset by Best-set Typesetter Ltd., Quarry Bay, Hong Kong.

9 8 7 6 5 4 3 2 1

ISBN-13: 978-1-4612-7800-9 e-ISBN-13: 978-1-4612-3110-3
DOI: 10.1007/978-1-4612-3110-3

Preface

In Chapter 1, Rose Gergerich and Howard Scott review their most recent research on the mechanism of virus transmission by leaf-feeding beetles. Based on these studies, the authors conclude that vector specificity is determined by virus-plant interactions that occur after virus in beetle regurgitant is deposited at a feeding-wound site. This form of vector specificity appears unique to beetle-borne viruses in that it is ultimately controlled by virus-plant rather than virus-vector interactions. An important step in the unraveling of the mystery surrounding the transmission process was the development of a gross-wound inoculation technique. The latter produces a wound site and introduces virus in a manner similar to the feeding process of viruliferous beetles. By combining this technique with gross-wound inocula containing purified virus and beetle regurgitant or RNase, Gergerich and Scott were able to demonstrate that beetle regurgitant, and specifically the RNase in regurgitant, can selectively prevent infection by viruses not transmitted by beetles. Beetle transmissible viruses can translocate (via the xylem) from gross-wound sites and, subsequently, infect unwounded plant cells, whereas non-beetle transmissible viruses cannot. Future research efforts will be directed at determining the bases for these differences and the mechanism by which beetle-transmissible viruses initiate cell infection following translocation.

Patricia Nuttall, Linda Jones and Clive Davies discuss, in Chapter 2, the role of arthropod vectors in arbovirus evolution. The co-evolution of arthropod-borne viruses of vertebrates (arboviruses) with their arthropod vectors may span at least 100 million years. Today some 500 viruses are listed in the "International Catalogue of Arboviruses." Many of the arthropod vectors of these viruses also act as resevoir hosts, maintaining the arbovirus infection for relatively long periods. These considerations—evolutionary history, arbovirus diversity, and maintenance of arbovirus infections—indicate that arthropod vectors play a major role in arbovirus evolution.

The authors consider that the evolutionary role of the arthropod can be distinguished at two levels: as a medium in which genetic changes (the building blocks of evolution) occur, and as a selective pressure that drives the course of arbovirus evolution. Changes in viral genotype take place during virus replication. The foci of infection within the arthropod vector represent the anatomical basis of arbovirus evolution. For example, the gut of mosquitoes and ticks is implicated as the site of virus reassortment (a means of rapid virus evolution through the exchange of viral genes). Target sites of infection within the arthropod vector also act as selection pressures, e.g., the gut barrier, gut release barrier, salivary gland barrier, etc. Such barriers must be overcome by the infecting virus as a prelude to successful virus transmission to a new host. The importance of transmissibility implies selection for arboviruses of relatively low virulence in their vector and comparatively high virulence in their vertebrate host. This contrasts with the established view that evolution favors reduced virulence. Other examples of vector-mediated selection pressures relate to interspecific and intraspecific vector variation. For example, vectors having a high threshold of infection will select for virus strains that induce high levels of viremia. Comparisons of the roles of vector and vertebrate hosts suggest that the arthropod vector has more opportunities than the vertebrate host to influence the course of arbovirus evolution.

In Chapter 3, Motoyoshi Mogi and Teiji Sota discuss the many parameters of integrated control of mosquitoes and mosquito-borne diseases in ricelands. The flooded land required for the optimal growth of high-yield rice varieties also provides mosquito vectors of human diseases such as malaria, filariasis, and viral encephalitis with extensive larval habitats. The authors present their treatise in three parts, beginning by pointing out similarities and dissimilarities between integrated control of economic pests and human disease vectors. Next, they describe the characteristics of rice agroecosystems as mosquito habitats and briefly review methods for riceland mosquito control. In the final section, Mogi and Sota focus on livestock management, hopefully to stimulate additional research into this very important but least explored component of integrated control of mosquitoes and mosquito-borne diseases in ricelands. The authors close by noting that the persistence of mosquito-borne diseases in ricelands is a consequence of the overall effects of environmental components and human factors which together provide for all essential links in a pathogen transmission cycle. Thus, although certainly worldwide in scope, mosquito-borne disease problems in ricelands are also distinctly local and require a full awareness of local situations for successful resolution.

Bob Wirtz and Thomas Burkot present, in Chapter 4, a comprehensive overview of traditional and more recent methodologies for detecting malarial parasites in mosquitoes. The identification of sporozoite-infected mosquitoes is an integral part of many malaria epidemiological studies. Historically, this has been accomplished by dissection of freshly killed mosquitoes and examination of the salivary glands—a labor intensive, time-consuming, costly process requiring experienced technicians which still does not permit species identification of the parasite. The development of new biotechnology-based methods has significantly reduced both time and cost factors while simplifying and improving our ability to detect and identify sporozoites.

The latter is best exemplified by the production and use of species-specific, anti-circumsporozoite protein monoclonal antibodies (MAbs) in immunofluorescent antibody or immunohistochemical assays. Immunofluorescent antibody assays permit species identification of salivary gland sporozoites from field collected mosquitoes, whereas immunohistochemical assays make such tests possible in many more laboratories by eliminating the need for a fluorescent microscope. Coupling MAbs with enzyme-linked immunosorbent assays (ELISAs) and immunoradiometric assays permits the testing of large numbers of dried mosquitoes and lessens the logistic burden associated with many field studies. Indeed, the distribution of ELISA kits to scientists without resources to develop their own assays is one of the most successful examples of the transfer of biotechnology to developing countries, greatly facilitating comparisons of data from different geographic regions. However, before such assays are used on field-collected mosquitoes, it is essential to verify that the target epitope of the MAb, present on the sporozoite, is conserved in new study areas. The authors are confident of a continuing increase in the use of nucleic acid probes in malaria research. Ribosomal RNA (rRNA) probes offer tremendous potential for the development of diagnostic systems for the quantitative and species-specific detection of both mosquito vectors and malaria parasites. DNA probes will continue to be valuable but await adaptation to nonradioisotopic detection systems to become routinely useful in field laboratories. Wirtz and Burkot also note that, except for transmission studies, establishing the vector status of an anopheline mosquito requires the combined use of traditional and more recent technologies for sporozoite detection and identification.

In Chapter 5, Mary Miller and Dennis Brown review the study of alphavirus infection in vertebrate and mosquito cell culture. They summarize recent reports on virus entry into vertebrate cells and replication of viral RNA during the early stages of infection. Evidence of host cell participation in both vertebrate and invertebrate cells is reviewed with emphasis on the differences in host cell response between the two phylogenetically distinct systems. Molecular genetic approaches to understanding the process of alphavirus infection are also described. The authors end their chapter with a discussion of viral morphogenesis and cytopathic response to infection in mosquito cells, and the establishment of the persistently infected state in insect culture. Their emphasis is on the importance of characterizing alphavirus infection in insect cells as models for controlling the pathogenic viruses that insects vector.

Advances in triatomine bug ecology in relation to Chagas' disease are discussed in Chapter 6. Since all of the approximately 116 species of

Triatominae are directly or indirectly of interest in the study of Chagas' disease, Toby Barrett, the author, begins by considering the individual species according to their taxonomic groupings. This unbiased arrangement reveals that ecology and distribution are often well correlated with systematics. Additionally, it calls attention to those groups for which our ecological knowledge is most inadequate and avoids the danger of confusing degrees of synanthropy with stages of an evolutionary trend. Barrett discusses recent developments in the population dynamics of domestic vectors along with work on the influence of human ecology on vector populations. The author provides a synopsis of the current status of research, with directions to the literature on the different aspects of a rather wide topic, while examining critically some of the conclusions that have been drawn from previous work. The possible effects of environmental alterations on triatomine populations are briefly considered, as are the implications of advances in population genetics and molecular taxonomy for ecological studies.

Past achievements and recent advances in the pathogenesis and etiology of tick paralyses are discussed in Chapter 7. The authors, Rainer Gothe and Albert Neitz review the past 60 years of progress in research and list 60 tick species belonging to 10 genera as potential paralysis inducers. Pathomechanisms and etiology of tick paralyses, however, are only investigated in the disease syndrome caused by *Argas (Persicargas) walkerae, Dermacentor andersoni* and *D. variabilis, Rhipicephalus evertsi evertsi* and *Ixodes holocyclus*. But these tick species are of medical importance: *I. holocyclus* of Australia and *D. andersoni* and *D. variabilis* of North America in human medicine, and these same species as well as *R. evertsi evertsi* and *A. walkerae* of the Ethiopian faunal region in veterinary medicine.

I thank the authors for their outstanding contributions and their patience and support while working with me to bring Volume 8 of *Advances in Disease Vector Research* to a successful and rewarding conclusion. And, as always, the encouragement and technical assistance of the members of the Editorial Board and the staff of Springer-Verlag are humbly acknowledged and sincerely appreciated.

Kerry F. Harris

Contents

Contributors

Toby V. Barrett
Departamento da Ciências de Saúde, Instituto Nacional de Pesquisas da Amazônia, 69083 Manaus-AM, Brazil

Dennis T. Brown
Cell Research Institute and Department of Microbiology, The University of Texas at Austin, Austin, Texas 78713, USA

Thomas R. Burkot
Tropical Health Program, Queensland Institute of Medicial Research, Bramston Terrace, Herston, Brisbane, Queensland 4006, Australia

Clive R. Davies
Department of Medical Parasitology, London School of Hygiene & Tropical Medicine, UK

Rose C. Gergerich
Department of Plant Pathology, University of Arkansas, Fayetteville, Arkansas 72701, USA

Rainer Gothe
Institute for Comparative Tropical Medicine and Parasitology, University of Munich, W-8000 Munich 40, Germany

Linda D. Jones
NERC Institute of Virology & Environmental Microbiology, Oxford, OX 1 3SR, UK

Mary L. Miller
Cell Research Institute and Department of Microbiology, The University of Texas at Austin, Austin, Texas 78713, USA

Motoyoshi Mogi
Division of Parasitology, Department of Microbiology, Saga Medical School, Nabeshima, Saga 849, Japan

Albert W.H. Neitz
Department of Biochemistry, University of Pretoria, Pretoria 0002, Republic of South Africa

Patricia A. Nuttall
NERC Institute of Virology & Environmental Microbiology, Oxford, OX 1 3SR, UK

Howard A. Scott
Department of Plant Pathology, University of Arkansas, Fayetteville, Arkansas 72701, USA

Teiji Sota
Division of Parasitology, Department of Microbiology, Saga Medical School, Nabeshima, Saga 849, Japan

Robert A. Wirtz
Department of Entomology, Walter Reed Army Institute of Research, Washington D.C. 20307, USA

Contents for Previous Volumes

Volume 1

Volume 2

Volume 3

Volume 4

Volume 5

Volume 6

Volume 7

1
Determinants in the Specificity of Virus Transmission by Leaf-feeding Beetles

Rose C. Gergerich and Howard A. Scott

Introduction

Vector specificity is a well-recognized characteristic of plant viruses. The plant viruses that are transmitted by leaf-feeding beetles are in four virus groups and cannot be transmitted by other commonly recognized virus vectors such as aphids, leafhoppers, or nematodes. The basis for vector specificity has been elucidated for some virus–vector combinations, and in many cases the interaction between the vector and virus is determined by virus coat proteins or by nonstructural proteins, as with the aphid-transmitted potyviruses and caulimoviruses (16, 17). These viral proteins have been shown to mediate a specific, definitive interaction of the virus particle with some surface of the vector. Sites of virus binding to vector surfaces that play a role in vector specificity have been identified for nematode, fungal, aphid, and leafhopper vectors (2, 16, 17). In some cases, virus coat proteins are involved in interactions with and transport across vector membranes as in the case with luteovirus passage through the aphid gut wall and accessory salivary gland cells (15).

This chapter is a review of research that has been conducted in our laboratory on the mechanism of virus transmission by leaf-feeding beetles. Vector specificity for beetle-transmitted viruses appears to be controlled by the interaction of virus particles with the host plant following beetle feeding and delivery of the virus to the plant in regurgitant. This is a unique type of virus–vector specificity controlled by virus–plant interactions rather than the virus–vector interactions characteristic of other plant virus transmission systems.

Rose C. Gergerich, Department of Plant Pathology, University of Arkansas, Fayetteville, Arkansas 72701, USA.
Howard A. Scott, Department of Plant Pathology, University of Arkansas, Fayetteville, Arkansas 72701, USA.

Readers are referred to numerous reviews of the types of plant viruses and the beetles that transmit them as well as the epidemiology of these viruses (5–8). Many of the procedures used in vector research with leaf-feeding beetles have also been reviewed (14). This chapter will be concerned with the proposed mechanism of vector specificity of plant virus transmission by leaf-feeding beetles.

Association of Plant Viruses with Beetle Vectors

Regurgitant

Initial explanations of virus transmission by leaf-feeding beetles postulated a simple mechanical process involving contaminated mouthparts (39). Early investigators (25) also suggested that the ability of beetles to transmit viruses is related to the regurgitation of infective virus from the foregut. Although beetles regurgitate during feeding, they do not have typical salivary glands. Cephalic glands, however, are present but their functions are unknown (40). Mexican bean beetles, *Epilachna varivestis* Muls., that had fed on bean leaves infiltrated with bromphenol blue, deposited dye when they attempted to feed on filter paper disks that had been soaked in 10% sucrose (R. Gergerich and H. Scott, unpublished observations), or if they fed on etiolated bean leaves, the blue dye could be seen along the edges of the feeding areas (21). Various stimuli will induce viruliferous beetles to regurgitate and the collected regurgitant can be analyzed for virus and other components of regurgitant (11).

Our studies indicate that beetles deposit virus in regurgitant on the surface of the leaf during feeding. Both a transmitted virus, the cowpea strain of southern bean mosaic (CP-SBMV), and a nontransmitted virus, the cowpea strain of tobacco mosaic virus (CP-TMV), are found in beetle regurgitant on the leaf surface either when the viruses are acquired through feeding on infected tissue or following injection of purified virus into the hemocoel (35). These two viruses also were detected in emitted regurgitant from beetles that had fed on infected bean leaves indicating that the source of the virus on the bean leaves is from regurgitant and not just contaminated mouthparts (21, 35).

Regurgitant components apparently do not destroy the infectivity of plant viruses. The activity of southern bean mosaic virus (SBMV) or CP-TMV when mixed with regurgitant remained at the same level as that in plant sap when both were stored for 7 days at room temperature (8). When cowpea chlorotic mottle virus (a bromovirus) and zucchini yellow mosaic virus (a potyvirus), were mixed with regurgitant and then re-isolated from virus/regurgitant mixtures by CsCl density gradients, they were still infective (26). Although regurgitant contains numerous proteases

(22) and high levels of ribonuclease (13), plant viruses apparently are not inactivated by these enzymes in virus-regurgitant mixtures. A likely exception to this is cucumber mosaic virus, which is destroyed when mixed with ribonuclease at concentrations much lower than that found in beetle regurgitant (3).

Proteolytic enzymes in beetle regurgitant partially digest the coat proteins of intact virus particles of several comoviruses. This digestion results in a change in the overall charge on the virus particle, but it does not inactivate the virus (22). Proteolytic conversion of comoviruses such as bean pod mottle (BPMV), cowpea mosaic (CPMV), and squash mosaic (SqMV) is highly specific and for CPMV has been shown to be restricted to the carboxyl terminal portion of the smaller of the two capsid proteins (28). Trypsin is one of the enzymes known to digest comovirus coat proteins (28). Beetle regurgitant exhibits strong proteolytic activity and a portion of this activity is trypsin-like (22). The limited digestion of comoviruses by the beetle during the transmission process is a unique type of interaction between a vector and a plant virus. Although this modification apparently is not necessary for the infectivity of the virus, it may play some necessary role in the interaction of the virus with the beetle.

Hemolymph

Viruses that are acquired by beetle feeding on virus-infected leaves are found in the hemolymph of the beetle vector. Freitag (4) first demonstrated that beetle-transmitted SqMV could be found in the hemolymph of viruliferous striped cucumber beetles, *Acalymma trivittata* (Mann.). Several other viruses have been recorded in the hemolymph of beetles that had fed on virus-infected tissue including the beetle-transmissible SBMV (35), CP-SBMV (38), CPMV (37), and the non-beetle-transmissible CP-TMV (35). Slack and Fulton (37) reported that tobacco ringspot virus (TRSV) and BPMV were not present in the hemolymph of viruliferous beetles, but they used undiluted hemolyph in their infectivity tests. The subsequent demonstration that hemolymph contains an inhibitor (8) and that a dilution of at least 200-fold of the hemolymph is necessary to overcome the inhibitor suggest that their results with undiluted hemolymph should be reevaluated.

Ingested virus appears very rapidly in hemolymph of beetles (8), and virus injected into the hemocoel can be transmitted by the beetle (33, 35). The site of transfer from the gut into the hemocoel and from the hemocoel into the regurgitant is unknown. CP-SBMV was detected in the hemolymph of bean leaf beetles, *Cerotoma trifurcata* Forst., for 7 days after they fed on infected plants for 24 h. The concentration of virus in the hemolymph and the ability of the beetle to transmit the virus were reduced with time (38). This decrease in concentration suggests that multiplication of the virus in the beetle does not occur.

Beetles apparently respond actively to injection of plant viruses into the hemocoel. Injection of CP-SBMV, a beetle-transmissible virus, and CP-TMV, a non-beetle-transmissible virus, into the hemocoel of bean leaf beetles led to active phagocytosis of these viruses by beetle hemocytes. In large phagosomes, the CP-TMV particles were tightly packed forming paracrystalline bodies that survived up to 2 weeks after injection (19, 20). The beetle response when virus particles are introduced into the hemocoel by the more natural process of virus acquisition through beetle feeding on infected leaves is not known.

Detailed studies on virus in the hemolymph were based on the assumption that association of virus with the hemolymph might be a factor in explaining transmission and specificity. However, a non-beetle-transmissible virus also moved into the hemolymph after acquisition by feeding on infected leaves and the association of virus with the hemolymph was in many ways similar to a beetle-transmissible virus (35). The hemocoel appears to be involved in retention of virus for several days or weeks but does not seem to be a factor in vector specificity.

Beetle Regurgitant as a Determinant in Virus Transmission

Although non-beetle-transmissible viruses are not inactivated by beetle regurgitant (26) and are deposited as infective virus on the surface of the leaf during feeding (35), no transmission occurs. The original assumption was that regurgitant components inhibited the transmission of viruses, but when dilutions of regurgitant were mixed with virus and mechanically inoculated, the dilution end point at which regurgitant no longer had an effect on local lesion formation was the same for a beetle-transmissible virus, SBMV, and a non-beetle-transmissible virus, TRSV (11).

Mechanical inoculation of Carborundum-dusted leaves produces damage that is quite different from that produced by beetles during feeding. The gross-wound inoculation technique was developed to mimic beetle feeding damage on leaves. When virus/regurgitant mixtures were inoculated using this technique, the presence of undiluted regurgitant prevented transmission of non-beetle-transmissible viruses but did not interfere with infection by beetle-transmissible viruses (11, 26). The gross-wound inoculation technique uses the fractured edge of a glass cylinder (cut from a Pasteur pipet) to bore a leaf disk out of the leaf to be inoculated (11). The glass cylinder is dipped into an inoculum mixture prior to cutting the disk. This technique mimics beetle feeding in that entire areas of the leaf are removed and many types of cells are damaged as the cylinder cuts through the leaf. Also, the inoculum mixture bathes these wounded cells much like regurgitant does when the beetle damages cells with its mandibles while regurgitating onto the leaf.

The role of regurgitant in virus transmission was dramatically demonstrated using the gross-wounding technique. Although all viruses tested were infectious when inoculated with the gross-wounding technique, the addition of regurgitant to the inoculum mixture prevented infection of all but the beetle-transmissible viruses. Regurgitants from three different leaf-feeding beetles, the bean leaf beetle, the Mexican bean beetle, and the spotted cucumber beetle, *Diabrotica undecimpunctata howardii* (Barber), produced this selective inhibitory effect when inoculated in combination with several beetle-transmissible and non-beetle-transmissible viruses (11, 26). An important feature of this inhibitory effect is that its selective nature is only evident if the gross-wounding method of inoculation is used.

The effect of regurgitant on virus transmission is not due to inactivation of non-beetle-transmissible viruses nor to irreversible binding of some regurgitant component to virus particles. When a mixture of regurgitant and a non-beetle-transmissible virus was diluted (11), or viruses were repurified from mixtures of regurgitant and virus by CsCl density gradients (26), the viruses were infective when inoculated with the gross-wounding technique or with mechanical inoculation. The lack of evidence for direct inactivation of the non-beetle-transmissible viruses suggests that the inhibitor in regurgitant must function by affecting either the host itself or the interaction of the virus with the host.

Role of Regurgitant Ribonuclease in Specificity of Transmission

Investigation into the component(s) of beetle regurgitant responsible for its selective inhibitory effect on non-beetle-transmissible viruses revealed that the factor(s) is heat labile, has a molecular weight of more than 50,000 daltons, and is stable below −20°C (11). The factor is not present or is found only in low concentration in plant sap as plant sap in gross-wound inoculation mixtures did not inhibit virus transmission.

Beetle regurgitant contains numerous enzymes, such as proteases (22), nucleases (13), and cellulases (R. Gergerich, unpublished observations). The introduction of several types of proteases into inoculum mixtures did not reproduce the selective inhibitory effect of regurgitant (R. Gergerich unpublished observations). However, when pancreatic ribonuclease (RNase) was added to the inoculum mixture at activity levels equivalent to those found in the regurgitant of three types of leaf-feeding beetles, the specific inhibitory effect of beetle regurgitant on non-beetle-transmissible viruses was reproduced (13). This inhibitory effect was noted at activities of RNase much lower than that found in regurgitant. For instance, transmission of CP-TMV and TRSV was inhibited at RNase activities one-twentieth of that found in Mexican bean beetle regurgitant. In contrast, the beetle-transmissible SBMV and BPMV were transmitted when the concentration of pancreatic RNase in the inoculum was fivefold higher than that in Mexican bean beetle regurgitant (13). The RNase activity in regurgitant of different leaf-feeding beetles ranged from a high of 2600 Kalnitsky units for the Mexican bean beetle to 195 Kalnitsky units for the spotted cucumber beetle. For comparison purposes, bovine pancreatic RNase at 1 mg/ml had an activity of 2400 Kalnitsky units (13). The RNase activity in plant sap was only 20 to 30 Kalnitsky units indicating that most of the RNase activity in beetle regurgitant is probably derived from the beetle. Our experiments using pancreatic RNase indicate that the inhibition of transmission of viruses during beetle feeding or by gross wounding is because of the presence of RNase in regurgitant. However, our experiments do not eliminate the possibility of other regurgitant components that may affect virus transmission.

Experimental evidence suggests that the selective inhibitory effect of pancreatic RNase is due to the enyzmatic action of this protein. Three types of RNases differing in their modes of cleaving ribonucleic acid (RNA) prevented transmission of non-beetle-transmissible viruses when mixed with these viruses and inoculated by the gross-wound procedure (9). Also, pancreatic RNase that had been oxidized to eliminate its enzymatic activity did not prevent gross-wound transmission of non-beetle-transmissible viruses (H. Scott, unpublished observations). The ability of RNase to digest RNA apparently is responsible for its effect on transmission when viruses are inoculated by gross wounding or beetle feeding. The effect of RNase, however, must take place after inoculation of the virus because non-beetle-transmissible viruses are not inactivated by exposure of these viruses to regurgitant in a test tube. RNase may block some early event in virus infection of plant cells by digesting RNA. The failure of RNase to affect beetle-transmissible viruses suggests that the manner in which these viruses infect plants differs in some key way from that of non-beetle-transmissible plant viruses.

Unique Properties of Beetle-Transmissible Viruses that May Explain Their Transmissibility

Early experiments to determine how the beetle-transmissible viruses infect cells despite the presence of RNase at the inoculation site were based on the premise that these viruses somehow escape from the feeding site that contains the wounded cells and RNase. Evidence was obtained using the beetle-transmissible SBMV that the initial cells that are infected following gross-wound inoculation are not on the wounded edge of the inoculation site. When cells immediately surrounding the gross-wound site were killed by incorporating 1% sodium azide into the inoculum, SBMV was still transmitted (12). The azide killed a halo of tissue approximately 2 to 3 mm wide within 30 min after wounding; therefore, all cells wounded during inoculation apparently were dead and the infected cells were at a distance of at least 2 to 3 mm from the wounded edge. These results indicate that SBMV is translocated away from the site of inoculation into an area of unwounded cells where infection occurs. In contrast to the results with SBMV, two beetle-transmissible viruses, BPMV and black gram mottle virus, were as sensitive to the effects of sodium azide as were TRSV and CP-TMV, two non-beetle-transmissible viruses (R. Gergerich and H. Scott, unpublished observations). This suggests that members of the sobemovirus group are more mobile or infect in a different manner than do other viruses and thus overcome the effects of RNase in beetle regurgitant.

A comparison of the movement of purified virus particles of several beetle-transmissible and non-beetle-transmissible viruses in the xylem of cut stems of young bean plants indicates that beetle-transmissible viruses move in the xylem, whereas non-beetle-transmissible viruses do not (10). In these tests, young bean and cowpea plants, the first trifoliolate leaves of which were just beginning to expand, were severed at the base and then recut under water. The severed plants were placed in a concentrated suspension of purified virus (5 mg/ml) for 2 h. Beetle-transmissible viruses were found to be rapidly translocated to both the primary leaves and growing point of the test plants, as judged by virus infectivity assays of extracts from these plant parts. Non-beetle-transmissible viruses were not found in the primary leaves or growing points. However, when purified SBMV was successfully translocated in a similar manner into the primary leaves and the growing point of Pinto bean, a local lesion host, local lesions formed only in the young trifoliolates and not in the expanded primary leaves (R. Gergerich, unpublished observations). This suggests that SBMV cannot infect all plant parts to which it is translocated.

The ability to establish infection in unwounded plant cells appears to be a property of viruses that are transmitted by beetles. We used an experimental system described by Caldwell (1) and Schneider and Worley (34) to determine whether viruses can translocate through steam-killed sections of bean stems and subsequently infect unwounded cells above the steam-killed area. Only beetle-transmissible viruses established infection above the steam-killed stem sections when injected into the stem below the steam-killed area (10). Several non-beetle-transmitted viruses that we tested (10) and that were tested in a similar system (31, 32) did not infect systemic hosts above steam-killed areas. These observations suggest that two general characteristics of beetle-transmissible viruses are translocation in the xylem of plants and infection of unwounded cells.

Results of our research suggest that viruses transmitted by beetles differ from other viruses in translocation and in the manner in which they initiate primary infection. This difference is apparent when the viruses are inoculated by beetle feeding, by gross wounding in the presence of beetle regurgitant or RNase, or by injection of virus into stems below steam-killed areas. In the last case, the viruses must be translocated and initiate infection in unwounded cells. In the case of beetle feeding or gross-wound inoculation, the presence of regurgitant or RNase at the feeding site or gross wound appears to prevent infection of wounded cells at the point of introduction, and only those viruses that can be translocated and infect unwounded cells are successful under these inoculation conditions.

The differences in translocatability between beetle-transmissible and non-beetle-transmissible viruses raise the interesting question of what governs translocation of virus particles in plants. The simplest explanation would be a specific binding between some plant component, such as the cell wall or cell membrane, and the virus particle resulting in immobilization of the non-beetle-transmissible viruses. If non-beetle-transmissible viruses are bound, the beetle-transmissible viruses probably have a mechanism or surface property that prevents or at least limits their being bound to plant cell components.

Non-translocatability of a virus and the inability of the virus to infect unwounded cells may be closely related. If non-beetle-transmissible viruses are immobilized (not translocated) because of binding to some external component of the plant cell, this same interaction may prevent movement and entry of these viruses into unwounded cells where they initiate infection. Recently, evidence indicates that intact virus particles enter the cell and uncoat inside the cell through cotranslational disassembly (42). Immobilization of non-beetle-transmissible viruses on external cellular structures would prevent this type of infection. However, cotranslational disassembly has been observed only in cells wounded by mechanical inoculation of Carborundum-dusted leaves.

Sites of Infection of Beetle-Transmitted Viruses

Virus-specific fluorescent antibody staining has been used to detect virus-infected cells (24) in leaves following gross wounding or feeding by viruliferous beetles (29, 30). Immunofluorescent staining of leaf pieces that had been gross wounded revealed fluorescence only in association with veins when the inoculum consisted of purified preparations of SBMV, BPMV, and the non-beetle-transmissible CP-TMV and TRSV. No fluorescence was detected when TRSV and CP-TMV were mixed with regurgitant or RNase and inoculated.

The patterns of fluorescent staining observed for SBMV and BPMV were quite different. Fluorescence associated with SBMV infection was seen in the veins of the leaf and appeared to increase with time after inoculation. However, even 8 days postinoculation the fluorescence was still restricted to veins leading from the gross-wound edge. Control experiments in which Carborundum-dusted leaves were mechanically inoculated with SBMV indicated that SBMV-infected mesophyll cells were readily detected by the fluorescent antibody staining procedure. In contrast, the fluorescence of BPMV was associated with the veins leading from the feeding site but spread to the mesophyll cells surrounding the vein near the wound edge within 48 h of inoculation. The presence of regurgitant or RNase did not affect the pattern of infection of SBMV or BPMV. Gross-wound inoculation with purified TRSV and CP-TMV, two viruses not transmitted by beetles, in the absence of regurgitant or RNase produced a pattern of infection similar to that seen for BPMV. Fluorescence was not seen when TRSV and CP-TMV were inoculated in the presence of regurgitant or RNase.

Research on the detection of infection sites following gross wounding or beetle feeding on leaves did not provide a complete explanation. For instance, why is infection, as detected by fluorescent antibody staining, always associated with the veins of the leaf? The association is present even with infection by non-beetle-transmissible viruses when purified virus is inoculated by gross wounding. It does not appear to be due to a limitation of the fluorescent antibody staining technique, because control experiments with mechanically inoculated leaves clearly revealed virus infection of mesophyll cells. A possible answer is that with this particular kind of inoculation the only susceptible cells are found in the leaf veins. Equally puzzling is the apparent limitation of SBMV infection to veins in the inoculated leaf without spread into adjacent mesophyll cells. If this is a true tissue specificity related to the type of inoculation method, does the virus escape from the veins at some location in the plant, and, if so, where? More extensive studies with fluorescent antibody staining are needed to answer these questions.

Screening for Resistance to Beetle-Transmitted Viruses Using Gross-Wound Inoculation

Experiments to validate the gross-wounding procedure as an inoculation method that mimics transmission by beetle feeding revealed that some hosts were not susceptible to virus inoculation by gross wounding even though they were always infected when mechanically inoculated with these viruses. When these hosts were tested using actual beetle transmission trials, they were found to be much more resistant to virus transmission than comparable susceptible hosts. For example, Black Valentine bean is not infected by CPMV when it is inoculated by gross wounding with purified virus but every plant is infected when mechanically inoculated with infectious sap. Transmission trials with single bean leaf beetles resulted in 2% of Black Valentine bean plants becoming infected compared to 20% transmission to Monarch cowpea, a more susceptible host (R. Gergerich, et al., unpublished observations).

The most practical method of control for diseases caused by plant viruses is the use of resistant plants. The usual method for screening for resistance uses mechanical inoculation of Carborundum-dusted leaves with infectious sap or exposure of plants to natural spread by vectors in the field or under controlled conditions. The latter method can be extremely cumbersome, and evidence from controlled transmission tests in the laboratory (18, 27) and natural spread of virus by vectors in the field (23, 41) suggests that mechanical inoculation may cause infection of plants that are actually resistant to infection by vector transmission.

The resistance of certain hosts to virus infection by beetle feeding or gross wounding may be related to the relative susceptibility of these hosts to virus infection. Comparison of infectibility of hosts that are susceptible or resistant to gross-wound transmission indicates that those hosts that are more resistant to gross-wound inoculation are also more resistant to mechanical inoculation with dilutions of purified virus. For example, cowpea severe mosaic virus (CSMV) is more readily transmitted to cowpea than to bean by beetles and gross wounding. Mechanical inoculation with CSMV at a concentration of 0.01 mg/ml caused infection in cowpea (40%) but not in bean (R. Gergerich et al., unpublished observations). When bean and cowpea plants are mechanically inoculated with CSMV at higher concentrations, such as that found in infectious sap, all of the bean and cowpea plants become infected. If the concentration of virus for mechanical inoculation is low enough, it is possible to reproduce the results of transmission with gross wounding or beetle feeding, that is, infection of cowpea, but no infection of bean. These results suggest that transmission by beetle feeding or gross-wound inoculation is less efficient than transmission by mechanical inoculation.

The use of gross-wound inoculation in screening programs for detection of resistance to beetle-transmitted viruses offers several advantages. This technique mimics results with beetle transmission trials but is less cumbersome and more defined than inoculation with beetles. Inocula can be easily prepared and a standard amount of inoculation damage can be produced as opposed to the variability associated with beetle-feeding trials.

This screening procedure may prove to be useful for certain virus–host combinations where screening for resistance using standard mechanical inoculation has not succeeded. A good candidate for this type of screening could be BPMV in soybean, where mechanical inoculation has not identified resistance to this virus (36).

Conclusions

Studies regarding virus transmission by leaf-feeding beetles led to the conclusion that specificity is determined by the interaction of the virus with the plant after deposition of the virus in beetle regurgitant at the feeding wound. An important step toward understanding the role that regurgitant and RNase play in the transmission process was the development of the gross-wound inoculation technique. This technique produces a wound site and introduces virus in a manner similar to the feeding process of viruliferous beetles. The addition of regurgitant or RNase to purified virus in gross-wound inocula demonstrated that regurgitant, and specifically the RNase in regurgitant, can selectively prevent the infection of those plant viruses not transmitted by beetles. The gross-wound inoculation technique also mimics beetle feeding in that susceptible plants (as judged by mechanical inoculation) that are resistant to gross-wound inoculation are also resistant to beetle transmission. Thus, this inoculation technique may have application in identifying plant resistance that is specific to beetle transmission of viruses.

Beetle-transmissible viruses are translocated readily in the xylem of plants and can infect (after translocation) unwounded plant cells. Fluorescent antibody staining of leaves inoculated with virus by gross wounding or beetle feeding indicates that beetle-transmitted viruses move into the xylem, but little is known about the process of infection after translocation in the xylem. Future research efforts will be directed at determining why non-beetle-transmissible viruses do not translocate in the xylem and how beetle-transmissible viruses initiate infection after xylem translocation.

References

1. Caldwell, J., 1930, The physiology of virus diseases in plants. I The movement of mosaic in the tomato plant, *Ann. Appl. Biol.* **17**:429–443.
2. Childress S.A., and Harris, K.F., 1989, Localization of virus-like particles in the foreguts of viruliferous *Graminella nigrifrons* leafhoppers carrying the semi-persistent maize chlorotic dwarf virus, *J. Gen. Virol.* **70**:247–251.
3. Francki, R.I.B., 1968, Inactivation of cucumber mosaic virus (Q strain) nucleoprotein by pancreatic ribonuclease, *Virology* **34**:694–700.
4. Freitag, J.H., 1956, Beetle transmission, host range, and properties of squash mosaic virus, *Phytopathology* **46**:73–81.
5. Fulton, J.P., and Scott, H.A., 1977, Bean rugose mosaic and related viruses and their transmission by beetles, *Fitopathologia Brasileira*, **2**:9–16.
6. Fulton, J.P., Gergerich, R.C., and Scott, H.A., 1987, Beetle transmission of plant viruses, *Annu. Rev. Phytopathol.* **25**:111–123.
7. Fulton, J.P., Scott, H.A., and Gamez, R., 1975, Beetle transmission of legume viruses, Bird, J. and Maramorosch, K. (eds): Tropical Diseases of Legumes, Academic Press, New York, pp. 123–131.
8. Fulton, J.P., Scott, H.A., and Gamez, R., 1980, Beetles, Maramorosch, K. and Harris, K. (eds): Vectors of Plant Pathogens, Academic Press, New York, pp. 115–132.
9. Gergerich, R.C., and Scott, H.A., 1988a, The enzymatic function of ribonuclease determines plant virus transmission by leaf-feeding beetles, *Phytopathology* **78**:270–272.

10. Gergerich, R.C., and Scott, H.A., 1988b, Evidence that virus translocation and virus infection of non-wounded cells are associated with transmissibility by leaf-feeding beetles, *J. Gen. Virol.* **69**:2935–2938.
11. Gergerich, R.C., Scott, H.A., and Fulton, J.P., 1983, Regurgitant as a determinant of specificity in the transmission of plant viruses by beetles, *Phytopathology* **73**:936–938.
12. Gergerich, R.C., Scott, H.A., and Fulton, J.P., 1986a, Some properties of beetle-transmitted viruses that may explain their transmissibility, *Phytopathology* **76**:1122.
13. Gergerich, R.C., Scott, H.A., and Fulton, J.P., 1986b, Evidence that ribonuclease in beetle regurgitant determines the transmission of plant viruses, *J. Gen. Virol.* **67**:367–370.
14. Gergerich, R.C., Scott, H.A., and Fulton, J.P., 1986c, Evaluation of *Diabrotica* beetles as vectors of plant viruses, Krysan, J. and Miller, T. (eds): Methods for the Study of Pest *Diabrotica*, Springer-Verlag, New York, pp. 227–249.
15. Gildow, F.E., 1982, Coated-vesicle transport of luteoviruses through salivary glands of *Myzus persicae*, *Phytopathology* **72**:1289–1296.
16. Harris, K.F., 1990, Aphid transmission of plant viruses, Mandahar, C.L. (ed): in Plant Viruses, Vol. II: Pathology, CRC Press, Boca Raton, FL, pp. 177–204.
17. Harrison, B.D., and Murant, A.F., 1984, Involvement of virus-coded proteins in transmission of plant viruses by vectors, Mayo, M. and Harrap, K. (eds): in Vectors in Virus Biology, Academic Press, Orlando, FL, pp. 1–36.
18. Hobbs, H.A., and Kuhn, C.W., 1987, Differential field infection of cowpea genotypes by southern bean mosaic virus, *Phytopathology* **77**:136–139.
19. Kim, K.S., 1981, Ultrastructure of bean leaf beetle (*Ceratoma trifurcata*) hemocytes and their phagocytic activities on tobacco mosaic virus, a non-beetle-transmitted virus, *J. Ultrastruct. Res.* **75**:300–313.
20. Kim, K.S., Scott, H.A., and Robison, M.D., 1978, Ultrastructural responses of bean leaf beetle hemocytes to beetle-transmitted and non-transmitted plant viruses, *Proc. Amer. Phytopath. Soc.* **4**:130.
21. Kopek, J.A., and Scott, H.A., 1983, Southern bean mosaic virus in Mexican bean beetle and bean leaf beetle regurgitants, *J. Gen. Virol.* **64**:1601–1605.
22. Langham, M.A.C., Gergerich, R.C., and Scott, H.A., 1990, Conversion of comovirus electrophoretic forms by leaf-feeding beetles, *Phytopathology* **80**: 900–906.
23. Lecoq, H., Labonne, G., and Pitrat, M., 1980, Specificity of resistance to virus transmission by aphids in *Cucumis melo*, Ann. Phytopathol. **12**:139–144.
24. Lei, J.D., and Agrios, G.N., 1986, Detection of virus infection and spread by immunofluorescent staining of enzyme treated leaves, *Phytopathology* **76**: 1031–1033.
25. Markham, R., and Smith, K.M., 1949, Studies on the virus turnip yellow mosaic, *Parasitology* **39**:330–342.
26. Monis, J., Scott, H.A., and Gergerich, R.C., 1986, Effect of beetle regurgitant on plant virus transmission using the gross wounding technique, *Phytopathology* **76**:808–811.
27. Moyer, J.W., Kennedy, G.G., and Romanow, L.R., 1985, Resistance to watermelon mosaic virus II multiplication in *Cucumis melo*, *Phytopathology* **75**:201–205.

28. Niblett, C.L., and Semancik, J.S., 1969, Conversion of the electrophoretic forms of cowpea mosaic virus *in vivo* and *in vitro*, *Virology* **38**:685–693.
29. Patterson, C.A., 1989, Detection of the primary infection sites of beetle-transmitted plant viruses, M.S. Thesis, University of Arkansas, Fayetteville, Arkansas.
30. Patterson, C., and Gergerich, R., 1989, Primary infection loci of two viruses transmitted by leaf-feeding beetles, *Phytopathology* **79**:376.
31. Roberts, D.A., 1970, Viral infection of apparently uninjured leaves as influenced by particle morphology and host species, *Phytopathology* **60**:1310.
32. Roberts, D.A., and Price, W.C., 1967, Infection of apparently uninjured leaves of bean by the viruses of tobacco necrosis and southern bean mosaic, *Virology* **33**:542–545.
33. Sanderlin, R.S., 1973, Survival of bean pod mottle and cowpea mosaic viruses in beetles following intrahemocoelic injections, *Phytopathology* **63**:259–261.
34. Schneider, I.R., and Worley, J.F., 1959, Upward and downward transport of infectious particles of southern bean mosaic virus through steamed portions of bean stems, *Virology* **8**:230–242.
35. Scott, H.A., and Fulton, J.P., 1978, Comparisons of the relationships of southern bean mosaic virus and the cowpea strain of tobacco mosaic virus with the bean leaf beetle, *Virology* **84**:207–209.
36. Scott, H.A., Van Scyoc, J.V., and Van Scyoc, C.E., 1974, Reactions of *Glycine* spp. to bean pod mottle virus, *Plant Dis. Rep.* **58**:191–192.
37. Slack, S.A., and Fulton, J.P., 1971, Some plant virus-beetle vector relations, *Virology* **43**:728–729.
38. Slack, S.A., and Scott, H.A., 1971, Hemolymph as a reservoir for the cowpea strain of southern bean mosaic virus in the bean leaf beetle, *Phytopathology* **61**:538–540.
39. Smith, C.E., 1924, Transmission of cowpea mosaic by the bean leaf beetle, *Science* **60**:268.
40. Srivastava, U.S., 1959, The maxillary glands of some Coleoptera, *Proc. Royal Soc. Lond.* (A) **34**:57–62.
41. Thongmeearkom, P., Paschall II, E.H., and Goodman, R.M., 1978, Yield reductions in soybeans infected with cowpea mosaic virus, *Phytopathology* **68**:1549–1551.
42. Wilson, T.M.A., 1988, Structural interactions between plant RNA viruses and cells, *Oxford Surv. Plant Molec. & Cell Biol.* **5**:89–144.

43. [illegible]

2
The Role of Arthropod Vectors in Arbovirus Evolution

Patricia A. Nuttall, Linda D. Jones, and Clive R. Davies

Introduction

Arboviruses spend most of their time in their arthropod vectors. Their foray into a vertebrate host is usually a short-term expedient for amplification and consequent acquisition by more vectors. Thus arthropods have ample opportunity to influence the evolution of the arboviruses that they transmit. Evolution consists of a change in genotype with the ensuing creation of a new phenotype. Natural selection acts on the phenotypic differences resulting in the predominance of a particular genotype within a niche. The arthropod vector provides a milieu in which changes in the arboviral genotype occur, and exerts selection pressures on the different arboviral phenotypes.

The third edition of the "International Catalogue of Arboviruses" lists over 500 viruses that are definite, probable, or possible arboviruses (73). They vary greatly in size and structure, belonging to various families and genera. However, they are united by their ability to replicate in a blood-sucking arthropod and to infect a vertebrate host when the arthropod vector feeds on that host; following infection of the vertebrate host, the virus replicates producing viremia (162). Acquisition of the virus by another susceptible arthropod occurs during feeding on the viremic vertebrate. This form of vector-borne transmission is known as "biological" transmission as it depends on virus replication in the vector. Besides acting as a vector, the arthropod may also be the critical reservoir host of the

Patricia A. Nuttall, NERC Institute of Virology & Environmental Microbiology, Oxford, England, UK.
Linda D. Jones, NERC Institute of Virology & Environmental Microbiology, Oxford, England, UK.
Clive R. Davies, Department of Medical Parasitology, London School of Hygiene & Tropical Medicine, UK.

virus, particularly when the virus is transmitted vertically to succeeding generations. Hematophagous arthropods that transmit arboviruses are mosquitoes, ticks, phlebotomine flies, *Culicoides* midges, and certain species of bugs. Most arboviruses isolated from field-collected vectors are from mosquitoes (56%) and ticks (24%) (73).

Mechanisms of Arbovirus Evolution

The molecular changes underlying the evolution of viruses occur at the level of the nucleotide sequence. They include point mutations resulting from single base changes, additions or deletions to bases, and deletions or duplications of nucleic acid sequences. Such changes in the genetic information of the virus result in "genetic drift." With very few exceptions, all arboviruses possess an RNA rather than DNA genome. The mutation rates of RNA and DNA viruses of eukaryotes are much higher than those of their hosts (63, 117, 136). Because of such high mutational rates, a "virus" may best be considered a pool of variants (even when derived from a single viral plaque) in which certain genotypes are dominant. Thus a virus population is in a state of dynamic equilibrium, responding to intrinsic and extrinsic pressures. Small changes in this equilibrium, probably arising from the accumulation of point mutations, result in genetic drift. In general, viruses isolated at about the same time from different individuals within any local outbreak of disease have similar oligonucleotide maps, whereas viruses from earlier or later outbreaks exhibit increasing divergence; the different isolates are related by gradual mutational changes that can be drawn as an evolutionary tree (63).

A more rapid form of evolution, referred to as "genetic shift," results from either recombination, reassortment of genomic segments, or acquisition of exogenous host DNA. Recombination has been described as covalently linked genome rearrangement and, as such, is distinguished from reassortment of genome segments in which, probably, no covalent joining occurs (63). In poliovirus, recombination occurs by a copy-choice mechanism during RNA replication (76); it is assumed that all recombination occurs this way. The mechanism by which genome segments reassort is unknown and awaits a better understanding of viral morphogenesis. Evidence of true recombination among arboviruses is sparse. A notable example is that of Western equine encephalitis (WEE) virus, a recombinant of an eastern equine encephalitis (EEE)-like virus and a Sindbis (SIN)-like virus (58). In contrast to recombination, reassortment has been demonstrated in vitro for all the "vertebrate" multisegmented RNA virus families: Arena-, Bunya-, Orthomyxo-, and Reoviridae. As most (66%) of the classified arboviruses (including members of the Quaranfil serogroup, provisionally classified as arenaviruses) are represented by these families, that is, possess a segmented genome, the potential for rapid evolution of arboviruses through genome segment exchange is relatively high. Intertypic reassortment of arboviruses has been demonstrated in vitro for bunyaviruses of the Bunyamwera and California serogroups (53, 67), and orbiviruses of the Kemerovo serogroup (106). Reassortment is apparently limited to closely related viruses within a serogroup and does not occur between all members of a serogroup (116). Thus, recombination may be more important than reassortment as an evolutionary mechanism for arboviruses because it allows for the genetic interaction of viruses that have greater genotypic (and phenotypic) differences. Indeed, the success of WEE virus indicates that recombination may play an important role in the evolution of arboviruses even though this mechanism of rapid evolution appears to be a rare event. Although reassortment has been demonstrated extensively in vitro, its prevalence and significance in nature are unknown. Several studies have reported evidence of intra- and intertypic reassortment in arthropod vectors following artificial routes of infection by inoculation, or by feeding on blood pledglets, through membranes, or via capillaries containing virus–blood mixtures (Table 2.1). Reassortment of arboviruses under natural conditions of transmission (i.e., involving a viremic host) has been reported for Thogoto (THO) virus, a candidate orthomyxovirus. When uninfected ticks were exposed to two different temperature-sensitive (*ts*) mutants by interrupted feeding on viremic hamsters, reassortant viruses were detected in the engorged ticks; these ticks transmitted the reassortant viruses to uninfected hamsters during a subsequent feed (35). Conversely, when ticks infected with one of two *ts* THO virus mutants were allowed to cofeed on hamsters, reassortment occurred in a viremic hamster (71). In both scenarios the incidence of reassortment was low, despite the use of differential growth temperatures to select for reassortants, indicating that reassortment in nature is probably a rare event.

An alternative means of rapid evolution involves the movement of genetic information (transposons) into and out of the viral genome. This

TABLE 2.1. Intra- and intertypic reassortment of arboviruses within arthropod vectors.

Virus family	Parental viruses	Source of infection	Reference
Bunyaviridae	La Crosse × Snowshoe hare	Inoculation; artificial bloodmeal	8, 26
	La Crosse × La Crosse	Artificial bloodmeal	10
	Rift Valley fever × Rift Valley fever	Viremia	154
Reoviridae	Colorado tick fever × Colorado tick fever	Inoculation	88
	Bluetongue 10 × Bluetongue 17	Artificial bloodmeal	130
Unclassified	Thogoto × Thogoto	Viremia	35

"modular evolution" has been described for DNA viruses although an equivalent mechanism may exist in RNA viruses (139). It remains to be determined whether arboviruses can acquire exogenous nucleic acid from their arthropod vectors, and vice versa.

The role of the arthropod vector in providing a milieu in which recombination and reassortment occur depends on the opportunities for mixed infections. Studies on mosquito- and tick-borne viruses demonstrated that the potential for superinfection of arthropod vectors is limited by interference (9, 32, 33, 111, 147). Inhibition of superinfection occurs when genetically compatible viruses are acquired in the same feeding stage (intrastadially), in consecutive feeding stages (interstadially), or when infection by one virus occurs vertically. Interference inhibited reassortment between genetically compatible bunyaviruses when there was a delay of 24 h or more between the initial and subsequent infective bloodmeals of the vector mosquitoes (10). However, complete interference is not expressed in all mixedly infected vectors (9, 111). For example, in ticks superinfected with THO virus, either intra- or interstadially, 22% of infected nymphs failed to demonstrate complete interference (33). Hence, the potential for reassortment of THO virus existed even in ticks infected during consecutive feeding stages. The situation in the vertebrate host is more difficult to analyse because of the influence of immunity. Reassortment of THO virus in hamsters was not apparent if superinfection occurred 24 h after the initial infection (71). Thus the role of the arthropod vector in facilitating reassortment in the vertebrate host depends on the rate of virus transmission by infected vectors to susceptible vertebrate hosts.

Evidence of Arbovirus Evolution in Nature

Evolutionary relationships between different virus families have been proposed on the basis of sequence similarities and overall genome organization. Thus, for example, arboviruses of the Togaviridae (e.g., EEE and SIN viruses) show similarities with several groups of plant viruses, whereas members of the Flaviviridae, for example, yellow fever (YF) and dengue (DEN) viruses are related to the non-arthropod-borne pestiviruses (139). Comparison of tick-borne and mosquito-borne flaviviruses reveals evidence of close evolutionary relationships (113). In contrast, the tick-borne orbiviruses show significant divergence from the insect-borne members of the genus (101, 106). Intriguingly, Dhori and Thogoto viruses appear to be influenza viruses (51, 137) that have adapted to ticks by deriving their viral glycoprotein from an insect or an insect virus (baculovirus) gene (Morse, Marriott, and Nuttall, unpublished observation).

Sequencing the genomes (or by extrapolating from oligonucleotide fingerprints) of a variety of isolates collected from different sites and in different years has provided a picture of the genetic drift experienced by arboviruses. For example, DEN-1 isolates collected over 8 years demonstrated a 1.8% to 1.9% change in nucleotides (28); Kunjin (KUN) isolates (from Ord River, Australia) experienced a maximum sequence divergence of 1.5% over 10 years (50); Murray valley encephalitis (MVE) isolates from Australia differed by up to 1.7% of their nucleotide sequence, but up to 10% when compared with isolates from Papua New Guinea (30); and the nucleotide sequence of Egyptian Rift Valley fever (RVF) isolates differed from those from Zimbabwe by 4.5% (5). These data indicate that the rate of nucleotide substitutions of arboviruses is within the medial range of the 0.03% to 2.0% per year reported for RNA viral genomes (136).

Some evidence suggests that the evolutionary rate of arboviruses may be significantly lower than that of non-vector-borne viruses. However, most of the data relates to viruses passaged in the laboratory (4, 13). One study of evolution in the field was based on selective sequence analysis of 3 isolates of Ross River virus (RRV) obtained during a 10 month epidemic in the Pacific islands; only a single nucleotide change was detected in 1.6 kilobases (0.06%) of one of the isolates (23).

As mentioned above, evidence of genetic shift among arboviruses has been demonstrated for WEE virus, a naturally occurring recombinant (58). A similar mechanism (or one involving genetic drift) has been considered for the origin of O'nyong-nyong virus, an *Anopheles*-transmitted alphavirus that is closely related to the *Aedes*-transmitted Chikungunya (CHIK) virus (112). Evidence of intratypic recombination has been reported for an isolate of African swine fever virus (ASF), which has a DNA genome (38). Genetic shift resulting from exchange of genomic segments has been studied by fingerprint analyses of field isolates. Putative intratypic reassortants have been identified for La Crosse (LAC) virus (77) and for members of the Patois serogroup of bunyaviruses (155). Comparison of the genomic RNA segments and viral-induced polypeptides of bluetongue virus (BTV) serotypes 10 and 11 indicated that BTV-11 originated by reassortment between an ancestral BTV-11 serotype and BTV-10 (141). It is evident from these studies that arboviruses are undergoing both genetic drift and genetic shift.

Anatomical Basis of Evolution

Changes in the genotype of a virus (genetic drift and genetic shift) occur during viral replication. The role of the arthropod in acting as both a site for such changes and a selection pressure, depends on the anatomical basis of infection in the arthropod.

Most of the work on localization of arboviruses within their vectors has been undertaken with mosquito-borne viruses (36, 96). Although ticks differ fundamentally from hematophagous insects in their life history, feeding behavior and digestive physiology (107), the initial barrier to infection in both ticks and insects is the midgut or mesenteron. If a virus imbibed in a bloodmeal is subsequently transmitted horizontally (via salivary fluid) or vertically (via the egg or sperm), the ingested virus must first infect and replicate in the arthropod's midgut epithelial cells, and progeny virus must then disseminate via the hemocoel to the salivary glands. The ability of an arthropod to sustain an infection and subsequently deliver the virus during feeding is a measure of vector competence, the "combined effect of all the physiological and ecological factors of vector, host, pathogen, and environment that determine the vector status of a given arthropod population" (90). Intrinsic vector competence includes both physiological factors that govern infection of the vector and ability to transmit the virus, and innate behavioral traits such as host preference and probing activity. Řeháček (121) considered that "the ability of an arthropod to become a biological vector is principally determined genetically," whereas Smith (135) proposed that "ecological factors play an important role in determining the species of an arthropod host." A genetic basis for vectorial competence of arboviruses in mosquitoes and biting midges has been established, although the mode of inheritance and mechanisms of action have not been elucidated (55, 59, 96).

Successful infection of the midgut depends partly on the amount of virus in the host's blood and the volume of blood imbibed. The concept of "minimum dose" or "infection thresholds" permeates the literature on virus–vector systems (21, 102, 105, 121). The concentration of virus necessary to overcome the threshold of infection varies for different viruses in the same arthropod species, for the same virus in different arthropod species, and ultimately for individuals of the same arthropod or viral species (59, 36). This may not be the case for viruses that are transmitted vertically (148), produce unusually high levels of viremia in their vertebrate host (20, 125), or are transmitted via a "non-viraemic" host (70). Nevertheless, for most arboviruses the ability to penetrate the midgut is their first exposure to selection pressures within the arthropod vector.

The gut represents the first of a series of barriers that the virus must overcome (59). The gut barrier is thought to reflect the ability of gut epithelial cells to support viral replication (21, 102). However, as viral replication has been observed in epithelial cells following parenteral inoculation, other factors are implicated such as viral fusion or virus receptors. WEE virus appears to penetrate midgut cells by fusion (66). Studies with La Crosse virus indicate that binding of the virus to mosquito midgut cells depends on proteolytic cleavage of the G1 viral glycoprotein and consequent exposure of the G2 glycoprotein on the surface of the virion (86). The G2 protein may then fuse to midgut cells or bind to specific receptors on the cells. In hematophagous insects, blood digestion takes place rapidly and occurs in the lumen of the intestine; the proteases that are present in the gut may facilitate the necessary cleavage of viral glycoproteins. In contrast, blood digestion in ticks is a slow intracellular process; the properties of tick proteases indicate that viruses are not immediately exposed to proteolytic enzymes within the gut (1). Thus, the first step in the infection process for arboviruses may differ markedly in insects and ticks. This level of vector-mediated selection may explain why few tick-borne viruses are also transmitted by insects and, to a slightly lesser degree, the paucity of tick vectors for insect-borne viruses.

Following infection, viral titers in the midgut cells initially decrease (the "eclipse" phase) and then increase rapidly to reach maximum levels within a few days. Viral titers then usually decrease tenfold and either remain at this level or continue to decrease. These patterns of replication were observed in *Aedes albopictus* females infected per os with DEN-2 virus, and *Culex tritaeniorhynchus* and *C. pipiens* infected with Japanese encephalitis (JE) virus; viral antigens were observed in most of the cells in the posterior portion of the midgut after a few days (39, 40). Similar patterns were observed at the ultrastructural level with St. Louis encephalitis (SLE) virus in *C. pipiens* (161) and Eastern equine encephalitis virus in *Aedes triseriatus* (102) but only a relatively small proportion of the midgut epithelial cells were observed to be infected (1:5 and 1:3 cells, respectively). In ticks, relatively few midgut cells were infected with Dugbe (DUG) virus following per os infection of *Amblyomma variegatum* (16). The significance of these observations with regard to opporunities for mixed infection of midgut cells, and hence for recombination or reassortment of viruses, is undetermined. Studies in mosquitoes and ticks indicate that the midgut is the anatomical site of viral interference, thus implicating the midgut as the site of reassortment for arboviruses with segmented genomes. These investigations were carried out with LAC and Tahyna (TAH) viruses in *A. triseriatus* (142), and using temperature-sensitive mutants of THO virus in the tick vector, *R. appendiculatus* (72). However, the frequent observations of viral interference in mosquitoes dually infected by inoculation (9, 32, 129) indicate that interference in mosquitoes does not occur exclusively in the midgut. Chandler and colleagues (26) postulated that the ovaries may serve as a site for the evolution of new viral genotypes by genetic reassortment.

The next barrier to infection is the basal lamina. This barrier is often referred to as the "midgut escape barrier" or "salivary gland infection barrier" (59). Studies with LAC virus in *A. triseriatus* collected from different geographic regions demonstrated the importance of the midgut escape barrier: a significant proportion of the mosquitoes with infected midguts did not develop disseminated infections and were therefore incapable of virus transmission (108). In *C. tarsalis* infected with WEE virus, the salivary gland infection barrier was overcome in some of the females after an extended incubation period (82). Hence, these barriers appear to be both time and dose dependent. The infecting virus must pass through the basal lamina of the midgut into the hemocoel. Although the mechanism of viral penetration is unknown, mature SLE virions have been observed in the basal lamina of *C. pipiens* (161). Recent studies on Rift Valley fever virus have shown that virus can also disseminate via the cells at the foregut/midgut junction into the intussuscepted foregut (126).

In some virus–vector associations, a "leaky gut" has been described whereby the virus passes into the hemocoel more rapidly than if replication occurred. Short extrinsic incubation periods have been observed for Whataroa (WHA) virus in *A. australis* (92), Uganda S virus in *A. aegypti* (14), RVF virus in *C. pipiens* (47), and Venezuelan equine encephalitis (VEE) virus in *C. taeniopus* (159). The passive movement of virus from the gut lumen to the hemocoel may relate to potentially explosive cycling and vertebrate epizootics, and reflect a response of the virus to changes in selection pressures.

Following release into the hemocoel, the virus may infect virtually all mosquito or tick organs (27, 54, 59, 109, 110). Hemocytes play an important role in the internal dissemination of some arboviruses, as demonstrated for African swine fever (ASF) virus in *Ornithodoros moubata* (54) and DUG virus in *A. variegatum* (16). Salivary glands may be infected by a virus carried in the hemolymph, or alternatively, transfered via hemocytes by cell to cell contact, or by invasion of salivary gland tissue by a process of diapedesis (16); a neural pathway has been proposed for WHA virus in *A. australis* mosquitoes (92) and JE virus in *C. tritaeniorhynchus* (85).

Ultimately, the virus must overcome the "salivary gland barrier." This barrier has been reported for *A. hendersoni* orally infected with LAC virus. Infective virus was detected in the salivary glands of *A. hendersoni*, but the mosquitoes were unable to transmit by the bite (108).

Secondary amplification of virus in extramesenteronal cells and tissues is a prerequisite for infection of the salivary glands of some arboviruses. For viruses transported by hemocytes and not detected in acellular hemolymph, the ability to infect and replicate in hemocytes may be a key selection pressure. An infection threshold, similar to that described for the midgut, has been postulated for salivary glands (25). If low concentrations of virus are ingested, amplification may be necessary to overcome the salivary gland barrier. For example, secondary amplification of JE virus can occur in the fat body cells adjacent to the mesenteron, prior to infection of the salivary glands and other susceptible tissues (39, 40). In *R. appendiculatus* ticks, dissemination of THO virus occurred within 6 days of an infective bloodmeal, but infection of the salivary glands was not observed until 25 days postengorgement (15); the site of secondary amplification was the neural cortex of the synganglion. Thus, the requirement for secondary amplification, and the site of such replication, depend on the strategy of infection of the arthropod vector by a particular arbovirus, which, in turn, will be influenced by selection pressures exerted by the arthropod on the virus.

Unlike mosquitoes, ticks usually moult before taking their next bloodmeal. Hence, following infection of a tick, the virus must survive transstadially in order to be transmitted in salivary fluid when the succeeding stage feeds. During the transstadial period, a decrease in virus titer just prior to metamorphosis, followed by an increase in virus titer after ecdysis, have been reported for several tick–virus systems (11, 94, 128). These observations probably reflect the histological changes that occur at this time (3). The extensive histolysis associated with metamorphosis represents a strong selection pressure. The strategy adopted by different tick-borne viruses in surviving this period shows remarkable versatility. For example, THO virus persists in the neural cortex surrounding the synganglion, one of the few organs that does not undergo hystolysis (15). In contrast, DUG virus establishes an infection in the tick hemocytes and does not infect nervous tissue (16). The flavivirus, tick-borne encephalitis (TBE) virus, establishes a more widespread infection in the tick, with virus present in the hypodermis, salivary glands, and dermal glands, as well as nondifferentiated epithelial cells of the intestine (103).

The successful perpetuation of arboviruses ultimately depends on the successful transmission of the virus, by the infected vector, to a susceptible vertebrate. For certain virus–vector host associations, the stimulus of probing or attachment is required before the virus disseminates to the salivary gland. Examples of this are *R. appendiculatus* ticks infected with THO virus (15) and *A. variegatum* ticks infected with DUG virus (16). In both cases virus was not detected in the salivary glands until feeding had commenced.

One of the most important factors influencing the vector potential of hematophagous arthropods is the "transmission rate." There is evidence to suggest that arboviruses may manipulate their arthropod vectors to achieve maximum transmission. *Aedes triseriatus* mosquitoes infected with LAC virus tended to probe more and engorge less than uninfected mosquitoes, and transmission rates increased as the level of probing increased (56). Infection of the vertebrate host may also affect the vector, as demonstrated by the ability of mosquitoes to locate blood more rapidly on RVF virus-infected hosts (127). These observations suggest that the virus may exert a positive effect on the arthropod in terms of enhanced host-seeking behavior or reduced vector–host contact, with the benefit to the virus of an increased rate of transmission. In these situations there are obvious possibilities for arboviruses to influence the evolution of their arthropod vectors.

The time taken between acquisition of virus in a bloodmeal and transmission of the virus during feeding is known as the "extrinsic incubation period" (EIP). During this period the vector is incapable of biological transmission because insufficient time has elapsed for the virus to establish an infection of the salivary glands. Hence, the EIP is an important factor in the epidemiology and epizootiology of arthropod-borne viruses, as it dictates how long the vector must survive before it is a competent transmitter. Extrinsic conditions, such as ambient temperature, can affect the

EIP (75, 152, 158). Obviously, the selection pressure on insect-borne viruses is to ensure that the EIP does not exceed the lifespan of the insect otherwise the vector will die before the virus is transmitted to a vertebrate host; vertical transmission overcomes such pressure. For tick-borne viruses this is not a problem because of the comparative longevity of ticks.

Various mechanisms exist to ensure the survival of virus populations in their natural foci of infection. Transstadial persistence in ticks is regarded as such, however, in this case it is crucial for the transmission of the infecting virus, as ticks normally feed only once before moulting. Another maintenance mechanism is vertical transmission, "the direct transfer of infection from a parent organism to his, her or its progeny" (48). Vertical transmission of arboviruses includes transovarial, transovum, and transveneral passage. Transovarial and transvenereal transmission provide protection for the virus within the egg (the stage most suited to withstand adverse conditions) and shelter the virus from many of the selection pressures experienced during horizontal transmission (see Vector-Mediated Selection Pressures below). The ability of arboviruses to be transmitted vertically by their arthropod vectors has been recorded for many mosquito- and tick-borne viruses (120, 145).

The anatomical basis of infection of the egg is poorly understood (84, 124). Differences in vertical transmission rates in female ticks infected parenterally by inoculation, as opposed to per os, led Rehacek (121) to postulate the existence of an "ovary barrier" to infection. Evidence of such a barrier is derived from the fact that some vector species are unable to tansmit an arbovirus transovarially whereas others can. Inter- and intraspecific differences in mosquitoes can influence transovarial transmission. Similarly, differences in the rates of transmission of different strains of an arbovirus have been recorded (36, 84). For TBE virus, the transovarial and filial infection rates depend on when the ticks fed and the level of viremia in the vertebrate host at the time of feeding (80, 81, 120). Thus, both intrinsic and extrinsic selection pressures act on the virus at the level of vertical transmission. Stabilized infections have been demonstrated in a number of arbovirus-vector associations (36, 148). They occur when all the female germinal cells are infected irrespective of their stage of development, and the virus is transmitted to all of the offspring (84). In theory, the virus could be maintained in the vector population soley by maternal inheritance. Presumably, the costs to the virus of this strategy of maintenance are too high otherwise the virus would no longer be an arbovirus (i.e., capable of infecting a vertebrate host) (24).

Determination of the anatomical basis of infection in the vector is important in understanding the role of the arthropod in arbovirus evolution. Target cells or organs within the arthropod are the most likely sites of genetic shift and genetic drift of the virus. Phenotypic variants thus generated will be exposed to vector-mediated selection, such as the ability to disseminate from the midgut (i.e., to overcome the midgut release barrier), and ability to infect the reproductive organs (selection for vertical transmission). New routes of transmission may expose arboviruses to dramatic changes in selection pressure. For example, concurrent ingestion of midgut-puncturing microfilariae has been demonstrated in a number of virus–vector associations (91, 150, 153). The microfilariae facilitate entry of the virus directly into the hemocoel. A similar route of infection occurs in tick species that exhibit cannibalism, that is, the feeding of one tick on the bloodmeal of another (62, 104). These unusual routes of infection bypass the gut barriers and thus may introduce arboviruses to new potential vectors and concomitant selection pressures.

Vector-Mediated Selection Pressures

How do selection pressures on arboviruses differ from those experienced by directly transmitted viruses? Obviously, arboviruses are selected for their ability to survive and replicate in arthropod cells. For efficient transmission by their preferred vector, the course of infection in arthropods following feeding demands that viruses are able to surmount a number of barriers (see above). Vectors may also influence the selection pressures on the arbovirus within its vertebrate host. In particular, the different modes of transmission of arboviruses and directly transmitted viruses will determine the selection pressures on virulence, that is, "the negative effect on host fitness resulting from the parasitism" (45). Traditionally, parasitologists have argued that selection on both host and parasite acts to minimize virulence. For example, Reid (122) wrote that "it is axiomatic that in a stable host-parasite ecosystem, natural selection favors less virulent viruses and relatively resistant "essential" hosts, and unusual virulence for a vertebrate indicates the recent introduction of virus or host into that area." This view is now untenable, following the recognition that the evolutionary endpoint of host–parasite coevolution is not necessarily one in which the parasite does little harm to its host; instead, the "optimal" virulence of a parasite will depend on its transmissibility (2, 87). Parasite severity at equilibrium will lie between the host's optimum (no disease or very slight disease, depending on the costs of defence) and the optimum for the parasite.

Ewald (43) used the comparative method (*sensu* 29) to support the hypothesis that vector-borne parasites should be more virulent than directly transmitted parasites. In a review of human infectious diseases, a significant association was demonstrated between arthropod-borne transmission and virulence in vertebrate hosts. Selection will favor high virulence in vector-borne parasites, such as arboviruses, because the costs are relatively low (arboviruses can be transmitted readily from immobilized vertebrate hosts) and the benefits are relatively high (hosts infected with highly virulent arboviruses should be more infective for potential arthropod vectors). In support of this hypothesis, significant correlations have been demonstrated between virulence and viremia titers (17, 122), and between viremia titers and the percentage of vectors infected (34, 59). In contrast to the response in the vertebrate host, selection will act on vector-borne parasites to minimize any negative effects on vector fitness caused by extensive multiplication, because immobilized vectors cannot transmit parasites. Thus, arboviruses should evolve towards relatively low virulence in their vector and relatively high virulence in their vertebrate host (44). In general, this appears to be the case and deleterious effects of virus infection on the vector are not apparent (15, 16, 83, 85). However, several exceptions have been noted in the laboratory. For example, degeneration of the salivary glands was observed in *A. aegypti* infected with Semliki Forest (SF) virus (95); mosquitoes infected with LAC or RVF viruses showed a reduced ability to refeed and decreased fecundity (46, 56, 151); and larvae infected transovarially with KUN, YF, or California Encephalitis (CE) viruses required more time to develop to the pupal stage than did uninfected siblings (7, 144, 149). The significance of these observations with regard to infections of arbovirus vectors in nature needs to be determined.

If the benefit to an arbovirus of high virulence accrues from its mode of transmission, virulence will decrease when arboviruses are maintained by direct transmission (either between vertebrates or between arthropods) as the costs of high virulence outweigh the benefits. This hypothesis can be tested by examining the effect of extended replication of the virus in either the vertebrate or arthropod system in (1) cell culture/laboratory animals, (2) different ecosytems, (3) different hosts, and (4) at different times.

Cell Culture/Laboratory Animals

In the laboratory, repeated subculturing of an arbovirus in either vertebrate or invertebrate cell lines leads to changes in phenotype such as increased frequencies of temperature-sensitive and small-plaque mutants, and defective interfering particles (18, 37, 41). Such changes may be accompanied by reduced virulence (12, 138). For ASF virus, decreased virulence after cell culture passage correlated with various rearrangements in the genomic DNA, including large deletions (143). Passaging arboviruses in a vertebrate system may also lead to a decrease in infectivity for the vector. For example, one strain of YF virus, when passaged five times in mouse brains and seven times in BHK-21 cells, showed a decline in its ability to infect *Aedes aegypti* mosquitoes from 62% to 35% and a decline in transmission rate from 64% to 45% (93). A concurrent 2% change in oligonucleotide fingerprints indicated that the change in phenotype corresponded with genetic changes. Although these observations are essentially artificial, they indicate that there is a cost associated with high infectivity for vectors, and thus this trait is only maintained when the virus has the opportunity to replicate in arthropods.

Different Ecosystems

African swine fever virus is found in two different ecosytems—a tick-transmitted cycle involving warthogs, and a directly transmitted cycle involving domestic pigs. Virus isolates from ticks (*Ornithodoros moubata*) in warthog burrows demonstrate great diversity, as detected by restriction enzyme analysis (38); variation was most extreme between isolates from different areas, but genetic differences were also observed between isolates from the same warthog burrow. In contrast, restriction enzyme analysis of ASF isolates from domestic pigs demonstrated a high degree of conservation, in particular over a central region of 125 kb, even when comparing isolates from Europe, the Caribbean, and Cameroon collected over 30 years (160). Large deletions of DNA close to the left-hand terminus of the genome, characteristic also of ASF virus maintained continuously in vertebrate cell culture (see above), were observed in ASF virus isolates from domestic pigs, but not in isolates from warthog burrows, suggesting that this part of the genome contains genes specifically required for tick transmission. The explanation for greater genetic diversity in warthog burrows is possibly due to the greater genetic heterogeneity of warthog populations compared to domestic pigs. However, an additional explanation may involve the greater ability of new virus strains to persist in a tick-transmitted cycle; this is due to the limited gene flow between warthog burrows caused by minimal tick dispersal, and also to the ticks' ability to transmit ASF virus vertically and transvenereally (114, 115), thus reducing the strength of the vertebrate host-mediated selection pressures.

Interestingly, ASF virus is highly pathogenic in domestic pigs but avirulent for warthogs. This observation apparently conflicts with the hypothesis that vector-borne transmission favors higher virulence than direct transmission. However, the picture for ASF virus is confounded by the equivocal data on the mechanism of virus transmission, the immune response to infection, and the significance of vertical transmission of the virus in ticks.

Different Hosts

Comparison of the genotype or phenotype of viruses isolated from vertebrate hosts and arthropod vectors in the same locality provides additional clues regarding the selection pressures experienced by arboviruses. For example, oligonucleotide fingerprints of JE isolates from humans in a Thai village in 1962 to 1963 demonstrated little variation compared to isolates from mosquitoes in the same village (22); isolates from pigs showed intermediate variation. A possible explanation is that only highly virulent JE virus strains are able to infect humans, so selecting out much of the genetic variation that can persist in mosquitoes (which can also transmit JE virus vertically). As pigs are more susceptible to infection than man, the selection pressure to maximize virulence is less extreme.

Thus, this study indicates that vectors may effectively maintain genetic diversity in a virus population.

When variation between Colorado tick fever (CTF) virus isolates, collected over several years from the same geographical area, was analyzed by cross-neutralization tests, isolates from ticks (*Dermacentor andersoni*) and wild mammals showed less antigenic variation than did isolates from humans (74). CTF virus is unusual amongst arboviruses in that it induces viraemia of long duration in infected vertebrate hosts, and has even been isolated from infected hosts at a time when homologous antibody was present (42). Thus, the host immune response may provide the selection pressures which lead to the greater diversity of human isolates. Such diversity is probably due to the selection of variants already present in low frequencies rather than the generation of novel viral genotypes during replication. This was indicated by an analogous study of bluetongue, which, like CTF virus, can induce prolonged viremia. Calves were infected with plaque-purified strains of BTV; virus isolates collected over 2 months from the infected calves were genetically stable, as determined by oligonucleotide fingerprinting analysis and monoclonal antibody mapping (61).

Two factors may account for the generally high conservation of genes in CTF viruses, as detected by polyacrylamide gel electrophoresis (19). One is the fact that *Dermacentor andersoni* ticks are unable to transmit the virus vertically (49). The other is the considerable gene flow between virus populations at different sites due to host migration, as indicated by the same degree of genetic heterogeneity between sites as within sites (19). Thus the role of the vectors in maintaining genetic diversity in an arbovirus population will depend on the ecological characteristics of the vector, such as whether they favor a restricted or generalized habitat (see below).

Different Times

Finally, the specific selection pressures associated with vectors can be identified by comparing virus strains isolated from the same locality during different seasons. Many arboviruses overwinter in inactive (possibly dormant) vector populations (118). Thus, for many months of the year arboviruses will experience a life cycle that does not involve the vertebrate host. By comparing the phenotype of an arbovirus population before and after overwintering in their vectors, one can infer the selection pressures induced solely by replication in arthropod cells. For example, WEE virus (an alphavirus transmitted by *Culex tarsalis* in California) is thought to overwinter in the vector population; virus strains isolated from January to March characteristically demonstrate low pathogenicity for mice as compared with strains isolated during the summer season of arbovirus transmission amongst vertebrate hosts (119). These results indicate that continuous replication of WEE virus in mosquitoes selects for variants of low pathogenicity towards vertebrate hosts. Thus, arboviruses can experience a cost (in terms of fitness) associated with high pathogenicity for vertebrates, when infecting arthropods.

Interspecific Vector Variation

Arboviruses are often transmitted by more than one vector species, the geographic ranges of which may or may not overlap. An extreme case is illustrated by Crimean-Congo hemorrhagic fever (CCHF virus), which has been isolated from at least 27 tick species or subspecies (65), although not all of these are necessarily vectorially competent for CCHF virus. Vector species differ in a number of traits that have significant implications for the selection pressures that they induce on the viruses they transmit. These traits can be divided into two groups: (1) traits involving vector–virus interactions, and (2) traits involving vector–host interactions.

Vector–Virus Interactions

The key characteristic of vectors is their competence for a given arbovirus. Comparative tests of arbovirus infections in the laboratory demonstrate that viruses are specifically adapted for infecting particular vector species. In general, the natural vector species of an arbovirus are more competent for that virus than are potential vector species, which do not overlap in their geographic range with the virus. Thus, for example, *Culex taeniopius*, the vector of VEE virus (subtype 1E) in Guatemala, is highly susceptible to infection by its sympatric virus type, but refractory to infection with allopatric VEE virus isolates (133). Clearly, in the field there is selection on viruses to maximize the efficiency with which they infect a vector. The greater this efficiency, the lower is the infection threshold of the vector, and hence vertebrate hosts with viremias of lower titer are able to infect a greater percentage of the vectors that feed on them (34).

The corollary is that if an arbovirus evolves greater virulence, potentially more hosts can develop high-titred viremias, and a greater number of potential vector species become competent to transmit the virus. This is illustrated by VEE virus, which exists in two geographically overlapping, but biologically distinct, forms throughout northern South America, Central America, Mexico, and Florida: a persisitent enzootic form, and a periodic epizootic form. For example, enzootic VEE virus in Columbia experienced genetic drift in the 1960s (identified by oligonucleotide fingerprints) that led to the evolution of highly virulent epizootic forms (123). In Central America, where a major epizootic took place from 1969 to 1972, the enzootic cycle is maintained by a single mosquito species, *C. taeniopius* (132), whereas the epizootic variant was transmitted by up to six species (although, curiously, not by *C. taeniopius*) (131). Epizootics of VEE virus are self-limiting because the number of susceptible hosts is exhausted.

Interspecific variation in vector competence can lead to selection of variants in virus virulence. For example, SLE virus has three biotypes—of high, intermediate, or low virulence—and these are genetically distinct by oligonucleotide fingerprint analysis (146). Most isolates from Central and East U.S.A. are highly virulent, whereas those from the West are of intermediate virulence. Thus, SLE virus is a more serious disease, and epidemics are more frequent, in the East than in the West. The explanation for this geographic distinction lies with the interspecific variation of the vector (98). In the East, SLE virus is transmitted by *C. tarsalis*, a highly efficient vector that transmits virus strains which induce only low-titerd viremia in avian hosts (and thus, incidentally, are less pathogenic for man); in the East, *C. tarsalis* is replaced by *C. pipiens*, a less competent vector, which therefore selects for virus strains causing high viremia in birds (and also greater severity for man).

Interspecific variation in vector competence also may be significant for viruses introduced to new areas, where different potential vector species are present. For example, in 1979, Ross River virus spread east from its previously limited region of Australia, New Guinea, and the Solomon Islands, to Fiji, American Samoa and—in 1980—to the Cook Islands. In Rarotonga, the most populous of the Cook Islands, the majority of the inhabitants became infected, and the levels of viremia in humans were unusually high (125). The severity of this epidemic may have been solely due to the high susceptibility of the native population. An additional explanation is that a phenotypic change was induced in the virus by the presence of a different vector species in the Cook islands (*A. polynesiensis*) compared to Australia (*C. annulirostris* and *A. vigilax*). This notion needs to be tested by comparing the virulence of isolates from the Cook Islands and Australia, and by comparing the competence of the different vector species. Similar hypotheses have been proposed to explain the unusually severe epidemic of RVF virus in Egypt when the virus appeared there for the first time in 1977 (5), and for the apparently greater virulence of YF virus in South America than in Africa where YF virus originated (97).

Vector species also differ in their ability to transmit viruses vertically. Viruses that are vertically transmitted may be sheltered from some of the selection pressures induced by vertebrate hosts, and so (as suggested above for JE virus) vertical transmission will act to increase genetic diversity. Additionally, vertical transmission in a relatively nondispersive vector population will reduce gene flow between small virus populations, and so increase the potential for new genotypes to become established.

Vector–Host Interactions

The feeding preferences of vectors (i.e., vector–host interactions) also have significance for arboviruses in that different hosts will vary in their susceptibility to the virus. For example, the maintenance hosts of West

Nile (WN) virus are wild birds, and the vector of WN virus in Africa and the Middle East is *C. univittatus*, which specializes on birds (and is also anthrophilic). Thus in South Africa, the infection rate of this mosquito species is high, with a minimum of 25:1000 females infected. In contrast, in the Indian subcontinent, the main vector appears to be *C. tritaeniorhynchus*, a cattle-feeder that only rarely feeds on birds or man. Here the infection rate is very low, with a minimum of 0.1:1000 females infected (60).

The optimum virulence of viruses transmitted by vectors that feed on refractory hosts will be higher than that of viruses transmitted by vectors feeding on more susceptible hosts. This may explain the speed with which highly virulent strains can evolve during an epidemic/epizootic, such as for VEE virus in Central America. In this case, the transmission cycle changes from an enzootic cycle involving *C. taeniopius* feeding on viremic wild rodents and marsupials (which are susceptible to enzootic VEE virus strains) to an epizootic cycle involving different mosquito species, such as *A. taeniorrhynchus* and *Psophora comfinnis*, feeding on viremic horses and man (and possibly dogs), which are relatively refractory to enzootic VEE virus strains (132, 140). Highly virulent strains will be selected during the epizootic cycle because of the feeding preferences of the mosquito species involved.

Vector species also differ in their ability to disperse. For example, Hoogstraal (64) divided tick vectors into species living in restricted habitats and those living in generalized habitats. Restricted habitats involve shelter-seeking ticks adapted to feeding throughout their life cycle only on animals inhabiting burrows, trees, or ground-level colonies; whereas generalized habitats involve ticks that feed on wandering hosts. A firm prediction would be that viruses transmitted by restricted habitat ticks are likely to be the most genetically diverse. This may explain the high genetic diversity of ASF virus, transmitted by soft ticks living in the restricted habitat of a warthog burrow, compared to the genetic homogeneity of CTF virus, transmitted by immature hard ticks which live in generalized habitats and feed on small mammals. However, this distinction is complicated by the dispersal habits of the vertebrate hosts. Viruses may be transported vast distances, for example, by migrating birds (105, 134). Such a vehicle provides gene flow between geographically dispersed niches and may explain why, for example, tick-borne orbiviruses found in seabird colonies in the Northern and Southern hemispheres represent a single gene pool (100). In contrast, the extreme genetic heterogeneity of LAC virus is probably due to the limited gene flow between populations of the mosquito *A. triseriatus* isolated in small woodlots, which may be only 200 to 300 m apart (57). This is not only due to the inability of the mosquitoes to disperse, but also because the vertebrate hosts of LAC virus, the eastern chipmunk and the grey squirrel, are also restricted to woodlots (52).

Intraspecific Variation

Following the suggestion by Craig and Hickey (31) that there must be genetic variation in the ability of mosquitoes to transmit arboviruses, intraspecific variation in susceptibility to infection has been reported for populations of the vectors of numerous arboviruses, including CHIK, DEN, LAC, SLE, WEE, WN, and YF viruses (36, 59). Furthermore, genetic variation in transmission rates by infected mosquitoes has been reported for LAC virus in *A. triseriatus* (57) and for YF virus in *A. aegypti* (6). As for interspecific variation (see above), intraspecific variation in vector competence can be a major influence on the selection pressures on arbovirus virulence.

Perhaps the most studied example of intraspecific variation in vector competence is for *A. triseriatus*, the vector of LAC virus. The virus is only endemic within a limited region of the geographic range of the mosquito; there are large areas surrounding the endemic region where *A. triseriatus* is found but LAC virus is only rarely detected (108). Variation in the vector competence of *A. triseriatus* from different geographic regions has been reported, with vector populations in the endemic region having significantly lower transmission and infection rates than those in nonendemic regions (57). It has been postulated that in the region where LAC virus is endemic, mosquitoes are more frequently exposed to the virus, and selection favors resistance to infection (57). This argument is based on reports that oral infection by LAC virus (and other arboviruses) causes significant fitness costs to a mosquito, whereas vertically infected mosquitoes experience less deleterious effects and are refractory to superinfection by feeding on viremic hosts (108). Thus, in the endemic region LAC virus is maintained by vertical transmission, and mosquito fitness is maximized by having low susceptibility to oral infection.

A confounding effect that strengthens the correlation between the vector competence of *A. triseriatus* and LAC virus endemicity may involve geographic variation in LAC virus virulence. In regions where mosquitoes have relatively low susceptibility to LAC virus there will be strong selection pressure on the virus population to maximize virulence (and so increase the level of viremia); in contrast, in regions where mosquitoes have very high susceptibility to infection, virus strains with relatively low virulence are able to be transmitted. Thus, the high prevalence of infection in the endemic region could be explained—at least partially—by the greater probability of virus isolation from infected hosts in that area, as a result of the relatively high virulence of local virus strains. Although considerable genetic heterogeneity amongst LAC viral isolates has been detected in oligonucleotide fingerprints (77), we are unaware of any attempt to identify phenotypic variation amongst LAC virus strains.

Intraspecific variation in other factors, such as host preference, may also have significance for arboviruses. For example, *C. univittatus*, the vector of

WN virus in South Africa, apparently varies in its degree of anthropophily. In endemic sites on the highveld, these mosquitoes feed primarily on birds, and are only slightly anthropophilic, whereas in the Karoo region, where a major epidemic was recorded, *C. univittatus* is very attracted to man (89). The difference in feeding behavior between these two populations may be intrinsic. Alternatively, host-mediated competition (157) caused by high population densities in the Karoo region may have led to host switching.

Differences in the densities of vector populations, per se, can influence selection pressures on arboviruses. At high densities, transmission frequencies are higher, so that the costs and benefits associated with virulence will be altered. When ecological parameters induce an increase in vector population density, the enhanced benefits of high virulence caused by the greater transmission frequency could outweigh the increase in costs due to host morbidity. Thus, competition between viruses within the host will lead to the evolution of higher virulence. This may explain why epidemics/epizootics of certain arboviruses, such as EEE and VEE viruses (99, 123), are commonly associated with the evolution of new strains. An epidemic is generated by an increase in vector population density (or at least an increase in vector/host contact), and this in turn changes the selection pressures on viruses so that relatively high virulence strains become favored. The combination of high vector density and highly virulent viruses leads to a significant increase in the number of hosts infected, and possibly to an increase in the host range (which may also allow new mosquito species to act as vectors) which, in turn, leads to genetic variability (as demonstrated by VEE virus). These examples illustrate the complex interactions between vector and vertebrate host that influence the selection pressures exerted upon arboviruses.

Relative Roles of Vector and Vertebrate Hosts in Arbovirus Evolution

Although this review is concerned with the roles of arthropod vectors in arbovirus evolution, it is relevant to consider how these roles compare with those of the vertebrate host. In terms of selection pressures, the most obvious difference is vertebrate immunity; the role of arthropod immunity in arbovirus evolution has not been explored. Based on the degree of antigenic variation of arboviruses, predictions have been made regarding the relative roles of vertebrate and invertebrate hosts in virus evolution (78, 79). Viruses that show high levels of serotypic variation are exposed to strong immune pressure and therefore are considered to depend on the vertebrate host for maintenance; for viruses that show little serotypic variation the vertebrate is a dead-end host and the vector the maintenance host. One problem with these predictions concerns the definition of viral species. For example, BTV is considered a single viral species comprising

24 serotypes; the virus appears to rely on vertebrate hosts (particularly cattle) for maintenance (79). By analogy, the Great Island group of tick-borne orbiviruses probably represents a single species of some 35 serotypes (100). The strong immune pressure to which GI viruses are exposed is exerted by seabirds; however, GI viruses rely on the tick vector for maintenance during the period when the seabirds vacate the breeding colony. Furthermore, if serotypically stable viral species do not require a vertebrate host for maintenance and transmission, then they must rely on vertical transmission by the vector in order to survive. Only 2 serotypes of CTF virus are recognized, indicating that this virus is sheltered from the immune pressures of the vertebrate hosts, and relies on the tick vector for maintenance. However, CTF virus is not transmitted vertically by ticks (42). Thus, in contrast to the predictions based on antigenic variation (see above), a virus may rely on its vector for maintenance but still be exposed to high levels of immune pressure, and alternatively, a virus may require amplification in the vertebrate host for maintenance despite evidence that it experiences relatively low levels of immune pressure.

Low levels of antigenic variation are also consistent with high virulence. If an arbovirus gives rise to high mortality rates in a vertebrate population, there will be a low or abnormal distribution of antibody prevalence in the vertebrate population (resulting from death of otherwise immune hosts) and a corresponding reduction in the degree of immune selection pressure.

Vertebrate hosts can also develop immunity to the arthropod vector, particularly to ixodid ticks (163, 164). Vector-borne virus transmission is impaired when the vertebrate host is immune to the vector species (69, 156). Furthermore, the potential for vertical transmission of arboviruses may be greatly reduced owing to the reduced fecundity of adult female ticks fed on tick-resistant hosts (68). The adverse effect on reproductive output may be one reason why tick-borne viruses that are transmitted vertically by ticks also rely on horizontal transmission for maintenance (see above).

Besides immune pressure, which largely acts at the level of genetic drift, the vertebrate host also differs from the arthropod vector in providing opportunities for genetic shift of arboviruses. The potential for genetic shift depends on the frequency of mixed infections of a single cell with genetically compatible viruses. Factors affecting this frequency are generalized in Table 2.2. In the vertebrate host, mixed infections are probably limited to those occasions when an animal is inoculated with more than one viral genotype by cofeeding arthropod vectors. This requires that multiple, genetically compatible viral types are circulating within an ecological niche. Recombination or reassortment may then occur if the genotypes coinfect cells of the vertebrate host. In the arthropod vector, the potential for reassortment (but not necessarily recombination) is limited by interference. The effect of interference is circumvented by interrupted feeding, a common event in insects but rare in ticks. Davies and colleagues (35)

TABLE 2.2. Factors influencing the probability of mixed viral infections in the vertebrate or invertebrate host.

Effect on the probability of mixed infections	Vertebrate host	Arthropod vector
Positive	High density of vector on host High viremia levels	Lifetime persistence of infection Vertical transmission Multiple bloodmeals (insects)
Negative	Short duration of viremia Infections induce immunity/death Interference?	Few bloodmeals (ticks) High mortality rates off the vertebrate host Interference Low levels of virus in infected vector

postulated that reassortment of tick-borne viruses is most likely to occur during epizootics in which the vertebrate hosts develop high viremic titers and die. These conditions would increase the likelihood of partially engorged infected ticks completing their bloodmeals on a second, virus-infected host.

The relative probabilities of recombination/reassortment in the vertebrate and invertebrate hosts need to be determined in order to assess the potential threat of new recombinant/reassortant viruses to human and veterinary health. Generally, the persistence of arbovirus infections in the arthropod vector is considered to provide greater opportunities for recombination and reassortment compared with the relatively short-term viremia in the vertebrate host (35, 58, 130).

Conclusions

In order to develop effective strategies for combating arboviral infections of humans and other animals, we need to understand (1) how arboviruses change in response to changing environmental factors, (2) how rapidly they change, and (3) to what type of selection pressures they are responding (139). As demonstrated in this review, all these factors involve the arthropod host of an arbovirus, either directly or indirectly. One selection pressure, only briefly discussed, is the effect of temperature on the development of arboviral infections within the arthropod vector. Micro- and macroclimatic conditions also affect the development and distribution of vector species, which in turn influence arboviral epidemiology, epizootiology, ecology, and biogeography. Thus, a major selection pressure for arboviruses in the near future (and even today) may be the impact of global warming and ensuing climatic changes.

Acknowledgments. Many thanks to Drs. J. Aaskov, C. Dye, E.A. Gould, J.S. Porterfield, and S. Randolph for critical reviews of the manuscript, and to S. Clarke for typing.

References

1. Akov, S., 1982, Blood digestion in ticks, Obenchain, F.D., and Galun, R. (eds): in Physiology of Ticks, Current Themes in Tropical Science Vol. 1, Pergamon Press, Oxford, pp. 197–211.
2. Anderson, R.M., and May, R.M., 1982, Coevolution of hosts and parasites. *Parasitology* **85**:411–426.
3. Balashov, Yu. S., 1968, Bloodsucking ticks (lxodoidea)—vectors of diseases of man and animals, Leningrad, Nauka. English translation in *Miscellaneous Publications of the Entomological Society of America* **8**:161–376 (1972).
4. Baldridge, G.D., Beaty, B.J. and Hewlett, M.J., Genomic stability of La Crosse virus during vertical and horizontal transmission, *Arch. Virol.* **108**: 89–99.
5. Battles, J.K., and Dalrymple, J.M., 1988, Genetic variation among geographic isolates of Rift Vally fever virus. *Am. J. Trop. Med. Hyg.* **39**: 617–631.
6. Beaty, B.J. and Aitken, T.H.G., 1979, In vitro transmission of yellow fever virus by geographic strains of *Aedes aegypti. Mosq. News* **39**:232–238.
7. Beaty, B.J., Tesh, R.B., and Aitken, T.H.G., 1980, Transovarial transmission of yellow fever virus in *Stegomyia* mosquitoes, *Am. J. Trop. Med. Hyg.* **29**:125–132.
8. Beaty, B.J., et al., 1981, Formation of reassortant bunyaviruses in dually infected mosquitoes, *Virology* **111**:662–665.
9. Beaty, B.J., et al., 1983, Interference between bunyaviruses in *Aedes triseriatus* mosquitoes, *Virology* **127**:83–90.
10. Beaty, B.J., et al., 1985, Evolution of bunyaviruses by genome reassortment in dually infected mosquitoes (*Aedes triseriatus*), *Science* **230**:548–550.
11. Benda, R., 1958, The common tick, *Ixodes ricinus* L., as a reservoir and vector of tick-borne encephalitis. I. Survival of the virus (strain B3) during the development of the tick under laboratory conditions. *J. Hyg. Epidemiol. Microbiol. Immunol.* **2**:314–330.
12. Bhatt, P.N., and Anderson, C.R., 1971, Attenuation of a strain of Kyasanur forest disease virus for mice. *Ind. J. Med. Res.* **59**:199–205.
13. Bilsel, P.A., Tesh, R.B. and Nichol, S.T., 1988, RNA genome stability of Toscana virus during serial transovarial transmission in the sandfly *Phlebotomus perniciosus. Virus Res.* **11**:87–94.
14. Boorman, J., 1960, Observations on the amount of virus present in the haemolymph of *Aedes aegypti* infected with Uganda S, yellow fever and Semliki forest viruses. *Trans. R. Soc. Trop. Med. Hyg.* **54**:362–365.
15. Booth, T.F., et al., 1989, Anatomical basis of Thogoto virus infection in BHK cell culture and the ixodid tick vector, *Rhipicephalus appendiculatus. J. Gen. Virol.* **70**:1093–1104.

16. Booth, T.F., et al., 1991, Dissemination, replication and trans-stadial persistence of Dugbe virus in the tick vector, *Amblyomma variegatum*. *Am. J. Trop. Med. Hyg.* (in press).
17. Bowen, G.S., et al., 1980, Geographic variation among St. Louis encephalitis virus strains in the viremic responses of avian hosts, *Am. J. Trop. Med. Hyg.* **29**:1411–1419.
18. Brown, D.T., and Condreay, L.D., 1986, Replication of alphaviruses in mosquito cells, Schlesinger, S., and Schlesinger, M.S. (eds): in The Togaviridae and Flaviviridae, Plenum Press, Ltd., New York, pp. 171–207.
19. Brown, S.E., et al., 1989, Co-circulation of multiple Colorado tick fever virus genotypes. *Am. J. Trop. Med. Hyg.* **40**:94–101.
20. Burgdorfer, W., 1960, Colorado tick fever. II. The behavior of Colorado tick fever virus in rodents, *J. Infect. Dis.* **107**:384–388.
21. Burgdorfer, W., and Varma, M.G.R., 1967, Trans-stadial and transovarial development of disease agents in arthropods, *Ann. Rev. Entomol.* **12**: 347–376.
22. Burke, D.S., and Leake, C.J., 1988, Japanese encephalitis, Monath, T.P. (ed.): in The Arboviruses: Epidemiology and Ecology, Volume 3, CRC Press, Inc., Boca Raton, Florida, pp. 63–92.
23. Burness, A.T.H., et al., 1988, Genetic stability of Ross River virus during epidemic spread in nonimmune humans, *Virology* **167**:639–643.
24. Chamberlain, R.W., 1982, Arbovirology—then and now, *Am. J. Trop. Med. Hyg.* **31**:430–437.
25. Chamberlain, R.W., and Sudia, W.D., 1961, Mechanism of transmission of viruses by mosquitoes, *Ann. Rev. Entomol.* **6**:371–390.
26. Chandler, L.J., et al., 1990, Heterologous reassortment of bunyaviruses in *Aedes triseriatus* mosquitoes and transovarial and oral transmission of newly evolved genotypes, *J. Gen. Virol.* **71**:1045–1050.
27. Chernesky, M.A., and McLean, D.M., 1969, Localisation of Powassan virus in *Dermacentor andersoni* ticks by immunofluorescence, *Can. J. Microbiol.* **15**:1399–1408.
28. Chu, M.C., O'Rourke, E.J., and Trent, D.W., 1989, Genetic relatedness among structural protein genes of dengue 1 virus stains. *J. Gen. Virol.* **70**: 1701–1712.
29. Clutton-Brock, T.H., and Harvey, P.H., 1984, Comparative approaches to investigating adaptation, Krebs, J.R., and Davies, N.B. (eds): in Behavioural Ecology. An evolutionary approach (2nd. Ed.), Blackwell Scientific Publications, Oxford pp. 7–29.
30. Coelen, R.J., and Mackenzie, J.S., 1988, Genetic variation of Murray Valley enephalitis virus. *J. Gen. Virol.* **69**:1903–1912.
31. Craig, G.B., Jr., and Hickey, W.A., 1967, Genetics of *Aedes aegypti*, Wright, J.W., and Pal, R. (eds): in Genetics of Insect Vectors of Disease, Amsterdam, Elsevier, pp. 67–131.
32. Davey, M.W., Mahon, R.J., and Gibbs, A.J., 1979, Togavirus interference in *Culex annulirostris* mosquitoes, *J. Gen. Virol.* **42**:641–643.
33. Davies, C.R., Jones, L.D., and Nuttall, P.A., 1989, Viral interference in the tick, *Rhipicephalus appendiculatus*. I. Interference to oral superinfection by Thogoto virus, *J. Gen. Virol.* **70**:2461–2468.

34. Davies, C.R., Jones, L.D., and Nuttall, P.A., 1990, A comparative study of the infection thresholds of Thogoto virus for *Rhipicephalus appendiculatus* and *Amblyomma variegatum. Am. J. Trop. Med. Hyg.* **43**:99–103.
35. Davies, C.R., et al., 1987, In vivo reassortment of Thogoto virus (a tick-borne influenza-like virus) following oral infection of *Rhipicephalus appendiculatus* ticks, *J. Gen. Virol.* **68**:2331–2338.
36. DeFoliart, G.R., Grimstad, P.R., and Watts, D.M., 1987, Advances in mosquito-borne arbovirus/vector research. *Ann. Rev. Entomol.* **32**:479–505.
37. Devi, P.S., 1966, Some biological properties of two variants of Kyasanur Forest disease virus. *Ind. J. Med. Res.* **54**:419–424.
38. Dixon, L.K., and Wilkinson, P.J., 1988, Genetic diversity of African swine fever virus isolates from soft ticks (*Ornithodoros moubata*) inhabiting warthog burrows in Zambia. *J. Gen. Virol.* **69**:2981–2993.
39. Doi, R., 1970, Studies on the mode of development of Japanese encephalitis virus in some groups of mosquitoes by the fluorescent antibody technique, *Jap. J. Exp. Med.* **40**:101–115.
40. Doi, R., Shiraska, H., and Sasa, M., 1967, The mode of development of Japanese encephalitis virus in the mosquito *Culex tritaeniorhynchus summorosus* as observed by the fluorescent antibody technique, *Jap. J. Exp. Med.* **37**:227–238.
41. Eaton, B.T., 1978, Persistent togavirus infection of *Aedes albopictus* cells, Kurstak, E., and Maramorosch, K. (eds): in Viruses and the Environment, Academic Press, New York, pp. 181–201.
42. Emmons, R.W., 1988, Ecology of Colorado tick fever virus, *Ann. Rev. Microbiol.* **42**:49–64.
43. Ewald, P.W., 1983, Host-parasite relations, vectors, and the evolution of disease severity. *Ann. Rev. Ecol. Syst.* **14**:465–485.
44. Ewald, P.W., 1987, Tranmission modes and evolution of the parasitism-mutalism continum, *Annals N.Y. Acad. Sci.* **503**:295–306.
45. Ewald, P.W., 1988, Cultural vectors, virulence, and the emergence of evolutionary epidemiology, P.H. Harvey (ed), in: Oxford Survey of Evolutionary Biology, Oxford University Press, Vol. 5, pp. 215–245.
46. Faran, M.E., et al., 1987. Reduced survival of adult *Culex pipiens* infected with Rift valley fever virus. *Am. J. Trop. Med. Hyg.* **37**:403–409.
47. Faran, M.E., et al., 1988, The distribution of Rift valley fever virus in the mosquito *Culex pipiens* as revealed by viral titration of dissected organs and tissues, *Am. J. Trop. Med. Hyg.* **39**:206–213.
48. Fine, P.E.M., 1975, Vectors and vertical transmission: An epidemiologic perspective, *Annals N.Y. Acad. Sci.* **266**: 173–194.
49. Florio, L., Miller, M.S., and Mugruge, E.R., 1950, Colorado tick fever. Isolation of the virus from *Dermacentor andersoni* in nature and a laboratory study of the transmission of the virus in the tick. *J. Immunol.* **64**:257–263.
50. Flynn, L.M., Coelen, R.J., and MacKenzie, J.S., 1989, Kunjin virus isolates of Australia are genetically homogeneous. *J. Gen. Virol.* **70**:2819–2824.
51. Fuller, F.J., Freedman-Faulstich, E.Z., and Barnes, J.A., 1987, Complete nucleotide sequence of the tick-borne, orthomyxo-like Dhori/Indian/1313/61 virus nucleoprotein gene. *Virology* **160**:81–87.

52. Gauld, L.W., et al., 1974, Observations on a natural cycle of La Crosse virus (California group) in southwestern California. *Am. J. Trop. Med. Hyg.* **23**:983–992.
53. Gentsch, J.R., et al., 1980, Evidence from recombinant bunyavirus studies that the M RNA gene products elicit neutralizing antibodies. *Virology* **102**:190–204.
54. Greig, A., 1972, The localisation of African swine fever virus in the tick *Ornithodoros moubata porcinus, Arch. ges. Virusforsch.* **39**:240–247.
55. Grimstad, P.R., 1983, Mosquitoes and the incidence of encephalitis. *Ad. Virus Res.* **28**:357–438.
56. Grimstad, P.R., Ross, Q.E., and Craig Jr., G.B., 1980, *Aedes triseriatus* (Diptera: Culicidae) and La Crosse virus. II. Modification of mosquito feeding behaviour by virus infection, *J. Med. Entomol.* **17**:1–7.
57. Grimstad, P.R., et al., 1977, *Aedes triseriatus* and La Crosse virus: Geographic variation in vector susceptibility and ability to transmit. *Am. J. Trop. Med. Hyg.* **26**:990–996.
58. Hahn, C.S., et al., 1988, Western equine encephalitis virus is a recombinant virus, *Proc. Natl. Acad. Sci. USA* **85**:5997–6001
59. Hardy, J.L., et al., 1983, Intrinsic factors affecting vector competence of mosquitoes for arboviruses. *Ann. Rev. Entomol.* **28**:229–262.
60. Hayes, C.G., 1988, West Nile Fever, Monath, T.P. (ed): in The Arboviruses: Epidemiology and Ecology, Vol. 5, CRC Press, Inc., Boca Raton, Florida, pp. 59–88.
61. Heidner, H.W., et al., 1988, Bluetongue virus genome remains stable throughout prolonged infection of cattle, *J. Gen. Virol.* **69**:2629–2636.
62. Helmy N., Khalil, G.M., and Hoogstraal, H., 1983, Hyperparasitism in *Ornithodoros erracticus, J. Parasitol.* **69**:229–233.
63. Holland, J., et al., 1982, Rapid evolution of RNA genomes. *Science* **215**:1577–1585.
64. Hoogstraal, H., 1973, Viruses and ticks, Gibbs, A.J. (ed): in Viruses and Invertebrates, North-Holland Publ., The Hague, pp. 351–390.
65. Hoogstraal, H., 1979, The epidemiology of tick-borne Crimean-Congo hemorrhagic fever in Asia, Europe and Africa. *J. Med. Entomol.* **15**:307–417.
66. Houk, E.J., et al., 1985, Western equine encephalomyelitis virus: In vivo infection and morphogenesis in mosquito mesenteronal epithelial cells, *Virus Res.* **2**:123–138.
67. Iroegbu, C.U., and Pringle, C.R., 1981, Genetic interactions among viruses of the Bunyamwera complex, *J. Virol.* **37**:383–394.
68. Jones, L.D., and Nuttall, P.A., 1988, The effect of host immunity on the transmission of tick-borne viruses, *Anim. Tech.* **39**:161–165.
69. Jones, L.D., and Nuttall, P.A., 1990, The effect of host resistance to tick infestation on the transmission of Thogoto virus by ticks. *J. Gen. Virol.* **71**: 1039–1043.
70. Jones, L.D., et al., 1987, A novel model of arbovirus transmission involving a nonviremic host, *Science* **237**:775–777.
71. Jones, L.D., et al., 1987, Reassortment of Thogoto virus (a tick-borne influenza-like virus) in a vertebrate host, *J. Gen. Virol.* **68**:1299–1306.

72. Jones, L.D., et al., 1989, Viral interference in the tick, *Rhipicephalus appendiculatus*. II. Absence of interference with Thogoto virus when the tick gut is by-passed by parenteral inoculation. *J. Gen. Virol.* **70**:2469–2473.
73. Karabatsos, N., 1985, International Catalogue of Arboviruses including Certain Other Viruses of Vertebrates, Third Edition, American Society of Tropical Medicine and Hygiene, San Antonio.
74. Karabatsos, N., et al., 1987, Antigenic variants of Colorado tick fever virus, *J. Gen. Virol.* **68**:1463–1469.
75. Kay, B.H., Fanning, I.D., and Mottram, P., 1989, Rearing temperature influences flavivirus vector competence of mosquitoes, *Med. Vet. Entomol.* **3**:415–422.
76. Kirkegaard, K., and Baltimore, D., 1986, The mechanism of RNA recombination in poliovirus, *Cell* **47**:433–443.
77. Klimas, R.A., et al., 1981, Genotypic varieties of La Crosse virus isolated from different geographic regions of the continental United Sates and evidence for a naturally occuring intertypic recombinant La Crosse virus. *Am. J. Epidem.* **114**:112–131.
78. Knudson, D.L., and Shope, R.E., 1985, Overview of the orbiviruses, Barber, T.L., and Jochim, M.M. (eds): in Bluetongue and related orbiviruses, Alan R. Liss Inc., New York, pp. 255–66.
79. Knudson, D.L., and Monath, T.P., 1990, Orbiviruses, Fields, B.N. et al.: in Virology, Raven Press, New York, pp. 1405–1433.
80. Kondrashova, Z.N., and Filippovets, R.V., 1970, Infection rate of *Ixodes persulcatus* ticks and certain questions of transovarial transmission after dosaged infection with tick-borne encephalitis virus, *Vop. Virusol.* **15**:703–708.
81. Korenberg, E.I., and Pchelkina, A.A., 1984, Tick-borne encephalitis virus titres in engorged adult *Ixodes persulcatus* ticks, *Parazitologiya, Leningrad* **18**:123–127. English translation, NAMRU-3 T1788.
82. Kramer, L.D., et al., 1981, Dissemination barriers for western equine encephalomyelitis virus in *Culex tarsalis* infected after ingestion of low viral doses, *Am. J. Trop. Med. Hyg.* **30**:190–197.
83. Kuberski, T., 1979, Fluorescent antibody studies on the development of Dengue-2 virus in *Aedes Albopictus* (Diptera: Culicidae), *J. Med. Entomol.* **16**:343–349.
84. Leake, C.J., 1984, Transovarial transmission of arboviruses by mosquitoes, Mayo, M.A. and Harrap, K.A. (eds): in Vectors in Virus Biology, Academic Press, London, pp. 63–91.
85. Leake, C.J., and Johnson, R.T., 1987, The pathogenesis of Japanese encephalitis virus in *Culex tritaeniorhyncus* mosquitoes, *Trans. Roy. Soc. Trop. Med. Hyg.* **81**:681–685.
86. Ludwig, G.V., et al., 1989, Enzyme processing of La Crosse virus glycoprotein G1: A bunyavirus-vector infection model, *Virology* **171**:108–113.
87. May, R.M., and Anderson, R.M., 1983, Epidemiology and genetics in the coevolution of parasites and hosts. *Proc. Roy. Soc. London* **B219**:281–313.
88. McCance, E.F., 1984, Genetics of Colorado tick fever virus, Ph.D. Thesis, Yale University, New Haven, Connectícut.

89. McIntosh, B.M., et al., 1976, Epidemics of West Nile and Sindbis viruses in South Africa with *Culex (Culex) univittatus* Theobald as vector. *S. Afr. J. Sci.* **72**:295–300.
90. McKelvey, J.J. Jr., Eldridge, B.F., and Maramorosch, K., eds., 1981, Vectors of Disease Agents, Praeger, New York, p. 243.
91. Mellor, P.S., and Boorman, J., 1980, Multiplication of bluetongue virus in *Culicoides nubeculosis* (Meigen) simultaneously infected with the virus and the microfilariae of *Onchocerca cervicalis* (Railliet & Henry), *Ann. Trop. Med. Parisotol.* **74**:463–469.
92. Miles, J.A.R., Pillai, J.S., and Maguire, T., 1973, Multiplication of Whataroa viurs in mosquitoes, *J. Med. Entomol.* **10**:176–185.
93. Miller, B.R., and Mitchell, C.J., 1986, Passage of yellow fever virus: Its effect on infection and transmission rates in *Aedes aegypti*, *Am. J. Trop. Med. Hyg.* **35**:1302–1309.
94. Miller, B.R., et al., 1985, Experimental studies on the replication and dissemination of Qalyub virus (Bunyaviridae: Nairovirus) in the putative tick vector, *Ornithodoros (Pavlovskyella) erraticus*, *Am. J. Trop. Med. Hyg.* **34**:180–187.
95. Mims, C.A., Day, M.F., and Marshall, I.D., 1966, Cytopathic effect of Semliki forest virus in the mosquito *Aedes aegypti*, *Am. J. Trop. Med. Hyg.* **15**:775–784.
96. Mitchell, C., 1983, Mosquito vector competence and arboviruses, Harris K. (ed): in Current Topics in Vector Research Vol. 1, Praeger, New York, pp. 63–92.
97. Monath, T.P., 1988, Yellow fever, Monath, T.P. (ed): in The Arboviruses: Epidemiology and Ecology, Vol. 5. CRC Press, Inc., Boca Raton, Florida, pp. 139–232.
98. Monath, T.P., and Tsai, T.F., 1987, St. Louis encephalitis: Lessons from the last decade, *Am. J. Trop. Med. Hyg.* **37**(Suppl.):40S–59S.
99. Morris, C.D., 1988, Eastern Equine Encephalomyelitis, Monath, T.P. (ed): in The Arboviruses: Epidemiology and Ecology, Vol. 2. CRC Press, Inc., Boca Raton, Florida, pp. 1–20.
100. Moss, S.R., Ayres, C.M., and Nuttall, P.A., 1988, The Great Island subgroup of tick-borne orbiviruses represents a single gene pool, *J. Gen. Virol.* **69**:2721–2727.
101. Moss, S.R., Fukusho, A., and Nuttall, P.A., 1990, RNA segment 5 of Broadhaven virus, a tick-borne orbivirus, shows sequence homology with segment 5 of bluetongue virus, *Virology* **179**:482–484.
102. Murphy, F.A., Whitfield, S.G., Sudia, W.D., and Chamberlain, R.W., 1975, Interaction of vector with vertebrate pathogenic viruses, Maramorosch, K., and Shope, R.E. (eds): in Invertebrate Immunity, Academic Press, New York, pp. 25–48.
103. Nosek, J., et al., 1986, Pecularities of tick-borne encephalitis virus reproduction in *Haemaphysalis inermis* and their explants, *Acta Virol* **30**:396–401.
104. Ntiamoa-Baidu, Y., 1986, Parasitism of female *Ixodes (Afrixodes) moreli* (Acari:Ixodidae) by males, *J. Med. Entomol.* **23**:484–488.
105. Nuttall, P.A., 1984, Transmission of viruses to wild life by ticks, Mayo, M., and Harrap, K.A. (eds): in Vectors in Virus Biology, Academic Press, London, pp. 135–159.

106. Nuttall, P.A., and Moss. S.R., 1989, Genetic reassortment indicates a new grouping for tick-borne orbiviruses, *Virology* **171**:156–161.
107. Obenchain, F.D., and Galun, R., eds., 1982, Physiology of Ticks, Pergamon Press, Oxford, p. 509.
108. Paulson, S.L., Grimstad, P.R., and Craig, G.B. Jr., 1989, Midgut and salivary gland barriers to La Crosse virus dissemination in mosquitoes of the *Aedes triseriatus* group, *Med. Vet. Ent.* **3**:113–123.
109. Pavlovsky, E.N., and Soloviev, V.D., 1940, Experimental study of the circulation of tick-borne encephalitis virus in the organism of the tick vector (*Ixodes persulcatus*), *Arh. Biol. Nauk.* **59**:111–117.
110. Pavlovsky, E.N., and Solovyov, V.D., 1941, On the circulation of spring-summer encephalitis virus in the organism of the tick vector, *Haemaphysalis concinna*, *Trudy voj. Med. Inst. Akad. Krasnoiarsk Armii S.M. Kirova* **25**: 9–18.
111. Peleg, J., 1975, In vivo behaviour of a Sindbis virus mutant isolated from persistently infected *Aedes aegypti* cell cultures, *Ann. N.Y. Acad. Sci.* **166**: 204–213.
112. Peters, C.J., and Dalrymple, J.M., 1990, Alphaviruses, Fields, B.N. (ed): in Virology, Plenum Press, Ltd., New York, pp. 713–761.
113. Pletnev, A.G., Yamshchikov, V.F., and Blinov, V.M., 1990, Nucleotide sequence of the genome and complete amino acid sequence of the polyprotein of tick-borne encephalitis virus, *Virology* **174**:250–263.
114. Plowright, W., Perry, C.T., and Peirce, M.A., 1970, Transovarial infection with African swine fever virus in the argasid tick *Ornithodoros moubata porcinus*, Walton, *Res. Vet. Sci.* **11**:582–584.
115. Plowright, W., Perry, C.T., and Greig, A. 1974, Sexual transmission of African swine fever in the tick *Ornithodoros moubata porcinus*, Walton. *Res. Vet. Sci.* **17**:106–113.
116. Pringle, C.R. et al., 1984, Restriction of sub-unit reassortment in the bunyaviridae, Compans, R.W., and Bishop, D.H.L. (eds): in Molecular Biology of Negative Strand Viruses, Academic Press, Orlando, pp. 45–50.
117. Reanney, D.C., 1982, The evolution of RNA viruses, *Ann. Rev. Microbiol.* **36**:47–73.
118. Reeves, W.C., 1974, Overwintering of arboviruses. *Progr. Med. Virol.* **17**:193–220.
119. Reeves, W.C., Bellamy, R.E., and Scrivani, R.P., 1958, Relationships of mosquito vectors to winter surival of encephalitis viruses. I. Under natural conditions. *Am. J. Hyg.* **67**:78–89.
120. Řeháček, J., 1962, Transovarial transmission of tick-borne encephalitis virus by ticks. *Acta Virol.* **6**:220–226.
121. Řeháček, J., 1965, Development of animal viruses and rickettsiae in ticks and mites, *Ann. Rev. Entomol.* **10**:1–24.
122. Reid, H.W., 1984, Epidemiology of louping ill, Mayo, M.A., and Harrap, K.A. (eds): in Vectors in Virus Biology, Academic Press, London, pp. 161–178.
123. Rico-Hesse, R., et al., 1988, Genetic variation of Venezuelan equine encephalitis virus strains of the ID variety in Columbia, *Am. J. Trop. Med. Hyg.* **38**:195–204.

124. Rosen, L., 1988, Further observations on the mechanism of vertical transmission of flaviviruses by *Aedes* mosquitoes, *Am. J. Trop. Med. Hyg.* **39**:123–126.
125. Rosen, L., Gubler, D.J., and Bennett, P.H., 1981, Epidemic polyarthritis (Ross River) virus infection in the Cook Islands. *Am. J. Trop. Med. Hyg.* **30**:1294–1302.
126. Rosomer, W.S., Faran, M.E., and Bailey, C.L., 1987, Newly recognised route of arbovirus dissemination from the mosquito (Diptera: Culicidae) midgut, *J. Med. Entomol.* **24**:431–432.
127. Rossignol, P.A., et al., 1985, Enhanced mosquito blood-finding success on parasitaemic hosts: Evidence for vector-parasite mutualism, *Proc. Natl. Acad. Sci. U.S.A.* **82**:7725–7727.
128. Rozeboom, L.E., and Burgdorfer, W., 1959, Development of Colorado tick fever virus in the Rocky mountain wood tick, *Dermacentor andersoni*, *Am. J. Hyg.* **69**:138–145.
129. Rozeboom, L.E., and Kassira, E.N., 1969, Dual infection of mosquitoes with strains of West Nile virus, *J. Med. Entomol.* **4**:407–411.
130. Samal, S.K., et al., 1987, Mixed infection of *Culicoides variipennis* with bluetongue virus serotypes 10 and 17: Evidence for high frequency reassortment in the vector, *J. Gen. Virol.* **68**:2319–2329.
131. Scherer, W.F., et al., 1982, Mesenteronal infection threshold of an epizootic strain of Venezuelan encephalitis virus in *Culex (Melanoconion) taeniopus* mosquitoes and its implications to the apparent disappearance of this virus strain from an enzootic habitat in Guatemala, *Am. J. Trop. Med. Hyg.* **31**:1030–1037.
132. Scherer, W.F., et al., 1985, Ecological observations of Venezuelan encephalitis virus in vertebrates and isolations of Nepuyo and Patois viruses from sentinel hamsters at Pacific and Atlantic habitats in Guatemala, 1968–1980. *Am. J. Trop. Med. Hyg.* **34**:790–798.
133. Scherer, W.F., et al., 1987, Vector competence of *Culex (Melanoconion) taeniopus* for allopatric and epizootic Venezuelan equine encephalomyelitis virus. *Am. J. Trop. Med. Hyg.* **36**:194–197.
134. Schmidt, J.R., and Shope, R.E., 1971, Kemerovo virus from a migrating common redstart of Eurasia, *Acta Virol.* **15**:112.
135. Smith, C.E.G., 1964, Factors influencing the behaviour of viruses in their arthropodan hosts, Taylor, A.E.R. (ed): in Host-parasite relationships in invertebrate hosts, Blackwell Scientific Press, Oxford, pp. 1–31.
136. Smith, D.B., and Inglis, S.C., 1987, The mutation rate and variability of eukaryotic viruses: An analytical review, *J. Gen. Virol.* **68**:2729–2740.
137. Staunton, D., Nuttall, P.A., and Bishop, D.H.L., 1989, Sequence analyses of Thogoto viral RNA segment 3: Evidence for a distant relationship between an arbovirus and members of the Orthomyxoviridae, *J. Gen. Virol.* **70**:2811–2817.
138. Stollar, V., 1980, Togaviruses in cultured arthropod cells, Schlesinger, R.W. (ed): in The Togaviruses, Academic Press, New York, pp. 583–621.
139. Strauss, E.G., Strauss, J.H., and Levine, A.J., 1990, Virus evolution, Fields B.N. et al. (eds): in Virology, Second Edition, Raven Press, Ltd., New York, pp. 167–190.

140. Sudia, W.D., and Newhouse, V.F., 1975, Epidemic Venezuelan equine encephalitis in North America: A summary of virus-vector-host relationships. *Am. J. Epidem.* **101**:1–13.
141. Sugiyama, K., Bishop, D.H.L., and Roy, P., 1981, Analyses of the genomes of bluetongue viruses recovered in the United States. I. Oligonucleotide fingerprint studies that indicate the existence of naturally occurring reassortant BTV isolates, *Virology* **114**:210–217.
142. Sundin, D.R., and Beaty, B.J., 1988, Interference to oral superinfection of *Aedes triseriatus* infected with La Crosse virus, *Am. J. Trop. Med. Hyg.* **38**:428–432.
143. Tabarés, E., et al., 1987, African swine fever virus DNA: Deletions and additions during adaptation to growth in monkey kidney cells. *Arch. Virol.* **97**:333–346.
144. Tesh, R.B., 1980, Experimental studies on the transovarial transmission of Kunjin and San Angelo viruses in mosquitoes, *Am. J. Trop. Med. Hyg.* **9**:657–666.
145. Tesh, R.B., 1984, Transovarial transmissions of arboviruses in their invertebrate vectors, Harris, K.F. (ed): in Current Topics in Vector Research, Vol. 2, Praeger Publishers, New York, pp. 57–76.
146. Trent, D.W., et al., 1981, Genetic heterogeneity among Saint Louis encephalitis virus isolates of different geographic isolates. *Virology* **114**:319–332.
147. Turell, M.J., Hardy, J.L., and Reeves, W.C., 1982, Sensitivity to carbon dioxide in mosquitoes infected with California serogroup arboviruses, *Am. J. Trop. Med. Hyg.* **31**:389–394.
148. Turell, M.J., Hardy, J.L., and Reeves, W.C., 1982, Stabilized infection of California encephalitis virus in *Aedes dorsalis*, and its implications for viral maintenance in nature, *Am. J. Trop. Med. Hyg.* **31**:1252–1259.
149. Turell, M.J., Reeves, W.C., and Hardy, J.L., 1982, Transovarial and transstadial transmission of California encephalitis virus in *Aedes dorsalis* and *Aedes melanimon*, *Am. J. Trop. Med. Hyg.* **31**:1021–1029.
150. Turell, M.J., et al., 1984, Enhanced arboviral transmission by mosquitoes that concurrently ingested microfilariae, *Science* **225**:1039–1041.
151. Turell, M.J., Gargan II, T.P., and Bailey, C.L., 1985, *Culex pipiens* (Diptera: Culicidae) morbidity and mortality associated with Rift Valley fever virus infection, *J. Med. Entomol.* **22**:332–337.
152. Turell, M.J., Rossi, C.A., and Bailey, C.L., 1985, Effect of extrinsic incubation temperature on the ability of *Aedes taeniorhynchus* and *Culex pipiens* to transmit Rift valley fever virus, *Am. J. Trop. Med. Hyg.* **34**: 1211–1218.
153. Turell, M.J., et al., 1987, Increased dissemination of dengue 2 virus in *Aedes aegypti* associated with concurrent ingestion of microfilariae of *Brugia malayi*, *Am. J. Trop. Med. Hyg.* **37**:197–201.
154. Turell, M.J., et al., 1990, Generation and transmission of Rift Valley fever viral reassortants by the mosquito *Culex pipiens*, *J. Gen. Virol.* **71**:2307–2312.
155. Ushijima, H., Clerx-Van Haaster, C.M., and Bishop, D.H.L., 1981, Analyses of Patois group bunyaviruses: Evidence for naturally occurring recombinant bunyaviruses and existence of immune precipitable and non-

precipitable nonvirion proteins induced in bunyavirus-infected cells. *Virology* **110**:318–332.

156. Voyakov, V.I., and Mishaeva, N.P., 1980, Investigation of a possibility of protecting vertebrates against transmissive infection with tick-borne encephalitis virus, *Vop. Virus.* **2**:170–172.
157. Waage, J.K., and Davies, C.R., 1986, Host-mediated competition in a bloodsucking insect community, *J. Anim. Ecol.* **55**:171–180.
158. Watts, D.M., et al., 1987, Effect of temperature on the vector efficiency of *Aedes aegypti* for Dengue 2 virus, *Am. J. Trop. Med. Hyg.*, **36**:143–152.
159. Weaver, S.C., 1986, Electron microscopic analysis of infection patterns for Venezuelan equine encephalomyelitis virus in the vector mosquito, *Culex (Melanoconion) taeniopus*, *Am. J. Trop. Med. Hyg.* **35**:624–631.
160. Wesley, R.D., and Tuthill, A.E., 1984, Genome relatedness among African swine fever virus field isolates by restriction endonuclease analysis. *Prev. Vet. Med.* **2**:53–62.
161. Whitfield, S.G., Murphy, F.A., and Sudia, W.D., 1973, St. Louis encephalitis virus: An ultrastructural study of infection in a mosquito vector, *Virology* **56**:70–87.
162. W.H.O., 1985, Arthropod-borne and rodent-borne virual diseases. *WHO Technical Report Series*, No. 719.
163. Wikel, S.K., 1982, Immune responses to arthropods and their products, *Ann. Rev. Entomol.* **27**:21–48.
164. Willadsen, P., 1980, Immunity to ticks, *Adv. Parasitol.* **18**:293–313.

3
Towards Integrated Control of Mosquitoes and Mosquito-borne Diseases in Ricelands

Motoyoshi Mogi and Teiji Sota

Introduction

Rice is the most important staple food supporting ca. 60% of the human population. Yet the higher production is needed to fill the demand from the increasing population. The flooded land required for the optimal growth of high-yield rice varieties provides mosquitoes, including vectors of human diseases, with extensive larval habitats.

Irrigated rice fields are a main larval habitat of ca. 40%, 20%, and 10% of major vector mosquitoes of malaria, filariasis, and viral diseases, respectively, at least locally (126). These figures are raised when we include species that prefer irrigation systems (canals, ponds) or their by-products (e.g., smaller, open ground pools formed from leaking water) rather than rice fields per se. Most of these species occur in tropical and subtropical regions. Introduction of paddy rice cultivation may be followed by an increase in mosquito-borne diseases (MBDs) (19, 43, 54, 105, 113). Thus, prevention of MBDs is an important component for achievement of sustainable agricultural development in developing countries.

In developed countries, MBDs associated with rice production have been reduced greatly or eradicated due to vector control efforts and, for some viral diseases, vaccination, in combination with changes in environments, housing conditions, and human behavior (34). However, riceland mosquitoes still abound and are a nuisance. Abundance levels or human-biting rates of these mosquitoes may increase under favorable weather (73) or by acquisition of insecticide resistance (46, 103, 116). Increase in international movements of humans and animals brings the risk of introduction of infectious sources and incidence of secondary transmission by indigen-

---

Motoyoshi Mogi, Division of Parasitology, Department of Microbiology, Saga Medical School, Nabeshima, Saga 849, Japan.
Teiji Sota, Division of Parasitology, Department of Microbiology, Saga Medical School, Nabeshima, Saga 849, Japan.

ous mosquitoes (9). Introduction of infective mosquitoes by airplanes can be another infectious source (21). Thus, MBD problems associated with rice production are actually or potentially worldwide.

This chapter consists of three parts. First, we make clear the similarity and dissimilarity between integrated control of economic pests and human disease vectors. Next, we describe the characteristics of rice agroecosystems as mosquito habitats and briefly review methods for riceland mosquito control. Then, we focus on livestock management, one of the least explored aspects despite its potential importance for mosquito and MBD control in ricelands. The first topic is general but particularly important with regard to riceland mosquito control, because of the necessity of effective coordination with rice pest control. Insofar as possible, we select literatures from riceland mosquito studies but with exceptions on necessity.

Integrated Control of Mosquito and Mosquito-borne Diseases: Conceptual Revalidation

Origin of Problems

Control of vector mosquitoes before the dichloro-diphenyl-trichloroethane (DDT) era was in reality integrated control (127). However, recent circulation of the integrated control concept in mosquito control has been attended by some confusion and ambiguity that arise from (1) influences of the concept established earlier for economic pest control, and (2) increasing diversity of mosquito pest status. Mosquitoes are detrimental to people as vectors of human diseases and as nuisances, pests deteriorating livestock productivity (as vectors and/or nuisances), or a combination of these (zoonotic human diseases). For control of mosquitoes as livestock pests, the concept developed for economic pest control may be applied (110). In some developed countries, mosquitoes are problems only as nuisances. Though methodologies for nuisance mosquito control have received increasing attention (27, 55), the scope of the following discussion is confined to control of mosquitoes transmitting human diseases.

Control of Economic Pests and Vectors: Similarity and Dissimilarity

The Food and Agriculture Organization of the United Nations (FAO) (31) defined *integrated pest control* as "a pest management system that, in the context of the associated environment and the population dynamics of the pest species, utilizes all suitable techniques and methods in as compatible a manner as possible and maintains the pest population at levels below those causing economic injury." This definition includes the rationale (consideration on environment and importance of ecology), the strategy (integration of all suitable methods), and the objective (pest suppression below the economic injury level). The World Health Organization (WHO) (127) defines *integrated vector control* (IVC) as "the utilization of all appropriate technological and management techniques to bring about an effective degree of vector suppression in a cost-effective manner." This definition also include the rationale (appropriateness with regard to environment), the strategy (cost-effective integration of all techniques), and the objective (the effective degree of vector suppression).

Differences between the above two concepts exist in (1) the object to be protected (a human being's belongings vs. a human being with free will), (2) the use of fund (investment for future returns vs. allocation of the limited fund), (3) the criterion for decision making (cost-benefit vs. cost-effectiveness), and (4) the decision maker (producers vs. public). Aside from much controversy on the definition of the economic injury level and practical procedures to use it (87), the final purpose of economic pest control is the maximization of profits under a given circumstance. The purpose of vector control is finally disease eradication and proximately substantial disease reduction, as indicated by "effective suppression" in WHO's definition. The degree of vector suppression is maximized when the limited fund is allocated in the most cost-effective manner. However, even the greatest suppression attainable within the available fund may not bring about substantial disease reduction. Namely, the purpose of vector control is often unattainable by vector control alone. Thus, "vector control should be considered as an integral part of a disease control programme" (127). This is another important difference between control of economic pests and human disease vectors.

Integrated Vector-borne Disease Control

A useful concept in the study of transmission dynamics of infectious diseases is the basic reproductive rate (R), which is defined as the expected number of secondary cases produced by an infectious individual in a large population of susceptibles. If $R > 1$, then the disease will be maintained in the population, though the equilibrium level may be lowered as R becomes smaller. If $R < 1$, the disease will eventually disappear from the population unless there is constant immigration of infectious hosts. In Dietz's malaria control model (4), for example,

$$R = ma^2gb\exp(-nv)/vr \qquad (1)$$

where m = mosquito density per human, a = human-biting rate of a single mosquito, b = proportion of infected mosquitoes that are actually infectious, g = proportion of infected people that are actually infectious, n = length of the extrinsic incubation period, v = mosquito death rate, and r =

recovery rate. Vector control can contribute to the reduction of R by reducing the vectorial capacity;

$$C = ma^2\exp(-nv)/v \tag{2}$$

which is a component of R consisting of entomological parameters alone (35). Clearly, the impact of vector control on disease prevalence is variable depending upon other parameter values, and vector control, even though not very effective solely, can contribute to substantial reduction of R in combination with measures that change other parameter values (e.g., personal protection from mosquito bites, chemoprophylaxis, vaccination, chemotherapy, mass drug administration). In the most successful case, the disease will eventually disappear through keeping R below unity, realizing a situation called *anophelism without malaria*. Although the definition of R will vary depending on the transmission cycle of each pathogen, the outline mentioned above could hold in the control of MBDs.

We define *integrated vector-borne disease control* (IVDC) as "a disease control strategy that uses the most cost-effective techniques available to reduce disease spread, with the least undesirable side effects on the environment." Thus, vector control is an integral part of IVDC. In IVDC, the required level of vector suppression may be alleviated due to inclusion of other control practices acting to reduce R, thus vector control may be simplified.

If vector control were a unique antidisease measure, then IVDC would be reduced to IVC. However, it is *always* possible to reduce human-biting rates through changes in human behavior by his or her own will. The only necessity is motivation, prompted through education. A slight change in human behavior may substantially reduce human-biting rates of vector mosquitoes (12), and importance of human factors in vector-borne disease transmission has been emphasized recently (39, 65). Vector control, as a part of IVDC, requires us to query whether vector control is the most cost-effective measure for disease control before considering which techniques are most cost-effective for vector control.

Rice Agroecosystems, Riceland Mosquitoes, and Mosquito-borne Diseases

Characteristics of Rice Agroecosystems

The rice agroecosystem is a human-modified, water-dependent system including people and their associates such as rice plants, crops other than rice, domestic animals, and indigenous or imported wild life thriving in or tolerating the human-induced modification (modified from 32). Its characteristics are influenced primarily by climate, geography, edaphic factors, and irrigation systems. The International Rice Research Institute recognized five types and 18 subtypes of rice-growing environments based mainly on water sustainability and climatic favorability (36). In addition, major differences exist in cropping systems and dependency on rice (e.g., synchrony vs. asynchrony, rice monoculture vs. rotation with other crops, with vs. without stock farming). Furthermore, rice cultivation procedures are diverse in tillering, seeding, water management, fertilization, pest/disease/weed control, the degree of mechanization, and so on. Human behavior and housing conditions are diverse also. Thus, the rice agroecosystem is a locally and seasonally diverse system that is prone to gradual or radical changes by human activities. This variability of rice agroecosystems inevitably brings about the variability of mosquito ecology (93) and epidemiological patterns (83). Flexibility in space and time is one of the most important qualifications for mosquito and MBD control systems in ricelands.

Rice Agroecosystems as Habitats of Larval Mosquitoes

Fundamental determinants of mosquito abundance are availability and characteristics of larval habitats and bloodmeal hosts. Despite the abovementioned variability, most rice agroecosystems have some common features with regard to larval habitats and bloodmeal hosts of mosquitoes.

Irrigated rice fields as mosquito larval habitats are characterized by extensive area and rich predator fauna. Extensive area makes larval control practical only when it is highly cost-effective. It must be emphasized that this extensive habitat has ample potential to support still larger populations of mosquitoes. Mogi (71) and Chubachi (15) suggested that *Culex*

TABLE 3.1. Density of *Culex tritaeniorhynchus* larvae in rice fields classified by sequential sampling[a]

Date	No. of rice fields with water	No. of rice fields where the density is		
		<43	Not determined	>947
July 2	28	26	2	
9	93	76	17	
22	91	65	21	5
29	91	47	39	5
Aug. 6	91	62	27	2
11	93	87	6	
20	90	84	6	
Sept. 1	93	93		
16	91	91		

[a]Based on Figure 2 of Ref. (76). However, only planted fields were included. Critical densities adopted for classification, 0.23/dip and 5.09/dip, were converted to absolute density/m^2 using a conversion coefficient (121).

tritaeniorhynchus populations are regulated through overcrowding effects among larvae. However, it does not imply that most larvae in rice fields suffer overcrowding. Figure 3.1 shows the relationship between pupation success and larval density in the laboratory (104), and Table 3.1 may give some idea about the density of *Cx. tritaeniorhynchus* in rice fields. Though density in the laboratory is not equivalent to density in the field with regard to the intensity of overcrowding because of differences in food concentration, water depth, and age structure, the above comparison suggests that larval densities in most rice fields usually remain far below the level at which the density-dependent mortality becomes evident.

Aquatic predators include arthropods and fish, both having longer generation time than mosquitoes do. Mortality among mosquito larvae in rice fields is high (usually >90%), the most important source being predation (Table 3.2). These estimates of predation mortalities were obtained from predator exclusion experiments, whereas Urabe et al. (118), based on precipitin tests and absolute density estimation of both the prey and the predator, estimated predation mortality of *Anopheles sinensis* by nymphs of a dragonfly, *Sympetrum frequens*, to be more than 90% in rice fields 1 month after transplanting. These facts imply that a small reduction in predation pressure for the aquatic stages may lead to a substantial increase in the adult abundance. Also, rice fields habor rich fauna of terrestrial (e.g., spider) and surface (e.g., water strider) predators that prey on adult mosquitoes (102). Maintenance of predator communities, both aquatic and terrestrial, should be a basic strategy for mosquito control in ricelands.

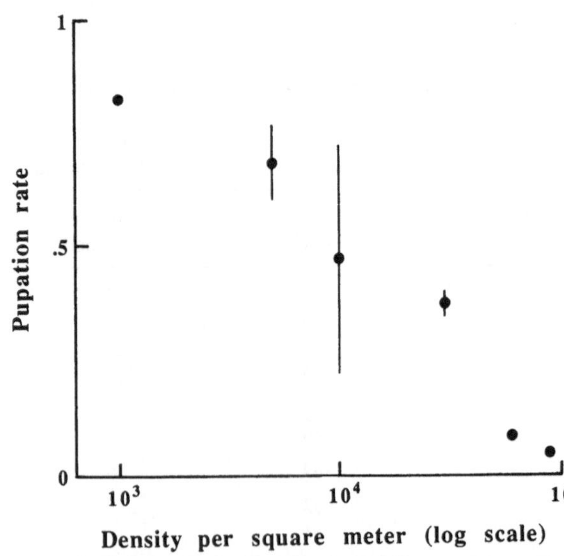

FIGURE 3.1. Relationship between larval density and pupation rate in *Culex tritaeniorhynchus* (From Ref. 104, Table 3.2).

TABLE 3.2. Mortality of mosquito immatures in rice fields

Taxa	Locality	Rice field state	No. of rice fields[a]	Mean mortality (%) PR	O	T	Adult emergence rate (%)[b]	Source
Culex tritaeniorhynchus	Japan	F, U	4			98	2	78
		P, U, S	10			97	3	79
		P, U, S	10			93	7	79
Culex[c]	Philippines	P, U	4	66	33	99	1	77
Anopheles gambiae s.l.	Kenya	P, S	*			84	16	102
		P, U	*			93	7	102
Anopheles[d]	Philippines	P, U	3			97	3	77
	Philippines	P, U	1	49	50	99	1	77
Anopheles[c]	Thailand	P, U	4	42	56	98	2	80
Psorophora columbiae	U.S.A.	P, U, S?	*	49	47	96	4	2

Note: F, fallow, P, planted, S, sprayed, U, unsprayed, PR, predation, O, others, T, total.
[a] Asterisk denotes that samples from multiple fields were combined.
[b] For *Ps. columbiae*, the survival rate is 5 days after hatch.
[c] Species belonging to the subgenus *Culex* or *Anopheles* were lumped together.
[d] Species belonging to the genus were lumped together.

Rice Agroecosystems as Habitats of Adult Mosquitoes

Rice agroecosystems for adult mosquitoes are characterized by the abundance of livestock kept as labor power or protein food sources. Mosquito bloodmeal identification studies include various species breeding in rice fields (for the latest review, see 122). Table 3.3 summarizes studies for *Cx. tritaeniorhynchus* and *Anopheles culicifacies* with domestic animal censuses. Clearly, these mosquitoes take most bloodmeals from one to two species of abundant livestock, and human blood indices are very low (5%>).

Abundance of livestock could influence mosquito abundance primarily through changes in host-finding rates and secondarily through overcrowding effects among biting flies at hosts. Host finding is a probabilistic process influenced by (1) distributions of hosts and of resting sites of mosquitoes, which are usually biased, (2) flight direction of mosquitoes, which is determined through complex interactions of wind direction and speed, innate optomoter response, topographical features, and so on (38, 59), and (3) attraction ranges of hosts, which may be less than 20 m from the host at the windward location (41). Though host-finding probabilities in nature are yet unknown, positive correlations are found between larval or adult mosquito density and cattle density in ricelands (1, 66a, 67), and between engorged or gravid rates of resting mosquitoes and bloodmeal host density in other

TABLE 3.3. Bloodmeal identification of *Cx. tritaeniorhynchus* and *An. culicifacies* in rice-growing areas of South and Southeast Asia with domestic animal census

	No. of hosts (% bloodmeal identified)[a]												
	1	2	3	4	5	6	7		8		9		10
Host	*Ct*	*Ct*	*Ct*	*Ct*	*Ct*	*Ct*	*Ct*	*Ac*	*Ct*	*Ac*	*Ct*	*Ac*	*Ac*
Man	29	20	500 (4)	1932 (1>)	27	Ca. 3,000 (1>)	6	(1>)	182	(1>)	115	(2)	5
Pig	16 (36)	8 (19)	10 (90)	626 (8)	3 (91)	66							
Bovid	8 (46)	1 (66)		556 (83)	2 (7)	1,387 (98)	30 (89)	(59)	284 (94)	(68)	36 (86)	(65)	68 (69)
Caprid	1 (6)	2 (1)				1,040		(1>)	39		(1>)		3
Camel							1	(1>)	1				2
Equine	(8)	2 (10)		(1>)		7	2 (1)	(1)	20	(1)		(1>)	2
Dog	3 (1)	5 (1>)	25 (5)	420 (1>)		?	6	(1)	52	(1)	24	(1)	20
Cat	3			92		?	6		19		7		
Galliformes	40 (1)		450 (1) (Galliformes and Duck)	4767 (1>)	10	736 (1>)[b] (Galliformes and Duck)	6		188	(1>)	29	(1>)	
Duck				700					19				
Passeriformes											(1>)		
Columbiformes										(1>)			
Mixed	(3)	(4)				(1)		(1>)					
Unidentified				(8)	(1)	(1)	(10)	(39)	(6)	(30)	(13)	(32)	(31)
FI[c]	>167	>1320	1125	>288	>819	>212	>18	>12	>60	>43	>275	>208	>5

Note: *Ct*, *Cx. tritaeniorhynchus*; *Ac*, *Anopheles culicifacies*. Bovid, cattle and buffalo; Caprid, goat and sheep; Equine, horse and donkey; Galliformes, chicken and guinea fowl; Passeriformes, wild perching bird; Columbiformes, wild dove and pigeon; Unidentified, mostly bovids or caprids.

[a] 1 and 2, Okinawa, Japan (88); 3, Sarawak, Indonesia (6); 4, Chiang Mai, Thailand (42), human and animal population statistics (44), (56); 5, Chiang Mai, Thailand (82); 6, North Arcot, India, no. hosts ($\times 10^3$) (14), human and animal population statistics (8); 7–10, Panjab, Pakistan (92).

[b] There is a possibility that this blood was from wild birds.

[c] FI of the primary bloodmeal host (bovids or pigs) to humans.

habitats (25). Usually, livestock are more accessible to mosquitoes than are humans and wild animals. Probably, abundance and distribution of livestock have significant influences on host-finding success of mosquitoes in ricelands, though direct evidence is absent.

Density-dependent reduction of feeding rates at hosts was observed in the laboratory (26) and also for *Cx. tritaeniorhynchus* at pigsties (33) and *Culex tarsalis* at chicken-baited traps (91). Significance of this phenomenon in dynamics of mosquito populations has yet to be studied.

Livestock may also influence mosquito abundance through habitat changes. Grazing cattle produce footprints that become preferred habitats of *Psorophora columbiae* larvae (10), while they remove tall/thick vegetation suitable for adult resting sites. Polluted water released from animal houses may also produce favorable larval habitats for some mosquitoes.

Effects of livestock on mosquito abundance are multilateral. Proper management of livestock could reduce mosquito abundance in ricelands effectively and should be another basic strategy for mosquito control in ricelands.

Transmission Cycles of Mosquito-borne Human Diseases in Ricelands

Transmission cycles of mosquito-borne human diseases in ricelands may be classified into either of two types. In malaria, bancroftian filariasis and nocturnally periodic brugian filariasis, only humans serve as reservoir hosts for pathogens (Fig. 3.2A). Nonhuman vertebrates, both domestic and wild, serve as bloodmeal hosts but do not allow development or multiplication of pathogens. The second type (Fig. 3.2B) includes viral diseases such as western equine encephalitis (WEE), St. Louis encephalitis (SLE), and Japanese encephalitis (JE). Viral pathogens of these diseases cause viraemia in nonhuman vertebrate hosts (amplifiers) but not in humans, although infected persons may suffer from the diseases (dead-end hosts). Amplifiers important as primary sources for human infection are wild birds for WEE, and domestic pigs for JE. Amplification of St. Louis virus primarily depends on wild birds but domestic fowl may be involved. Nocturnally subperiodic brugian filariasis and some viral diseases (yellow fever) belong to the third type of transmission cycles that may involve both human and nonhuman vertebrates as reservoirs (Fig. 3.2C). These diseases may exist in ricelands but are not immediate concerns of this chapter, because they are transmitted by mosquitoes utilizing water bodies other than rice fields (swamps, jars) as primary larval habitats.

Types of transmission cycles constitute the basic framework for establishment of MBD control strategies, as *R* could be reduced most effectively by proper management of reservoir hosts. Livestock that are pathogen reservoirs should be the primary target for MBD control (91).

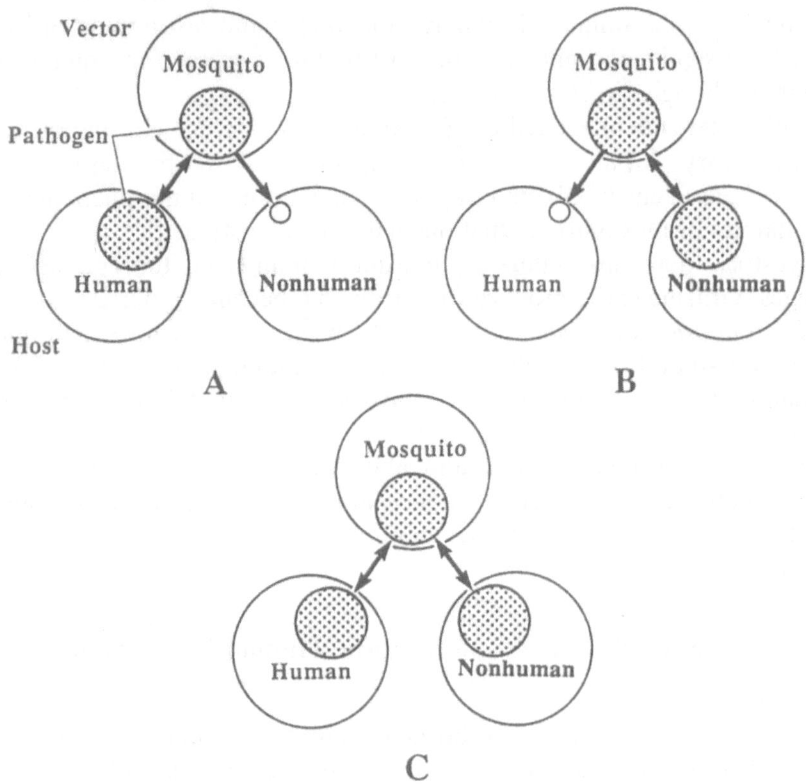

FIGURE 3.2. Transmission cycles of mosquito-borne diseases in ricelands. Small circles (dotted and open) indicate pathogens in vector mosquito and bloodmeal host populations. Bidirectional arrows indicate that mosquitoes and hosts can infect each other with pathogens, whereas unidirectional arrows indicate that mosquitoes may infect hosts with pathogens but hosts cannot infect mosquitoes with pathogens. For further details see text.

Options for Mosquito Control in Ricelands

Large-Scale Application of Wide-Spectrum Synthesized Insecticides

Repeated trials of application of wide-spectrum insecticides to a large area have shown that effectiveness measured as adult abundance is only transient due to adult immigration (101, 123, 124). Wide-spectrum insecticides destroy predator populations, and thus may increase abundance of rice field mosquito larvae (68, 85, 100) and adults (11). Large-scale application of insecticides for riceland mosquito control should be limited to those truly emergency cases. Establishment of organizations that ensure the prompt coordination of rice pest control and mosquito control on necessity could save cost and minimize undesirable side effects.

Larval Control

Field trials to improve techniques for application of narrow-spectrum or mosquito-specific agents, including insect growth regulators, microbial larvicides (*Bachilus thuringiensis* var. *israelensis*, *B. sphaericus*), and parasites (*Romanomermis culicivorax*, *Lagenidium giganteum*) remain active, especially in the United States under the auspices of the Riceland Mosquito Management Program (5). *Gambusia affinis*, a larvivorous poecilid fish, has been widely used in Californian rice fields, but the complicated impact of this generalist predator on aquatic arthropod communities has been revealed only recently (61, 62, 69). Probably, interaction among generalist predators is a factor deteriorating the reliability of *Gambusia affinis* as a mosquito control agent in rice fields (49).

A community-based trial in Indonesia that used poecilid fish (*Poecilia reticulata*) in combination with edible fish is an example of successful coordination of mosquito control with rice cultivation and protein food supply (84). Pisciculture aiming at mosquito control in rice fields is practiced also in some parts of China (64). Coordination with the necessity of using insecticides for rice pest control and drainage for optimal rice growth is essential to the success of rice field pisciculture for mosquito control.

Coverage of the water surface by an aquatic fern (*Azolla imbricata*), a natural fertilizer for rice plants (114), disturbs both oviposition and emergence of mosquitoes (63). Products containing active ingredients of the neem (*Azadirachta indica*), a cheap antifeedant protecting sprayed rice plants from injury by planthoppers (99), have been explored as an agent usable for simultaneous control of rice pests and mosquito larvae (90). These approaches have an advantage of facilitating the coordination between rice cultivation and vector control.

Water management accompanied with proper engineering has large potentiality for rice field mosquito control (106). Well-designed intermittent irrigation (48, 98) and wet irrigation (63) reduce mosquito production drastically without deteriorating rice yields. Flushing washes away mosquito larvae (72). However, the impact of drainage and flushing on aquatic predators has been little studied, and the impact of synchrony and asynchrony of rice cultivation in the tropical region on vector and predator populations also merits further studies (75). Water management for mosquito control has limitations and difficulties when it is planned in developed ricelands (74). To construct irrigation systems convenient for control practice, vector control personnel should explore the possibility of water management for mosquito control from the initial stage of riceland development projects and onward.

Adult Control

Residual house spraying with synthesized insecticides, used against endophagic/endophilic mosquitoes can reduce disease transmission rates substantially through the shortened life expectancy of infected mosquitoes (22). The findings of sibling species with different insecticide susceptibility and vector status may warrant the selective use of DDT which was previously abandoned (112), although pollution problems remain (23). However, residual house spraying is not a very effective and durable method for some riceland mosquitoes, because of exophily under the ready availability of daytime resting sites (e.g., among rice plant stands) and insecticide resistance often strengthened by insecticides used for rice pest control (46, 103, 116).

The impact of insecticide-impregrated mosquito nets on vector populations could be comparable to that of residual house spraying (129), because insecticides on nets have both repelling and killing effects (96, 128).

Livestock, as main bloodmeal hosts, can play the role of attractants to kill mosquitoes with appropriate methods. Residual pigsty spraying against *Cx. tritaeniorhynchus* was ineffective due to exophily of the mosquito and the open structure of pigsties (85), though the effectiveness may be improved in pigsties of a more enclosed design. Repellents or insecticides treated on animals can protect them from mosquito bites, but, as a method for controlling mosquitoes, killing effects are required. A fenchlorphos 1% emulsion treated on pigs reduced feeding rates of *Cx. tritaeniorhynchus* and killed substantial proportions of fed and unfed females collected from the nearby wall (70). The females of this species stay on hosts usually for 5 to 10 min (70, 109a), whereas contact with 1% fenchlorphos for 2.75 min yielded 50% mortality within 24 h in the laboratory (70). Safety for both livestock and consumers of the products is essential for animal treatment with insecticides.

When pigsties were covered with phenothrin impregnated 1 × 1 cm-mesh nets, a remarkably smaller number of *Cx. tritaeniorhynchus* invaded but mostly died until the next morning, including approximately 40% engorged individuals (62a).

Electric light traps operated at animal sheds have several advantages as a control method for *Cx. tritaeniorhynchus* in Japan (73), but field trials have not been conducted. Results of a village-scale trial in Thailand was inconclusive (89). The attraction range of a CDC (Center for Disease Control) miniature light trap was estimated to be less than 5 m (86). Improvement of light trap effectiveness with studies on mosquito behavior are desirable.

Sound traps set along rice fields caught *Cx. tirtaeniorhynchus* males efficiently (50), and improved traps set near pigsties caught unfed and gravid females as well (51). Fortnight removal of males by sound traps at an isolated weed stand reduced the insemination rate of resting females of *Cx. tarsalis* to 0% (52). Practicability of sound trapping for riceland mosquito control would depend on the size of attraction ranges.

Except for wide-spectrum insecticides, practicable options for adult control are still few. Potentiality of livestock management has been little explored. An advantage of livestock management for mosquito control is that it can increase livestock productivity (111) and, as such, will be acceptable by farmers. For immediate purposes, methods to treat livestock or livestock houses with insecticides for mosquito control need to be improved. However, development of resistance may be unavoidable if main bloodmeal hosts or enclosures are treated with insecticides extensively.

Livestock Management for IDVC in Ricelands

Problems and Research Necessities

From the viewpoint of IVDC, our primary concerns are to evaluate the role of the present livestock fauna in persistence of vector mosquitoes and MBDs, and to predict the impact of future changes in abundance and species composition of livestock on vector populations and disease prevalence. To include livestock management in IVDC programs, it is necessary that we explore further possibilities of (1) vaccination, isolation, or control of reservoir animal populations, (2) the use of livestock as baits to attract and kill mosquitoes, and (3) the use of nonreservoir animals kept around human dwellings to divert mosquito bites from people (zooprophylaxis) in a manner compatible with stock raising.

To meet these necessities, researchers must examine (1) mosquito host selection under various conditions, (2) the influence of host availability on mosqutio abundance, and (3) the relationship between disease dynamics and the former two. Knowledge of genetic structure of vector mosquitoes is essential as well, because host selection is, in part, a genetic trait with intraspecific variations (17, 40) and livestock management may favor particular genotypes with regard to host selection. This aspect has been little studied for culicine mosquitoes in ricelands.

Bloodmeal identification studies have made significant contributions to understanding host selection of riceland mosquitoes. However, there are no field data indicating the host-finding rate (Q in the following model) of mosquitoes. This is an important but almost ignored aspect in mosquito ecology. As a consequence, the relationship between host availability and mosquito population levels and its implication for disease prevalence have been little understood. Estimation of Q is quite difficult, and one possibility is to examine the relationship between host availability and parous rates that may reflect Q in some way. Detection of the relationship between host availability and mosquito abundance is not easy to undertake as well. Comparative studies or experiments in the field for this purpose are quite valuable and should be pursued insofar as possible. Still more difficult is to elucidate the complex interactions between mosquitoes and multiple bloodmeal hosts with regard to pathogen transmission in the field. One useful approach may be model simulation to fill the gap due to the lack of field data. Although the present knowledge is quite incomplete, attempt to construct model systems of such interactions may, in turn, provide a useful guidance for future field studies.

Livestock Density, Mosquito Abundance, and Human-biting Rates in Model Systems

Previous models for mosquito populations (18, 20, 24, 45, 81, 125) do not deal with the reproductive process as affected by bloodmeal host availability. Recently, Focks et al. (29, 30) developed a comprehensive simulation model for a riceland mosquito *Psorophora columbiae*, in which they incorporated interaction between female mosquitoes and cattle in the form of reduced adult survival with an increased number of female mosquitoes per cattle. Although they did not include the effect of cattle density on host-finding rates, the model simulation successfully mimicked the observed relationship between mosquito and cattle densities, and suggested the effectiveness of reducing cattle density or cattle treatment with residual insecticides for mosquito control (28).

The necessity of incorporating disease dynamics, in addition to the relationship between host availability and mosquito reproduction, may warrant the use of simpler, heuristic models. Sota and Mogi (108) attempted to make a simple model of mosquito population dynamics incorporating the probability of host finding. Suppose that there are H individuals of humans and L of one major animal species (say cattle), and mosquitoes find and feed at constant rates (biting efficiencies), a_1 and a_2, on man and cattle, respectively. The rate of successful blood feeding (Q) and proportion of biting from humans (P) in a unit time may be expressed in the following equations.

$$Q = 1 - \exp(-a_1H - a_2L). \tag{3}$$

$$P = a_1H/(a_1H + a_2L). \tag{4}$$

These equations reveal that, when the human density is fixed, increased cattle density raises the overall proportion of fed females (Fig. 3.3A) but reduces the proportion of biting from humans (Fig. 3.3B).

Based on the assumption that the mosquito population growth is limited by the rate of successful blood feeding (Q), the dynamics of the female mosquito population (M) may be expressed as

$$\mathrm{d}M/\mathrm{d}t = SEQM'f(EQM') - vM \tag{5}$$

where E = number of female eggs per fed female, S = density-independent larval survival rate, v = adult mortality rate, and M' denotes the female

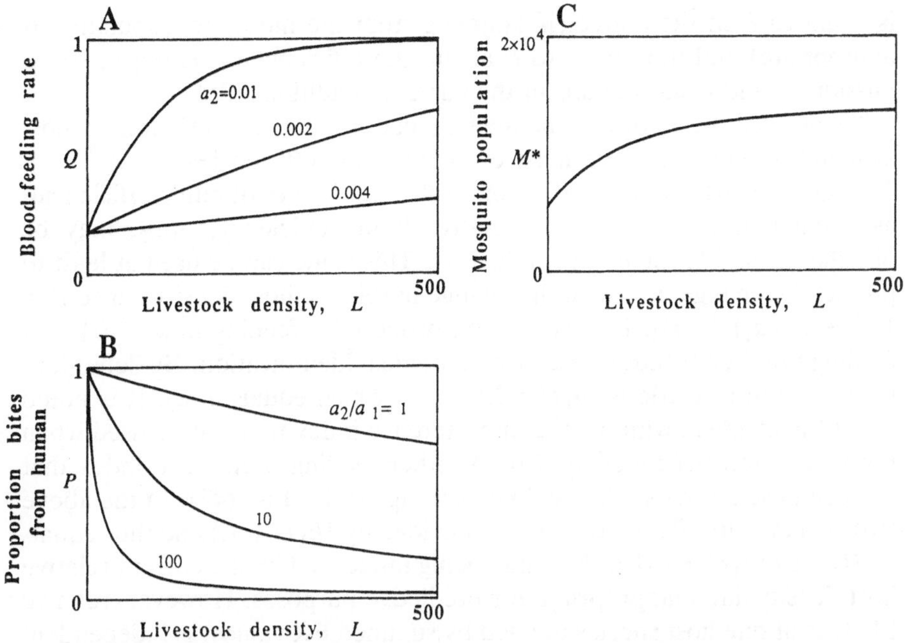

FIGURE 3.3. Influence of livestock density, L, on (A) rate of successful blood-feeding, Q (Eq. 3), (B) proportion of mosquito bites from humans, P (Eq. 4), and (C) mosquito population, M^* (Eq. 7). $H = 1000$; $a_1 = 0.0002$; $a_2 = 0.002$ (except for A and B); $E = 50$; $S = 0.05$; $v = 0.3$; $h = 10^{-5}$.

density lagged for the immature period (24). f is a density-dependent function that may affect larval survivorship. In a simple case,

$$f(EQM') = 1/(1 + hEQM'), \tag{6}$$

indicating the nonovercompensating density-dependence within the larval cohorts (h = constant). The equilibrium density (M^*) in this model is

$$M^* = (SEQ - v)/(hvEQ), \tag{7}$$

in which M^* increases with an increase in Q, thus M^* increases as a result of increased livestock density (Fig. 3.3C).

Indices of Mosquito Feeding Pattern in the Field

In a general multihost case, P may be expressed as $a_1H/\Sigma a_iN_i$, where a_i and N_i are biting efficiency for and density of ith host species. In ricelands, however, the number of important host species is limited (Table 3.3), then two (or three) host systems may be used without serious departure from reality. Human blood index (HBI) obtained from bloodmeal identification is equal to P in the above (if sampling from the mosquito population is appropriate) and important to evaluate the efficiency of pathogen transmission to and from humans in the current conditions (35).

To predict the variation in feeding pattern due to variation in host availability, however, one must evaluate biting efficiencies (a_1, a_2, . . .). Though it seems difficult to determine absolute values of biting efficiencies as defined in the model, the relative biting efficiency, a_1/a_2, may be obtained from bloodmeal identification. This value can be used at least to predict the change in P with the change in relative host density, since $P = 1/[1 + (a_2/a_1)(L/H)]$. Kay et al. (58) proposed a feeding index (FI) as a feeding preference index based on bloodmeal identification. By definition, FI of human to cattle is $(a_1H/a_2L)/(H/L)$ which equals a_1/a_2. It is noted that FI is identical with a general preference index that can be used when food depletion is negligible (16). Another feeding preference index that has been used in mosquito ecology is forage ratio (FR) (47). In the above two host system, FR of humans is P devided by $H/(H + L)$ and thus equals $a_1(H + L)/(a_1H + a_2L)$, the value being influenced by the current relative host density and inappropriate for predictive purposes. However, relative FR (FR of one host species divided by summed FR values) is independent from the current host density, and thus can be a useful index. In the above model system, the relative FR of humans equals $a_1/(a_1 + a_2)$, which is identical with Manly's β index of preference (13).

The biting efficiencies (a_1, a_2) and FI values depend not only on innate host preference but also greatly on accessibility (habitats and behavior) of the hosts (91, 94, 95, 117). In addition, the biting efficiency may vary with changes in host distribution pattern and/or attractiveness associated with density. The last row in Table 3.3 shows substantial variation of FI values even when the same mosquito species fed on the same combination of hosts. At present, we cannot say how local conditions and sampling problems contributed to such variations. Bloodmeal identification studies with domestic animal censuses under various conditions of host availability is essential to formulate the relationship between mosquito foraging pattern and extrinsic factors in ricelands.

Zooprophylaxis in Malaria Control

To combine the above system with a malaria transmission model (Eq. 1), PQ and M^*/H may be substituted for the human-biting rate (a) and mosquito density per person (m), respectively. This system was used to examine the effectiveness of zooprophylaxis in malaria control (108).

The aim of zooprophylaxis is to reduce R via reducing P by increasing L. The method depends on the opportunistic host selection of mosquitoes and cannot be effective against strictly anthropophilic species. Animals that can be reservoirs of other pathogens (pigs for JE virus) cannot be used if there is a possibility of the pathogen involvement. Domestic animals may have a_2/a_1 (FI) values much larger than unity (Table 3.3) and can be effective zooprophylaxis agents (7, 57, 60, 126, but see 97, 107). Though direct evidence for the effectiveness of zooprophylaxis for malaria control is virtually absent, lower HBI values in villages with larger numbers of domestic animals have been observed (7, 57). A suspected case of inverse evidences was reported from Guyana where reduction of the livestock density due to mechanization was followed by malaria epidemics probably due to the shift of primarily zoophilic anophelines to humans (37).

Despite the expected effectiveness, some problems and risks seem to be inevitable in the implementation of zooprophyraxis. (1) If the mosquito density increased due to increased livestock density, then malaria endemicity is not always reduced (Fig. 3.4). Application of zooprophylaxis should be considered in the area where the anopheline density is consistently high and further increase of mosquito density is not expected. However, in ricelands with ample larval habitats, such a situation may be rare. (2) Even if the endemic level is reduced by zooprophylaxis, then the malaria prevalence becomes more unstable (66, see also 3) because of the maintenance of high mosquito density, and the risk of malaria outbreak following slight changes in environmental conditions will persist. Thus, zooprophylaxis is not always a reliable strategy for malaria control, especially in ricelands.

Nevertheless, zooprophylaxis may be adopted in the absence of alternative methods to suppress high vector density and due to the compatibility with the necessity of domestic animals as labor power or food. It seems necessary to consider the reduction of a_1 (e.g., by bed-nets) and M^* (e.g., adult control at animal houses) in combination with zooprophylaxis to alleviate its risk. Reduction of a_1 always decreases P and R irrespective of host densities. If combined with such efforts, then zooprophyraxis can be a component in IVDC for malaria.

Livestock Management for JE Control

Except for regions where people never eat pork, pig farming requiring no pastures is quite suitable to riceland agroecosystems and apparently has been enlarged.

For JE control, the first consideration is isolation of pig farming from ricelands. Effectiveness of pig removal for JE control may be seen from the apparent absence or rareness of human JE cases in regions where vector mosquitoes exist but pig farming has not been developed due to religious reasons (115). However, such a decision may rarely be expected, because of the seasonal and epidemic nature of JE prevalence as well as economic importance of pigs (6a). Vaccination of susceptible pigs prior to the JE epidemic season has been tried at a few localities in Japan (120), but has not been adopted as an established method for JE control. A major difficulty arises from the high turnover rate of pigs and high costs. Pig

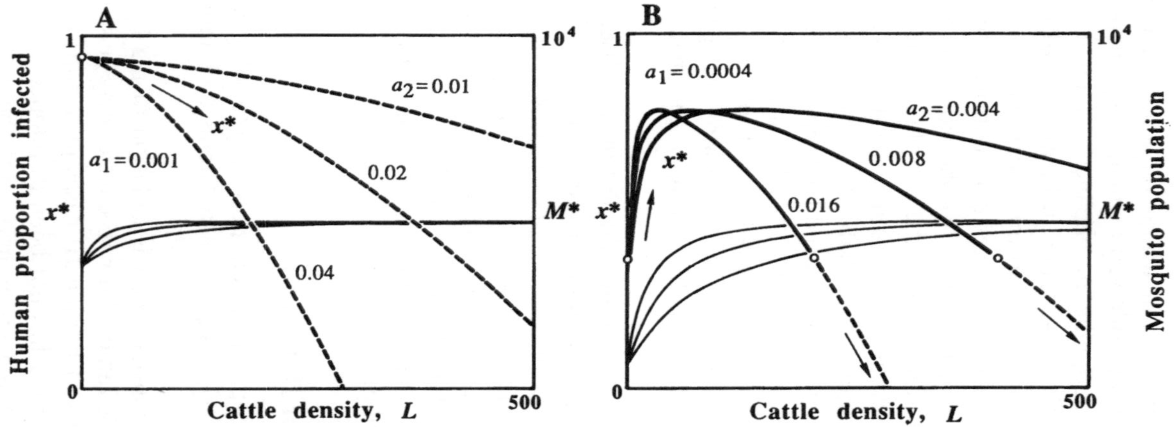

FIGURE 3.4. Changes in equilibrium mosquito population, M^* (Eq. 7), and proportion of malaria infection in humans, x^*, with changes in cattle density, L. In (A), M^* and x^* are already high at $L = 0$ because of high a_1 value ($= 0.001$), and x^* decreases with an increase in L, whereas in (B), M^* and x^* are initially low ($a_1 = 0.0004$), and x^* exceeds the initial level in the range indicated by thick solid line. $x^* = (R - 1)/(R + a/v)$ see 3, where R is given in Eq. (1) and $a = PQ$. $H = 1000$; $E = 50$; $S = 0.05$; $v = 0.3$; $h = 10^{-5}$; $r = 0.08$; $b = g = 1$; $n = 0$.

vaccination to prevent virus amplification may be more difficult in tropical regions where JE infection can occur throughout the year.

Wada (119) constructed a simulation model of a JE virus amplification cycle between pig and mosqutio populations and discussed the risk of human infection in terms of infective mosquito density. Alternatively, Sota and Mogi (109) applied the two-host system to analyze the effect of both pig and human densities on the human risk. Suppose that L is the pig density, then

$$P' = a_2L/(a_1H + a_2L), \tag{8}$$

which is the proportion of mosquito biting from pigs. The basic reproductive rate of the amplification cycle may be expressed as

$$R = (P'Q)^2(M^*/L)/[(u + r')v] \tag{9}$$

where u = instantaneous birth and death rate of the pig, and r' = the rate at which infected pig aquires immunity. The incidence of human infection was assumed to be not only proportional to infective mosquito density but also affected by PQ (Q is assumed to be a constant in ref. 109). Thus, the incidence of human infection per unit time may be proportional to the product (human risk factor, HRF): $(PQ) \times$ infective mosquito density, where P and Q are given in Eqs. (3) and (4).

Because high pig density favors mosquito population growth (Eq. 7) and virus amplification (Eq. 9), infective mosquito density increases with pig density (Fig. 3.5). However, HRF does not monotonically increase

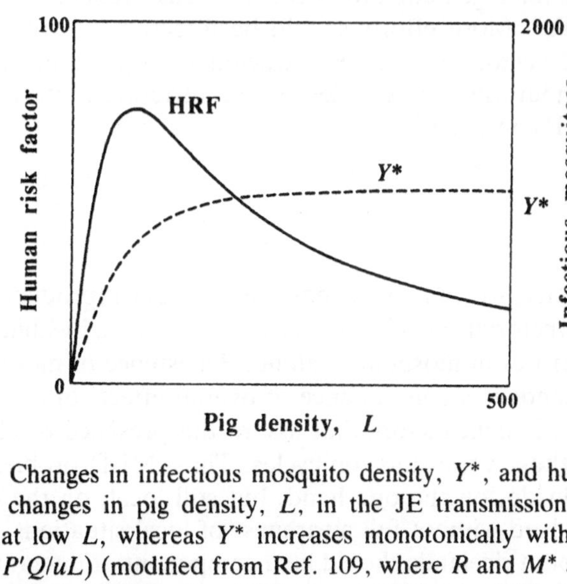

FIGURE 3.5. Changes in infectious mosquito density, Y^*, and human risk factor, HRF, with changes in pig density, L, in the JE transmission model. HRF is maximized at low L, whereas Y^* increases monotonically with L. $Y^* = (R - 1)(R/M^* + P'Q/uL)$ (modified from Ref. 109, where R and M^* are given in Eqs. (9) and (7). HRF = PQY^*. $H = 1000$; $a_1 = 0.0002$; $a_2 = 0.02$; $E = 50$; $S = 0.05$; $v = 0.3$; $h = 10^{-5}$; $r' = 0.2$; $u = 0.005$.

with L, being maximized at certain L, because P decreases with L, more rapidly with larger a_2/a_1 ratio. In fact, a_2/a_1, or FI of pig to human is very large (Table 3.3). When the increase in mosquito density with an increase in pig density is not significant, the model predicts that HRF is maximized when human and pig populations receive approximately equal numbers of mosquito bites ($a_1H \approx a_2L$). Thus, a situation where a small number of pigs are kept in the vicinity of human houses can yield a great risk. The distribution pattern of pigs, as well as its density, may be an important factor influencing HRF.

Presence of nonamplifier animals preferred by JE vectors, such as cattle, may have zooprophylaxis effects of reducing both P' and P. But if they contribute much to the increase in mosquito density by increasing Q, then HRF can be raised as mentioned in malaria zooprophylaxis.

In some Thai villages (A. Malainual et al. unpublished observations), people use screen nets to protect domestic animals, including pigs, from mosquito bites. This may effectively interrupt JE virus amplification via reduction of $P'Q$. In addition, the persistent and extensive use of nets may reduce mosquito density (M^*) and thus may contribute to the reduction of HRF. However, the animal houses are located usually very close to human houses. If the netting diverts attracted mosquitoes from animals to humans and if the human-biting rate (P) increases significantly, then HRF may increase at least temporarily. Overall effects of netting on JE prevalence in humans can be either desirable or undesirable, depending on local conditions.

Except for removal of pigs, present knowledge is far from sufficient to include livestock management into IVDC for JE as a reliable component to reduce R or HRF. More efforts should be directed to explore effective methods to kill vector mosquitoes attracted to pigs, if possible before feeding and without using insecticides. This contributes to the reduction of both R and HRF consistently.

Conclusion

Disease endemicity, which may be indicated by basic reproductive rates of diseases (R) or vectorial capacity (C), is not determined by abundance and innate characteristics of mosquitoes alone. Persistence of mosquito-borne diseases in ricelands is a consequence of overall effects of environmental components and human factors that assure the presence of all the links essential for pathogen transmission cycles. Thus, MBD problems in ricelands are worldwide, on the one hand, but still local, on the other, and would not be solved without full awareness of local situations.

Vector control in ricelands should be a component of integrated vector-borne disease control (IVDC), which, in turn, should be an essential component of regional development programs. Clearly, this cannot be realized without multilevel and multisectional consensus prevailing through central and regional governments, funding organizations, health departments, agriculture departments, nature conservancies, and so forth, and, most importantly, local community people. The Panel of Experts on Environmental Management (PEEM), established in 1981 by the World Health Organization (WHO), Food and Agriculture Organization of the United Nations (FAO), and the United Nations Environment Program (UNEP), has made efforts toward the establishment of such a consensus, with riceland development projects as a major target (53). A sustainable solution of MBD problems in ricelands will be attained only in the integrated program to create productive and healthy ricelands for our descendants.

References

1. Al-Azami, A., and Chew, R.M., 1959, Notes on the ecology of the dark rice field mosquito, *Psorophora confinnis* in Coachella Valley, California (Diptea: Culicidae), *Ann. Entomol. Soc. Am.* **52**:345–351.
2. Andis, M.D., and Meek., C.L., 1985, Mortality and survival patterns for the immature stages of *Psorophora columbiae*, *J. Am. Mosq. Control Assoc.* **1**:357–362.
3. Aron, J.L., and May, R.M., 1982, The population dynamics of malaria, Anderson, R.M. (ed): in Population Dynamics of Infectious Diseases, Chapman, New York, pp. 139–179.
4. Bailey, T.J., 1982, The Biomathematics of Malaria, Griffin, London, 210 p.
5. Bassi, D.G., 1987, Riceland mosquito management program-review of coordinated research, *J. Entomol. Sci. Suppl.* **1**:16–23.
6. Bendell, P.J.E., 1970, Japanese encephalitis in Sarawak: Studies on mosquito behaviour in a land dayak village, *Trans. R. Soc. Trop. Med. Hyg.* **64**: 497–502.
6a. Burke, D.S., and Leake, C.J., 1988, Japanese encephalitis, Monath, T.P. (ed): in The Arboviruses: Epidemiology and Ecology, vol. III, CRC Press, Boca Raton, Florida, pp. 63–92.
7. Burkot, T.R., 1988, Non-random host selection by anopheline mosquitoes, *Parasitol. Today* **4**:156–162.
8. Carey, D.E., Reuben, R., Myers, R.M., and George, S., 1968, Japanese encephalitis studies in Vellore, South India. Part IV. Search for virological and serological evidence of infection in animals other than man, *Indian J. Med. Res.* **56**:1340–1352.
9. Center for Disease Control (CDC), 1974, Introduced malaria in California, *Morbidity and Mortality* **23**:285–286.
10. Chambers, D.M., Steelman, C.D., and Schillings, P.E., 1979, Mosquito species and densities in Louisiana ricelands, *Mosq. News* **31**:658–668.
11. Chandler, J.A., and Highton, R.B., 1976, The breeding of *Anopheles gambiae* Giles (Diptera: Cilicidae) in rice fields in the Kisumu area of Kenya, *J. Med. Entomol.* **13**:211–215.

12. Charlwood, J.D., Paru, R., and Dagoro, H., 1984, Raised platforms reduce mosquito bites, *Trans. R. Soc. Trop. Med. Hyg.* **78**:141–142.
13. Chesson, J., 1983, The estimation and analysis of preference and its relationship to foraging models, *Ecology* **64**:1297–1304.
14. Christopher, S., and Reuben, R., 1971, Studies on the mosquitoes of North Arcot District, Madras State, India. Part 4: Host preferences as shown by precipitin tests, *J. Med. Entomol.* **8**:314–318.
15. Chubachi, R., 1979, An analysis of the generation-mean life table of the mosquito, *Culex tritaeniorhynchus summorosus*, with particular reference to population regulation, *J. Anim. Ecol.* **48**:681–702.
16. Cock, M.J.W., 1978, The assessment of preference, *J. Anim. Ecol.* **47**: 805–816.
17. Coluzzi, M., Sabatini, A., Petrarca, V., and Di Deco, M.A., 1979, Chromosomal differentiation and adaptation to human environments in the *Anopheles gambiae* complex, *Trans. R. Soc. Trop. Med. Hyg.* **73**:483–497.
18. Conway, G.R., 1970, Computer simulation as an aid to developing strategies for Anopheline control, *Miscellaneous publications Entomol. Soc. Am.* **7**: 181–191.
19. Coosemans, M.H., 1985, Comparaison de L'Endemie malarienne dans une zone de riziculture et dans une zone de culture de cotton dans la plaine de la Ruzizi, Burundi, *Ann. Soc. Belge Med. Trop.* Suppl. 2, **65**:187–200.
20. Cueller, C.B., 1969, A theoretical model of the dynamics of an *Anopheles gambiae* population under challenge with eggs giving rise to sterile males, *Bull. W.H.O.* **40**:205–212.
21. Curtis, C.F., and White, G.B., 1984, *Plasmodium falciparum* transmission in England: Entomological and epidemiological data relative to cases in 1983, *J. Trop. Med. Hyg.* **87**:101–114.
22. Das, M., Srivastava, B.N., Rao, C.K., Thapar, B.R., and Sharma G.K., 1987, Field trial of the effectiveness of indoor-spraying with pirimiphos-methyl emulsion for malaria control in a tribal area of Phulbani district, Orissa State, India, *Med. Vet. Entomol.* **1**:289–295.
23. Davies, J.E., Edmundson, W.F., and Raffonelli, A., 1975, The role of house dust in human DDT pollution, *Am. J. Public Health* **65**:53–57.
24. Dye, C., 1984, Models for the population dynamics of the yellow fever mosquito, *Aedes aegypti*, *J. Anim. Ecol.* **53**:247–268.
25. Edman, J.D., 1988, Disease control through manipulation of vector-host interaction: Some historical and evolutionary perspectives, Scott, T.W. and Grumstrup-Scott, J. (eds): in Proceedings of a Symposium: The Role of Vector-Host Interactions in Disease Transmission, *Miscellaneous publications Entomol. Soc. Am.* **68**:43–50.
26. Edman, J.D., Webber, I.A., and Kale, H.W., 1972, Effects of mosquito density on the interrelationship of host behaviour and mosquito feeding success, *Am. J. Trop. Med. Hyg.* **21**:487–491.
27. Farmer, F.L., Redfern, J.M., Meisch, M.V., and Inman, A., 1989, An evaluation of a community based mosquito abatement program: Residents' satisfaction, economic benefits and correlates of support, *J. Am. Mosq. Control Assoc.* **5**:335–338.
28. Focks, D.A., and McLaughlin, R.E., 1988, Computer simulation of management strategies for *Psorophora columbiae* in the rice agroecosystem, *J. Am. Mosq. Control Assoc.* **4**:399–413.

29. Focks, D.A., McLaughlin, R.E., and Smith, B.M., 1988a, A dynamic life table model of *Psorophora columbiae* in the southern Louisiana rice agroecosystem with supporting hydrologic submodel. Part 1. Analysis of literature and model development, *J. Am. Mosq. Control Assoc.* **4**:266–281.
30. Focks, D.A., McLaughlin, R.E., and Smith, B.M., 1988b, A dynamic life table model of *Psorophora columbiae* in the southern Louisiana rice agroecosystem with supporting hydrologic submodel. Part 2. Model validation and population dynamics, *J. Am. Mosq. Control Assoc.* **4**:282–299.
31. Food and Agriculture Organization (FAO), 1973, Report of the fourth session of the FAO panel of experts on integrated pest control, FAO, Rome, 35 p.
32. Food and Agriculture Organization (FAO), 1977, Report of the seventh session of the FAO panel of experts on integrated pest control, FAO, Rome, 45 p.
33. Fujito, S., Buei, K., Nakajima, S., Ito, S., Yoshida, M., Sonoda, H., and Nakamura, H., 1971, Effect of the population density of *Culex tirtaeniorhynchus* Giles on blood-sucking rates in cowsheds and pigpens in relation to its role in the epidemic of Japanese encephalitis, *Jpn. J. Sanit. Zool.* **22**:38–44 (in Japanese with English summary).
34. Gahlinger, P.M., Reeves, W.C., and Milby, M.M., 1986, Air conditioning and television as protective factors in arboviral encephalitis risk, *Am. J. Trop. Med. Hyg.* **35**:601–610.
35. Garrett-Jones, C., 1964, The human blood index of malaria vectors in relation to epidemiological assessment, *Bull. W.H.O.* **30**:241–261.
36. Garrity, D.P., 1988, Tropical rice agroecosystems: Characteristics, distribution, and future trends, in Vector-Borne Disease Control in Humans Through Rice Agroecosystem Management, IRRI, Manila, Philippines, pp. 13–28.
37. Giglioli, M.E.C., 1963, Ecological change as a factor in renewed malaria transmission in an eradicated area. A localized outbreak of *Anopheles aquasalis* transmitted malaria on the Demerara River estuary, British Guiana, in the fifteenth year of *A. darlingi* and malaria eradication, *Bull. W.H.O.* **29**:131–145.
38. Giglioli, M.E.C., 1965, The influence of irregularities in the bush perimeter of the cleared agricultural belt around a Gambian village on the flight range and direction of approach of a population of *Anopheles gambiae melas*, in Proceedings International Congress Entomol., 12th, London, 1964, pp. 757–758.
39. Gillett, J.D., 1985, The behaviour of *Homo sapiens*, the forgotten factor in the transmission of tropical disease, *Trans. R. Soc. Trop. Med. Hyg.* **79**: 12–20.
40. Gillies, M.T., 1964, Selection for host preference in *Anopheles gambiae*, *Nature* **203**:852–854.
41. Gillies, M.T., and Wilkes, T.J., 1970, The range of attraction of single baits for some West African mosquitoes, *Bull. Entomol. Res.* **60**:225–235.
42. Gould, D.J., Edelman, R., Grossman, R.A., Nisalak, A., and Sullivan, M.F., 1974, Study of Japanese encephalitis virus in Chiang Mai valley, Thailand. IV. Vector studies, *Am. J. Epidemiol.* **100**:49–56.
43. Gratz, N.G., 1988, The impact of rice production on vector-borne disease problems in developing countries, in Vector-Borne Disease Control in Humans Through Rice Agroecosystem, IRRI, Manila, Philippines, pp. 7–12.

44. Grossman, R.A., Gould, D.J., Smith T.J., Johnsen, D.O., and Pantuwatana, S., 1973, Study of Japanese encephalitis virus in Chiang Mai valley, Thailand. I. Introduction, *Am. J. Epidemiol.* **98**:111–120.
45. Haile, D.G., and Weidhass, D.E., 1977, Computer simulation of mosquito populations (*Anopheles albimanus*) for comparing the effectiveness of control technologies, *J. Med. Entomol.* **13**:553–567.
46. Herath, P.R.J., and Joshi, G.P., 1986, Factors affecting selection for multiple resistance in *Anopheles nigerrmus* in Sri Lanka, *Trans. R. Soc. Trop. Med. Hyg.* **80**:649–652.
47. Hess, A.D., Hayes, R.O., Tempelis, C.H., 1968, The use of the forage ratio technique in mosquito host preference studies, *Mosq. News* **28**:386–389.
48. Hill, R.B., and Cambournac, F.J.C., 1941, Intermittent irrigation in rice cultivation, and its effect on yield, water consumption and *Anopheles* production, *Am. J. Trop. Med.* **21**:123–144.
49. Hoy, J.B., Kauffman, E.E., and O'berg, A.G., 1972, A large-scale field test of *Gambusia affinis* and chlorphyrifos for mosquito control, *Mosq. News* **32**:161–171.
50. Ikeshoji, T., 1986, Distribution of the mosquitoes, *Culex tritaeniorhynchus*, in relation to disposition of sound traps in a paddy field, *Jpn. J. Sanit. Zool.* **37**:153–159.
51. Ikeshoji, T., and Ogawa, K., 1988, Field catching of mosquitoes with various types of sound traps, *Jpn. J. Sanit. Zool.* **39**:119–123.
52. Ikeshoji, T., Sakakibara, M., and Reisen, W.K., 1985, Removal sampling of male mosquitoes from field populations by sound-trapping, *Jpn. J. Sanit. Zool.* **36**:197–203.
53. International Rice Research Institute (IRRI), 1988, Vector-Borne Disease Control in Humans Through Rice Agroecosystem Management, IRRI, Manila, Philippines, 237 p.
54. Janssens, P.G., and Wery, M., 1987, Malaria in Africa south of the Sahara, *Ann. Trop. Med. Parasitol.* **81**:487–498.
55. John, K.H., Stoll, J.R., and Olson, J.K., 1987, An economic assessment of the benefit of mosquito abatement in an organized mosquito control district, *J. Am. Mosq. Control. Assoc.* **3**:8–14.
56. Johnsen, D.O., Edelman, R., Grossman, R.A., Muangman, D., Pomsdhit, J., and Gould, D.J., 1974, Study of Japanese encephalitis virus in Chiang Mai valley, Thailand. V. Animal infections. *Am. J. Epidemiol.* **100**:57–68.
57. Joshi, H., Vasantha, K., Subbarao, S.K., and Sharma, V.P., 1988, Host feeding patterns of *Anopheles culicifacies* species A and B., *J. Am. Mosq. Control Assoc.* **4**:248–251.
58. Kay, B.H., Boreham, P.F.L., and Edman, J.D., 1979, Application of the "feeding index" concept to studies of mosquito host-feeding patterns, *Mosq. News* **39**:68–72.
59. Kennedy, J.S., 1940, The visual responses of flying mosquitoes, *Proc. Zool. Soc. Lond.* **109**:221–242.
60. Kirnowordoyo, S., and Supalin, 1986, Zooprophylaxis as a useful tool for control of *A. aconitus* transmitted malaria in Central Java, Indonesia, *J. Comm. Dis.* **18**:90–94.
61. Kramer, V.L., Garcia, R., and Colwell, A.E., 1987, An evaluation of the mosquitofish, *Gambusia affinis*, and the inland silverside, *Menidia beryllina*,

as mosquito control agents in california wild rice fields, *J. Am. Mosq. Control Assoc.* **3**:626–632.
62. Kramer, V.L., Garcia, R., and Colwell, A.E., 1988, An evaluation of *Gambusia affinis* and *Bacillus thuringiensis* var. *Israelensis* as mosquito control agents in California wild rice fields, *J. Am. Mosq. Control Assoc.* **4**:470–478.
62a. Kurihara, T., Kamimura, K., and Arakawa, R., 1986, Phenothrin impregnation of wide-mesh net for potection from biting mosquitoes, *Jpn. J. Sanit. Zool.* **37**:261–262.
63. Lu B.L., 1988, Environmental management for the control of ricefield-breeding mosquitoes in China, in Vector-Borne Disease Control in Humans Through Rice Agroecosystem, IRRI, Manila, Philippines, pp. 111–121.
64. Luh, P.L., 1981, The present status of biocontrol of mosquitoes in China, Laird, M. (ed): in Biocontrol of Medical and Veterinary Pests, Praeger, New York, pp. 54–77.
65. MacCormack, C.P., 1984, Human ecology and behaviour in malaria control in tropical Africa, *Bull. W.H.O.* **62**(Suppl.):81–87.
66. Macdonald, G., 1957, The Epidemiology and Control of Malaria, Oxford University Press, London, 201 p.
66a. McLaughlin, R.E., and Focks, D.A., 1990, Effects of cattle density on New Jersey light trap mosquito captures in the rice/cattle agroecosystem of southwestern Louisiana, *J. Am. Mosq. Control Assoc.* **6**:283–286.
67. McLaughlin, R.E., and Vidrine, M.F., 1987, *Psorophora columbiae* larval density in southwestern Louisiana rice fields as a function of cattle density, *J. Am. Mosq. Control Assoc.* **3**:633–635.
68. Miura, T., Takahashi, R.M., and Mulligan, F.S. III, 1978, Field evaluation of the effectiveness of predacious insects as a mosquito control agent, *Proc. Calif. Mosq. Control Assoc.* **46**:80–81.
69. Miura, T., Takahashi, R.M., and Wilder, W.H., 1984, Impact of the mosquitofish (*Gambusia affinis*) on a rice field ecosystem when used as a mosquito control agent, *Mosq. News* **44**:510–517.
70. Mizutani, K., Suzuki, T., Ogata, K., and Tanaka, I., 1968, Control experiments of *Culex tritaeniorhynchus* by the spray of ronnel on pigs, *Jpn. J. Sanit. Zool.* **19**:67–72 (in Japanese with English summary).
71. Mogi, M., 1978, Population studies on mosquitoes in the rice field area of Nagasaki, Japan, especially on *Culex tritaeniorhynchus*, *Trop. Med. (Nagasaki)* **20**:173–263.
72. Mogi, M., 1979, Dispersal of *Culex tritaeniorhynchus* larvae (Diptera, Culicidae) by water currents in rice fields, *Trop. Med. (Nagasaki)* **21**:115–126.
73. Mogi, M., 1984, Mosquito problems and their solution in relation to paddy rice production, *Protection Ecol.* **7**:219–240.
74. Mogi, M., 1988, Water management in rice cultivation and its relation to mosquito production in Japan, in Vector-Borne Disease Control in Humans Through Rice Agroecosystem Management, IRRI, Manila, Philippines, pp. 101–109.
75. Mogi, M., and Miyagi, I., 1990, Colonization of rice fields by mosquitoes (Diptera: Culicidae) and larvivorous predators in asynchronous rice cultivation areas in the Philippines, *J. Med. Entomol.* **27**:530–536.

76. Mogi, M., and Wada, Y., 1973, Spatial distribution of larvae of the mosquito *Culex tritaeniorhynchus summorosus* in a rice field area, *Trop. Med.* (*Nagasaki*) **2**:69–83.
77. Mogi, M., Miyagi, I., and Cabrera, B.D., 1984, Development and survival of immature mosquitoes (Diptera: Culicidae) in Philippine rice fields, *J. Med. Entomol.* **21**:283–291.
78. Mogi, M., Mori, A., and Wada, Y., 1980, Survival rates of *Culex tritaeniorhynchus* (Diptera: Culicidae) larvae in fallow rice fields before summer cultivation, *Trop. Med.* (*Nagasaki*) **22**:47–59.
79. Mogi, M., Mori, A., and Wada, Y., 1980b, Survival rates of immature stages of *Culex tritaeniorhynchus* (Diptera: Culicidae) in rice fields under summer cultivation. *Trop. Med.* (*Nagasaki*) **22**:111–126.
80. Mogi, M., Okazawa, T., Miyagi, I., Sucharit, S., Tumrasvin, W., Deesin, T., and Khamboonruang, C., 1986, Development and survival of anopheline immatures (Diptera: Culicidae) in rice fields in northern Thailand, *J. Med. Entomol.* **23**:244–250.
81. Moon, T.E., 1976, A statistical model of the dynamics of a mosquito vector (*Culex tarsalis*) population, *Biometrics* **32**:355–368.
82. Mori, A., Igarashi, A., Charoensook, O., Khamboonruang, C., Leechanachai, P., and Supawadee, J., 1983, Virological and epidemiological studies on encephalitis in Chiang Mai area, Thailand. VII. Mosquito collection and virus isolation, in the year of 1982, *Trop. Med.* (*Nagasaki*) **25**:189–198.
83. Najera, J.A., 1988, Malaria and rice: Strategies for control, in Vector-Borne Disease Control in Humans Through Rice Agroecosystem Management, IRRI, Manila, Philippines, pp. 123–132.
84. Nalim, S., Boewono, D.T., Haliman, A., and Winoto, E., 1985, Control demonstration of the ricefield breeding mosquito *Anopheles aconitus* donitz in Central Java, using *Poecilia reticulata* through community participation: 3. field trial and evaluation. *Bull. Penelit. Kesehat.* **16**:6–11.
85. Nishigaki, J., 1970, Studies on the control of *Culex tritaeniorhynchus* by the larvicide application, *Trop. Med.* (*Nagasaki*) **11**:183–201.
86. Odetoyinbo, J.A., 1969, Preliminary investigation on the use of a light-trap for sampling malaria vectors in the Gambia, *Bull. W.H.O.* **40**:547–560.
87. Pedigo, L.P., Hutchins, S.H., and Higley L.G., 1986, Economic injury levels in theory and practice, *Annu. Rev. Entomol.* **31**:341–368.
88. Pennington, N.E., and Phelps, C.A., 1968, Identification of the host range of *Culex tritaeniorhynchus* mosquitoes on Okinawa, Ryukyu Islands, *J. Med. Entomol.* **5**:483–487.
89. Phan-Urai, P., Chansang, C., Malainual. A., and Thavara, U., 1990, Efficiency of mosquito light trap (FHK type) on JE vectors, in Abstracts Asia-Pacific Conference Entomol., 1st, Chiang Mai, p. 88.
90. Rao, D.R., and Reuben, R., 1989, Evaluation of neem cake coated urea as mosquito larvicides in rice fields, Uren, M.F., Blok, J., and Manderson, L.H. (eds): in Arbovirus Research in Australia-Proceedings Fifth Symposium, Brisbane, pp. 138–142.
91. Reeves, W.C., 1971, Mosquito vector and vertebrate host interaction: The key to maintenance of certain arboviruses, Fallis, A.M. (ed): in Ecology and Physiology of Parasites, Univ. Toronto Press, Toronto, pp. 223–231.
92. Reisen, W.K., Boreham, P.F.L., 1979, Host selection patterens of some Pakistan mosquitoes, *Am. J. Trop. Med. Hyg.* **28**:408–421.

93. Reisen, W.K., Aslamkhan, M., and Basio, R.C., 1976, The effects of climatic patterns and agricultural practices on the population dynamics of *Culex tritaeniorhynchus* in Asia, *Southeast Asian J. Trop. Med. Publ. Health* **7**:61–71.
94. Reuben, R., 1971, Studies on the mosquitoes of North Arcot District, Madras State, India. Part 2. Biting cycles and behavior on human and bovine baits at two villages, *J. Med. Entomol.* **8**:127–134.
95. Reuben, R., Mani, T.R., and Tewari, S.C., 1984, Feeding behaviour, age structure & vectorial capacity of *Anopheles culicifacies* Giles along the river Thenpennai (Tamil Nadu), *Indian J. Med. Red.* **80**:23–29.
96. Rozendaal, J.A., 1989, Impregnated mosquito nets and curtains for self-protection and vector control, *Trop. Diseases Bull.* **86**, No. 7, pp. 1–41.
97. Russell, P.F., 1934, Zooprophylaxis failure. An experiment in the Philippines, *Riv. Malariol.* **13**:610–616.
98. Russell, P.F., Knipe, F.W., and Rao, H.R., 1942, On the intermittent irrigation of rice fields to control malaria in South India, *J. Malar. Inst. India* **4**:321–340.
99. Saxena, R.C., Epino, P.B., Cheng-Wen, T., and Puma, B.C., 1983, Neem, chinaberry and custard apple: Antifeedant and insecticidal effects of seed oils on leafhopper and planthopper pests of rice, in Proceedings International Neem Conf., 2nd, Rauischholzhausen, pp. 403–412.
100. Schaefer, C.H., Miura, T., and Wilder, W.H., 1981, Mosquito production on a California rice field treated with a nonselective insecticide, *Mosq. News* **41**:791–793.
101. Self, L.S., Ree, H.I., Lofgren, C.S., Shim, J.C., Chow, C.Y., Shin, H.K., and Kim, K.H., 1973, Aerial applications of ultra-low-volume insecticides to control the vector of Japanese encephalitis in Korea, *Bull. W.H.O.* **49**: 353–357.
102. Service, M.W., 1977, Mortalities of the immature stages of species B of the *Anopheles gambiae* complex in Kenya: Comparison between rice fields and temporary pools, identification of predators, and effects of insecticidal spraying, *J. Med. Entomol.* **13**:535–545.
103. Shim, J.C., Ree, H.I., and Kim, C.L., 1982, Study on the susceptibility of insecticides against *Culex tritaeniorhynchus* larvae, *Korean J. Entomol.* **12**: 41–45 (in Korean with English summary).
104. Siddiqui, T.F., Aslam, Y., and Reisen, W.K., 1976, The effects of larval density on selected immature and adult attributes in *Culex tritaeniorhynchus* Giles, *Trop. Med. (Nagasaki)* **18**:195–202.
105. Smith, C.E.G., 1970, Studies on arbovirus epidemiology associated with established and developing rice culture, *Trans. R. Soc. Trop. Med. Hyg.* **64**:481–482.
106. Snellen, W.B., 1987, Malaria control by engineering measures: Pre-World-War-II examples from Indonesia, Annual Report International Institute for Land Reclamation and Improvement, 1987, pp. 8–21.
107. Snow, W.F., 1983. The attractiveness of some birds and mammals for mosquitoes in The Gambia, West Africa, *Ann. Trop. Med. Parasitol.* **77**: 641–651.
108. Sota, T., and Mogi, M., 1989, Effectiveness of zooprophylaxis in malaria control: A theoretical inquiry, with a model for mosquito populations with two bloodmeal hosts, *Med. Vet. Entomol.* **3**:337–345.

109. Sota, T., and Mogi, M., 1989. Models for JE transmission dynamics with vector mosquito dynamics, Uren, M.F., Blok, J., and Manderson, L.H. (eds): in Arbovirus Research in Australia-Proceedings Fifth Symposium, Brisbane, pp. 144–148.
109a. Sota, T., Hayamizu, E., and Mogi, M., 1991, Distribution of biting *Culex* tritaeniorhynchus (Diptera: Culicidae) among pigs: effects of host size and behavior, *J. Med. Entomol.* (in press)
110. Steelman, C.D., and Schilling, P.E., 1977, Economics of protecting cattle from mosquito attack relative to injury thresholds, *J. Econ. Entomol.* **70**: 15–17.
111. Steelman, C.D., White, T.W., and Schilling, P.E., 1976, Efficacy of Brahman characters in reducing weight loss of steers exposed to mosquito attack, *J. Econ. Entomol.* **69**:499–502.
112. Subbarao, S.K., Vasantha, K., and Sharma, V.P., 1988, Responses of *Anopheles culicifacies* sibling species A and B to DDT and HCH in India: Implications in malaria control, *Med. Vet. Entomol.* **2**:219–223.
113. Surtees, G., 1970, Effects of irrigation on mosquito populations and mosquito-borne diseases in man, with particular reference to rice field extension, *Int. J. Environ. Stud.* **1**:35–42.
114. Swaminathan, M.S., 1984, *Rice*, *Sci. Am.* **250**:63–71.
115. Takahashi, M., 1982, Differential transmission efficiency for Japanese encephalitis virus among colonized strains of *Culex tritaeniorhynchus*, *Jpn. J. Sanit. Zool.* **33**:325–333.
116. Takahashi, M., and Yasutomi, K., 1987, Insecticidal resistance of *Culex tritaeniorhynchus* (Diptera: Culicidae) in Japan: Genetics and mechanisms of resistance to organophosphorus insecticides, *J. Med. Entomol.* **24**:595–603.
117. Tewari, S.C., Mani, T.R., Suguna, S.G., and Reuben, R., 1984, Host selection patterns in anophelines in riverine villages of Tamil Nadu, *Indian J. Med. Res.* **80**:18–22.
118. Urabe, K., Ikemoto, T., Takei, S., and Aida, C., 1986, Studies on *Sympetrum frequens* (Odonata: Libellulidae) nymphs as natural enemies of the mosquito larvae, *Anopheles sinensis*, in rice fields. III. Esitmation of the prey consumption rate in the rice fields, *Jpn. J. Appl. Ent. Zool.* **30**:129–135.
119. Wada, Y., 1975, Theoretical considerations on the epidemic of Japanese encephalitis, *Trop. Med. (Nagasaki)* **16**:171–199.
120. Wada, Y., 1988, Strategies for control of Japanese encephalitis in rice production systems in developing countries, in Vector-Borne Disease Control in Humans Through Rice Agroecosystem Management, IRRI, Manila, Philippines, pp. 153–160.
121. Wada, Y., and Mogi, M., 1974, Efficiency of the dipper in collecting immature stages of *Culex tritaeniorhynchus summorosus*, *Trop. Med. (Nagasaki)* **16**:35–40.
122. Washino, R.K., and Tempelis, C.H., 1983, Mosquito host bloodmeal identification: Methodology and data analysis, *Annu. Rev. Entomol.* **28**:179–201.
123. Washino, R.K., Whitesell, K.G., Sherman, E.J., Kramer, M.C., and McKenna, R.J., 1972, Rice field mosquito control studies with low volume Dursban^R sprays in Colusa County, California. III. Effects upon the target organisms, *Mosq. News* **32**:375–382.
124. Weathersbee III, A.A., Meisch, M.V., Sandoski, C.A., Finch, M.F., Dame, D.A., Olson, J.K., and Inman, A., 1986, Combination ground and aerial

adulticide applications against mosquitoes in an arkansas riceland community, *J. Am. Mosq. Control Assoc.* **2**:456–460.

125. Weidhaas, D.E., 1974, Simplified models of population dynamics of mosquitoes related to control technology, *J. Econ. Entomol.* **67**:620–624.
126. World Health Organization (WHO), 1982, Manual on Environmental Management for Mosquito Control, with Special Emphasis on Malaria Vectors, WHO, Geneva, 283 p.
127. World Health Organization (WHO), 1983, Integrated vector control, WHO Technical Report Series, No. 688, Geneva, 72 p.
128. World Health Organization (WHO), 1989, The use of impregnated bednets and other materials for vector-borne disease control, *WHO/VBC/89.981*, WHO, Geneva, 45 p.
129. Xu J., Zao M., Luo X., Geng R., Pan S., and Liu S., 1988, Evaluation of permethrin-impregnated mosquito-nets against mosquitoes in China, *Med. Vet. Entomol.* **2**:247–251.

4
Detection of Malarial Parasites in Mosquitoes

Robert A. Wirtz and Thomas R. Burkot

Introduction

Malaria is the most important parasitic disease in the tropics, with indigenous transmission in over 100 countries or areas of the world (122, 123). The World Health Organization (WHO) estimates the global incidence of this mosquito-transmitted disease to be approximately 100 million cases annually (67); other estimates are in the 200 to 400 million range (57, 101). In 1984, nearly 400 million people, one-twelfth of the world's population, were living in areas where malaria is highly endemic and where no specific antimalarial measures were being applied. An additional 2700 million people, 56% of the world's population, live in areas where malaria is still endemic but where control measures have reduced its level of endemicity. In many of these areas malaria is increasing dramatically (67, 122, 123).

Malaria control programs designed to interrupt mosquito-human contact are restricted, in part, by our lack of knowledge about the vectors and the epidemiology of the disease. The application of recently developed biotechnology-based methods has the potential of greatly improving our understanding of malaria transmission. In this chapter we discuss the combined application of the traditional techniques with the new methods available to malariologists in their battle against malaria.

Human Malaria Parasites

There are four species of malarial parasites that commonly infect humans. *Plasmodium falciparum* is the most frequently occurring form throughout

Robert A. Wirtz, Department of Entomology, Walter Reed Army Institute of Research, Washington, D.C. 20307-5100, USA
Thomas R. Burkot, Tropical Health Program, Queensland Institute of Medical Research, Bramston Terrace, Herston, Brisbane, Queensland 4006, Australia.

the tropics and subtropics. It is also responsible for most malaria mortality. *Plasmodium vivax* covers the widest geographical area and is characterized by relapses caused by parasites that remain in the liver in a latent form. It is prevalent in many temperate as well as tropical and subtropical zones, but does not occur in large areas of tropical Africa. *Plasmodium malariae* is widely distributed but is much less common than *P. falciparum* and *P. vivax* are, and *P. ovale*, found chiefly in tropical Africa and Asia, is the least prevalent species.

There are nearly 100 other species of malarial parasites of mammals, birds, and reptiles. Simian malarias, some of which infect humans, are still present in isolated areas of the world (26, 39).

The human malarias are transmitted only by mosquitoes belonging to the genus *Anopheles*, as are some of the plasmodia infecting other animals. A susceptible mosquito becomes infected with human malaria by feeding on a gametocytemic person. The sexual forms of the parasite (gametocytes) are ingested by the mosquito during blood feeding. Asexual parasites usually predominate in parasitemic blood and are largely destroyed during digestion in the mosquito gut. Once in the mosquito midgut, the gametocytes undergo rapid maturation into the male and female gametes, which fuse to form a zygote. The zygote develops into a motile ookinete, which penetrates the midgut epithelium and settles under the basal laminal layer. The ookinete transforms into a spherical oocyst, projecting into the mosquito's hemocoel, in which the sporozoites develop and mature. Sporozoites emerge from ruptured oocysts into the mosquito hemocoel and are transported throughout the body cavity by the hemolymph and their moderate motility. A number of the sporozoites reach the salivary glands, penetrate and accumulate in the acinal cells, and some of those sporozoites pass into the salivary ducts. These enter the blood stream of the vertebrate host during a subsequent blood meal. Sporogonic development time is characteristic of each plasmodial species, varying between 7 and 15 days from the time of the infectious bloodmeal, and is directly dependent upon the ambient temperature (9, 47, 48, 98).

The number of oocysts on the midgut is usually less than 10 in field-collected mosquitoes, but in some instances can be over several hundred. Mature oocysts range in size from 40 to 80 μm in diameter. Estimates as to the number of sporozoites, or circumsporozoite (CS) protein equivalents, from a single oocyst range from 1000 to 10,000 (9, 14, 48, 57, 82, 83, 106).

The sporozoite is 10–14 μm long, 1.0 μm in diameter, and slightly curved with narrow ends. Their infectivity to man increases from a low degree in the mature oocyst, until they become highly infective shortly after entering the glands; the infectivity then declines with age (48). The number of sporozoites transmitted by an infectious anopheline is restricted to those flushed from the salivary duct during feeding, and appears to be fewer than 25, even from mosquitoes with heavily infected salivary glands (3, 93).

Sporozoites are covered with a circumsporozoite protein, which is immunodominant in the vertebrate host (25, 77). The repeat portion of the CS protein has been the target of the sporozoite vaccines and the immunological-based assays for detection and species identification of sporozoites in mosquitoes. Routine use of these assays is dependent on the CS proteins being conserved, at least in the area of study (92).

An understanding of the sporogonic developmental cycle in a vector mosquito is essential for proper interpretation of results obtained using dissection, immunological assays, and nucleic acid probe methods described later in this chapter.

The Mosquito Vector

There are over 400 described species of *Anopheles*, none of which are cosmopolitan, and most are not malaria vectors. Wernsdorfer (112) states that only 67 anophelines have been found to harbor sporozoites originating from natural infections, that approximately 30 additional species were found experimentally susceptible to infection with the human malarias, and only 27 anophelines are associated with a significant degree of malaria transmission. However, Gillies (51) states that approximately 45 species have been "seriously implicated" in transmission. Other studies indicate that up to 85 species should be regarded as vectors of human malarias (57, 114). The somewhat arbitrary classification of primary and secondary malaria vectors accounts for some of these discrepancies. Primary vectors have been associated with endemic malaria transmission, whereas secondary vector status was given to species that are able to maintain some transmission, at least in part of the study area. The term *incidental vector* has been used to describe anophelines of local importance that are generally thought to be incapable of maintaining extended transmission (9).

Most anophelines are not important natural malaria vectors because they are not physiologically susceptible to infection, are too short lived, or are not closely associated with humans. The most efficient vectors preferentially feed on humans. The degree of susceptibility to malaria infection for a mosquito species varies with the *Plasmodium* species and strain, and is considered to have a genetic basis. This partially explains why an anopheline species is viewed as an important vector in one geographic region and of little or no importance in another area (9, 47, 48).

Vector species lists have been compiled from studies based on observation of sporozoites in the salivary glands and oocysts on the guts of wild-caught anophelines. There is little doubt as to the primary vectors in many malarious areas of the world, especially where strong epidemiological evidence supports dissection results. However, in studies implicating secondary or incidental vectors where the salivary gland sporozoites were not identified, additional research must be conducted before vector status is confirmed.

Special consideration must also be given to studies in areas where ecological disruption has taken place, for example, refugee camps and deforested, reforested, or resettlement areas (1, 12, 55, 91). In these regions mosquitoes containing nonhuman salivary gland sporozoites may be collected feeding on humans. Anophelines capable of transmitting human malaria which normally feed on other animals may become important vectors with the elimination of their preferred bloodmeal source.

Some malaria vectors belong to groups of sibling species complexes, consisting of members that are morphologically indistinguishable using the current taxonomic keys. These species are reproductively isolated when they occur sympatrically, as they do not normally interbreed where mixed populations occur. Despite their morphological similarity, sibling species may exhibit ecological, behavioral, or physiological differences that can give rise to differences in vectorial capacity (102). The failure to recognize sibling species of *Anopheles* may result in the failure to distinguish between a vector and a nonvector species. For instance, the supposed behavioral changes recorded in malaria vectors under insecticide pressure were due to the differential survival of unknown sympatric sibling species (35). When possible, it is essential to distinguish between sibling species using nonmorphologic methods (32, 35, 114). The identification of a member of a species complex as a malaria vector may permit the development of a selective vector control strategy.

Measurement of Malaria Transmission

Human malaria parasites are transmitted only by anopheline mosquitoes and do not normally have reservoirs other than humans. Studying transmission would therefore seem to be relatively straightforward, involving measurements of the parasites in the human host and the local anopheline populations. Unfortunately, starting with Sir Ronald Ross in the late 1800s, each generation of malariologists has discovered that an accurate quantitative description of malaria transmission dynamics is exceedingly difficult to obtain. Measuring parasite prevalence or incidence in the human population is difficult because of similarities in parasite morphology, the presence of mixed infections, latent liver stages responsible for relapses, very low incidence rates, and low compliance among the human study population. Some of these problems are being overcome through the development and application of new methods in the fields of molecular biology, immunology, and sociology.

Historically, there have been three basic approaches to quantitating malaria transmission: parasitological, entomological, and mathematical (theoretical).

The parasitological approach is exemplified by the use of incidence and recovery rates, in particular, the infant conversion rate (71). Monitoring infants or young children for the first appearance of malaria blood stage parasites gives an estimation of the transmission rate. In areas of low endemicity the rate at which an infant changes from aparasitemic to parasitemic will approximate the rate at which infectious mosquitoes transmit sporozoites while blood feeding.

Quantitating malaria transmission also involves measuring the rate at which mosquitoes become infected from feeding on humans. Factors affecting the rate of mosquitoes acquiring infections from humans include gametocyte prevalence and density, transmission blocking or enhancing immunity, and variables associated with the mosquito vector (15, 22).

The entomological approach involves measuring the proportion of mosquitoes with sporozoites in their salivary glands (sporozoite rate) and the daily rate at which mosquitoes bite humans (daily human-biting rate). The product of these is the inoculation rate. The human-biting rate has traditionally been approximated by pyrethrum spray collections, exit traps on huts, or by landing catches in which humans collect mosquitoes landing on them. Landing catches tend to overestimate the true human-biting rate, whereas the other collection techniques usually underestimate the true biting rate (96, 120). Errors in accurately measuring sporozoite and human-biting rates are partially responsible for the discrepancy observed between the inoculation rate and the infant conversion rate (70, 78).

The concept of vectorial capacity (49, 50) was developed, in part, to overcome the problems associated with the traditional entomological approach. Vectorial capacity is an attempt to measure the transmission potential by relating the mosquito density, the human-biting habits of the vectors, and their survivorship. As none of the components of vectorial capacity involve parasitological measurements, vectorial capacity can be estimated in nonendemic as well as endemic areas. Unfortunately, each of the components of vectorial capacity is extremely difficult to measure accurately leading Dye (41) to urge the development of modified vectorial capacities in which key entomological parameters would be identified that could be correlated to either parasite prevalence or incidence in the human population. Recently, the concept of an individual mosquito vectorial capacity has been developed (95). The approach relies on measuring malaria parasite infections in mosquitoes collected in two of the following three ways: landing rates and indoor or outdoor resting mosquitoes. Obviously, these requirements limit this novel approach to endemic areas where large numbers of anophelines can be collected (54).

Parasite Detection Methods

Incrimination of an anopheline mosquito as a vector of human malaria requires that human malaria sporozoites be identified in the salivary glands of specimens collected in the field or that those mosquitoes be used to infect human volunteers. Neither the traditional examination of salivary glands for sporozoites or midguts for oocysts, nor the application of immunological assays or nucleic acid probes to whole mosquitoes can meet these criteria. Except for transmission studies, establishing vector status requires the combined use of these methods.

In Vivo Method

The *in vivo* method involves the feeding of infectious mosquitoes on suitable hosts. Malaria transmission by *Anopheles* was proven using this method, with the definitive studies conducted using human volunteers (8, 11, 47, 48). *In vivo* studies also have been used extensively to identify mosquitoes infected with human and simian malarias (26, 47, 88). Successful *in vivo* experiments can establish the vector status of a mosquito; however, negative feeding results may be difficult to interpret.

The identification of infectious mosquitoes, without injury to the specimens, is desirable for selection of individual insects to be used in vaccine challenge studies or the natural infection of hosts by mosquito bite. Such a method was described by Russell, West, Manwell, and MacDonald, (94) in which individual mosquitoes were confined in glass vials plugged with cotton wool. A small glass coverslip was attached to the cotton and a drop of sugar feeding solution was placed on the surface. If sporozoites were present in the salivary ducts, a number of them were released as the mosquito fed on the sugar solution. A harmless dye, such as food coloring, can be added to the sugar solution to easily determine if a particular mosquito has fed. Starved mosquitoes are more likely to feed rapidly when given access to the sugar solution, if direct observations of feeding are desired. Sporozoites on the coverslip can be counted directly or the preparations can be stained for easier observation. The immunological methods described below could then be used to determine the plasmodial species from field-collected anophelines.

The infection of humans by bites from field-collected anophelines or by injection of salivary gland sporozoites was the only method of establishing a mosquito species as a human malaria vector for over three-fourths of a century. This procedure remained essential for definitive vector incrimination studies until immunological methods were developed and incorporated into the testing of salivary gland sporozoites.

Dissection Method

The dissection method is used to incriminate malaria vectors and to establish sporozoite and oocyst rates in mosquitoes. The percentage of female anophelines of a given species caught in nature and found, on dissection within 24 h of capture, to contain sporozoites in the salivary glands is the sporozoite rate. The percentage with oocysts on the midgut is the oocyst rate (112). Sporozoite rates have and must continue to be determined by the dissection of individual specimens. The problem of accurate determination of sporozoite and oocyst rates is exacerbated by the extremely low infection rates found in many endemic areas. This is especially so in parts of Central and South America where studies in which thousands of mosquitoes were dissected resulted in very few (<0.01%) or no sporozoite or oocyst positives (109).

Detailed, illustrated instructions for removal of salivary glands and midguts from mosquitoes and their examination for sporozoites and oocysts, respectively, have been published in several texts. Books still in print, which contain this information, and references to earlier methods, include those by Bruce-Chwatt (9) and Vanderberg and Gwadz (104).

Field-collected mosquitoes must be identified to species using the appropriate taxonomic keys before dissections are conducted. Most keys are dichotomous, in that morphological characters are displayed in pairs or alternatives, and the worker proceeds from one couplet to another by a process of elimination and gradually narrows the number of possibilities for correct identification. An identification obtained from a key should be regarded as preliminary, especially in the case of unfamiliar species, and any doubtful specimens should be checked against a full description and confirmed by an authority on mosquito identification. Nonmorphological methods are available to identify members of some species complexes (32, 35).

Some researchers elect to examine all female *Anopheles* collected for parity, and only those mosquitoes with evidence of having oviposited at least once are examined for oocysts and salivary gland sporozoites. Routine use of this approach would eliminate the detection of sporozoites in anophelines where ovarian development does not follow a bloodmeal because of diapause or interrupted feeding (72) and some mosquito species require two or more blood meals for induction of egg production.

After the mosquito is identified, the salivary glands can be removed onto a microscope slide, crushed under a coverslip and examined with a compound microscope for the presence of sporozoites. Visual quantification of the degree of gland infection is difficult, and an estimation is usually used. A commonly used approach is the gland index, which divides the estimated degree of infection into five classes: 0 (no sporozoites), 1+ (1–10), 2+ (11–100), 3+ (101–1000) and 4+ (more than 1000 sporozoites). Several methods for more exact estimates of the number of sporozoites from macerated glands have been described, including the counting of sporozoites in suspension using standard or modified hemocytometers, Petroff–Hausser counting chambers, and counting stained sporozoites in a defined volume dried on a slide (104).

Morphologically, sporozoites of the four species of human malaria cannot be distinguished from each other or from most nonhuman plasmodial sporozoites. However, attention to sporozoite morphology can lead to studies that clarify the vector status in an area. This was exemplified by Wharton, Eyles, Warren, Moorhouse, and Sandosham (113) who identified some members of the *An. umbrosus* complex as vectors of primate malarias and others as vectors of *P. traguli*, a mouse deer malaria. This work was initiated, in part, because of reports of the abnormally thick and short (8 μm) *P. traguli* sporozoites found in the salivary glands and the large oocysts (120 μm) found on the guts of some complex members (47). These were likely incorrectly identified as primate malaria sporozoites in earlier studies.

The guts of female anopheline mosquitoes can also be removed and examined for oocysts. If present, oocysts should be counted and the size recorded and large oocysts saved for species identification of the developing CS protein (see Immunological Methods below). Shute and Maryon (97) reported species-specific differences in oocyst morphology for the human plasmodia. However, these differences were obscured in the later stage of oocyst development and are not routinely used as species indicators.

Freshly killed mosquitoes are normally dissected, however, frozen or fixed specimens have been used. Ward (108) reported that it was easier to dissect and examine the gut for oocysts in frozen specimens than for those in freshly killed *P. gallinaceum*-infected *Aedes aegypti*. He also found that salivary glands were slightly more difficult to remove from frozen specimens and that sporozoites have a tendency to adhere to the cells of the salivary glands.

A method in which the mosquito head, thorax, and abdomen were macerated, dired, fixed in methanol, and stained with Giemsa's stain was described by Gabaldon and Ulloa (45). Their procedure reduced the technician training and dissection time required to examine the salivary glands and gut, and resulted in a permanent slide. However, the method does not permit hemocoel sporozoites to be distinguished from those of the salivary glands when examining samples from the thorax, and the results are not equivalent to the sporozoite index, as suggested.

Ramsey, Bown, Aron, Beaudoin, and Mendez, (87) described a method in which up to 100 mosquitoes could be macerated, fixed with glutaraldehyde, and concentrated by centrifugation. A sample of the final filtrate was examined for sporozoites with a phase microscope. This method was evaluated in the laboratory using a minimum of 1000 sporozoites, and the lowest number detected in any batch of field-collected *An. albimanus* was 800 parasites. High fluorescent background of the glutaraldehyde-fixed material made species confirmation by immunofluorescent antibody assay difficult, but sporozoites from one batch of *An. albimanus* were reported as *P. vivax*.

Immunological Methods

Development of these methods required the production of immunological reagents, that their specificity be established, and that the appropriate methodology be incorporated into testing procedures. Inital studies were conducted using polyvalent antisera, however, monoclonal antibodies (MAbs) are now available to the CS proteins of the human malaria sporozoites and most other species studies as laboratory models. Not all MAbs are species-specific (118, 119) and some sporozoites of the same species have different CS proteins resulting in MAbs that do not react with all sporozoites of that species (28, 46, 92).

Immunofluorescent Antibody (IFA) Assay

Species confirmation by IFA usually involves testing sporozoites found during routine dissections of field-collected mosquitoes. Once sporozoites are observed, the coverslip is removed, and the slide is dried and stored for examination at a laboratory with a fluorescent microscope. Examining glands in the wells of a printed slide and using silicon-treated coverslips reduces parasite loss and makes subsequent IFA testing more productive.

The IFA assay is conducted by incubating the area containing the sporozoites with a solution of species-specific antibody, followed with a solution of fluorochrome-labeled secondary antibody. The slide is rinsed, a coverslip mounted, and the area examined for the fluorescing characteristic sporozoite form. Using fluorochrome-conjugated primary antibody eliminates the need for the labeled secondary antibody and reduces the likelihood of sporozoite loss associated with the additional incubation.

Immunofluorescence was used extensively for studies on blood stage malaria parasites in the early 1960s and Ingram, Otken, and Jumper, (60) used a fluorescent technique and antiserum produced against sporozoites to detect the erythrocytic stage of *P. gallinaceum*. Corradetti and coworkers (36) appear to be the first to have successfully applied the IFA technique to the problem of sporozoite identification. They produced rabbit antisera to *P. gallinaceum* sporozoites, conjugated the globulins to fluorescein, and demonstrated the specificity of the method when tested against *P. giovannolai*, an avian malaria species of the same genus. The authors reported that "Staining sporozoites of plasmodia with fluorescent antibodies opens the way to research which may have practical importance (36)." A major difficulty encountered by these investigators, and one which continues to plague researchers in the field, is the isolation of sufficient salivary gland sporozites for antibody production.

In 1964, Sodeman and coworkers (99, 100) demonstrated a lack of cross-reactivity between avian *P. gallinaceum* and antisera to *P. vivax*, *P.*

falciparum, and *P. cynomolgi*. They reported strong reactions with tagged homologous antisera and avian sporozoites, no reactions with fluorescent-labeled primate malarial antisera, and the use of Evans blue counterstain to control nonspecific staining of background material.

Nussenzweig, Montuori, Spitalny, and Chen, (76) used an IFA test for the identification of human malaria sporozoites. They produced antisera to *P. falciparum* sporozoites in rats and suggested that such reagents could be used to determine the strains and species of parasite found in vector mosquitoes. Nardin and coworkers (73, 74, 75) characterized rodent and primate sporozoite surface antigens using the IFA assay and defined stage and species-specific antimalarial antibodies in studies using sera of naturally infected human and simian hosts. Ramsey, Beaudoin, Bawden, and Espinal (85, 86) continued using this approach with investigations on the specificity of antisera and MAbs against the sporozoites of two species of rodent malaria. Krotoski and coworkers were the first to use the IFA method to immunostain developing oocysts (62). Ponnudurai et al. (80) used a fluorescein-conjugated *P. falciparum* MAb to determine the salivary gland sporozoite load of laboratory-infected *An. stephensi*.

A fluorescein-*P. falciparum* and rhodamine-*P. vivax* MAb system has been successfully evaluated using laboratory-infected mosquitoes. However, initial attempts to transfer the method to other laboratories for use on field-collected material met with limited success. Problems encountered included differences in microscope fluorescent filter systems required to distinguish between fluorescein and rhodamine, and weakly reacting sporozoites (R.A. Wirtz et al., unpublished data).

Immunohistochemical (IHC) Assay

The requirement for a fluorescent miscroscope and the limited number of easily distinguished fluorochromes restricts the use of the IFA procedure for species confirmation of salivary gland sporozoites. An IHC system is being developed by Golenda and coworkers (52) (C.F. Golenda, personal communication) which replaces the fluorochrome label with an enzyme, used in conjunction with a precipitating colored substrate. Alkaline phosphatase-*P. falciparum* and horseradish peroxidase-*P. vivax* labeled MAbs used with substrates producing red and brown products (Kirkegaard & Perry Lab. Inc., Gaithersburg, MD), respectively, have given promising initial results. A standard compound microscope can be used, the colors are easier to distinguish than the fluorescein-rhodamine combination and a permanent slide is produced. Other enzyme-substrate combinations are being considered for incorporation into the system. The goal of this project is the development of a simple IHC for the identification of three immunologically distinct sporozoites based on different colors produced from buffer-compatible enzyme-substrate combinations.

Immunoradiometric Assay (IRMA) and Enzyme-Linked Immunosorbent Assay (ELISA)

Two approaches have been used in the development of IRMAs and ELISAs for detection of CS proteins in mosquitoes. The most basic was an assay in which sporozoites or infected mosquitoes were triturated in a saline buffer, directly in a microtiter plate well. The CS protein, which bound in the well, was detected by the addition of unlabeled anti-CS antibody, followed by a labeled secondary antibody. This method was not quantitative, and sensitivity was inadequate as small amounts of CS protein competed for binding sites with soluble mosquito proteins present in higher concentrations. The primary advantage of this approach was that purified, labeled antibody was not required.

The two-site or "sandwich" method was used to develop a quantitative assay. An anti-CS capture antibody was first added to the well and allowed to bind. An aliquot of mosquito triturate was then added and the CS antigen, if present, bound to the capture antibody. A labeled anti-CS antibody was then added which completed the "sandwich" and permitted a quantitative estimation of the amount of CS protein in the test sample.

Wilkinson (115) appears to be the first to have applied these methods to the detection of sporozoites. He developed both a two-site IRMA and ELISA for detection of *P. berghei* sporozoites using purified rat anti-CS IgG and compared an ^{125}I-IRMA with alkaline-phosphatase- and horseradish-peroxidase-based ELISAs. Untreated or sonicated salivary gland sporozoites, individual infected mosquitoes, and single infected insects in pools of five or ten uninfected mosquitoes were evaluated in these systems. Sensitivity was in the range of 500 sporozoites per ml. Comparable positive/negative values were obtained with the IRMA and alkaline phosphatase ELISA, and these assays appeared more promising than did the peroxidase-based ELISA.

Zavala and coworkers (125) were the first to use MAb-based IRMAs for the detection of *P. berghei*, *P. knolesi*, *P. vivax*, and *P. falciparum* sporozoites in infected mosquitoes. Nonquantitative determinations of CS antigen were made by trituration and testing mosquitoes directly in microtiter plates, followed by ^{125}I-labeled MAb. A quantitative two-site, two-MAb IRMA was also described. Assays were conducted on fresh, frozen, and dried individual or pooled mosquitoes. The CS protein from fewer than 100 sporozoites could be detected in the two-site IRMA.

Monoclonal-antibody-based IRMAs for *P. knowlesi* and *P. cynomolgi*, two simian malarias, were evaluated by Collins and coworkers (31). Sporogonic development, testing pools of mosquitoes, simultaneous testing for two *Plasmodium* species using ^{125}I- and ^{131}I-labeled MAbs, and testing of desiccated mosquitoes were studied. A two-site, one MAb IRMA was used to define the immunodominant regions of CS proteins and to establish the presence of identical, multiple epitopes (124). The IRMAs have been used extensively in studies of the CS proteins, CS-like proteins, and efficacy testing of CS protein-based vaccines (25, 30, 37, 77).

The two-site IRMA was first used on field-collected mosquitoes when Collins et al. (34) determined the *P. falciparum* CS protein-positive and sporozoite equivalent loads of *An. gambiae* collected in The Gambia. Use of IRMAs and ELISAs in field research is summarized in the discussion section of this chapter.

Inherent with the use of an IRMA is the requirement for short-lived radioactive reagents, a sophisticated counting device for analysis, and the associated problems of shipment, storage, disposal, safety, and expense of radioisotopes. The ELISA technology was applied to the detection of CS proteins to circumvent these problems. The ELISAs use stable reagents and results may be read visually or quantified using a spectrophotometric microtiter plate reader.

Burkot et al. (21) developed a two-site single MAb ELISA for detection of *P. knowlesi* sporozoites in *An. dirus* with a sensitivity of ca. 100 sporozoites, comparable to that of an IRMA using the same MAb (T.R. Burkot et al., unpublished data). Burkot, Williams, and Schneider, (18) also reported the development of an ELISA for *P. falciparum*-infected mosquitoes with a similar level of sensitivity. Wirtz et al. (119) conducted a comparative study of ten MAbs from four laboratories for ELISA development which resulted in an assay with the sensitivity of 20–25 *P. falciparum* sporozoites. The sensitivity of a *P. vivax* ELISA (116) was improved to 20–40 sporozoites, after comparative testing and selection of a better MAb (118). Collins, Procell, Campbell, and Collins, (33) reported on a *P. malariae* two-site ELISA with a detection limit of approximately 50 sporozoites per well. The CS protein was detected in laboratory-infected mosquitoes stored at room temperature for 18 months. A similar assay for *P. ovale* CS protein was described by Procell and coworkers (84), making ELISAs available for detection of the four known human malaria CS proteins. An ELISA to detect the immunologically distinct *P. vivax* CS protein recently discovered in western Thailand is under development (92).

As with the IRMA, these ELISAs have been used extensively in laboratory and field studies to examine individual fresh, frozen, and dried mosquitoes, and pooled insects, and to monitor the development, location, and amount of detectable CS protein after an infectious bloodmeal or in conjunction with other variables.

Availability of positive control CS antigens is crucial for the routine use of the ELISAs and IRMAs. The assays were developed using salivary gland sporozoites and laboratory-infected mosquitoes; however, this was too labor-intensive to be considered for routine production of CS antigens. The sequencing of the repeat portions of the *P. falciparum*, *P. vivax*, and *P. malariae* CS proteins (25, 77) permitted production of synthetic or recombinant antigens for use as positive controls. The *P. ovale* CS repeat sequence is unknown, which severely restricts use of the assay because sporozoites for positive controls must be produced by feeding mosquitoes upon an infected chimpanzee. Efforts to sequence the *P. ovale* CS protein continue (G.H. Campbell, personal communication). The negative control samples used in the ELISAs and IRMAs will be dictated by the study and the statistical analysis used to determine cutoff values (2).

Not all MAbs are suitable for use in an ELISA. In comparative studies for assay development, MAbs were rejected because of cross-reactivity with other sporozoite species, low sensitivity, a requirement for high concentrations of capture MAb, high background absorbance, and loss of antibody activity during preparation of peroxidase conjugates (18, 116, 118, 119). Burkot, Wirtz, and Lyon (20) subsequently developed a method to identify MAbs suitable for conjugation to periodate-oxidized horseradish peroxidase. Labeling methods have also been evaluated by Tsang, Hancock, and Maddison (103) who found that conjugates prepared with glutaraldehyde were more useful in assays where a wide linear range is needed, whereas sodium periodate conjugates are more suited to assays where sensitivity is most important.

A biotin-streptavidin two-site ELISA using MAb 3Sp2 for *P. falciparum*-infected *An. stephensi* was described by Verhave et al. (106), with a lower limit of sensitivity of 100–350 sporozoites. The authors concluded that the ELISA could not be used for accurate sporozoite quantitation because of CS protein shedding. However, in the same report they estimated that a single oocyst could produce approximately 10,000 sporozoites, based on the CS protein detected by the ELISA, and later used the assay to examine the sporozoite load of *P. falciparum* infected *An. stephensi* with respect to multiple bloodmeals (89). This assay was also evaluated for sensitivity and specificity, in conjunction with mosquito dissections, using field-collected specimens (7).

The two-site sporozoite ELISA method (119) has been modified by different investigators in an effort to improve the assay or reduce the 5-h time period to complete the test. The ELISA was adapted to the F.A.S.T. (Falcon 3930, Becton Dickinson & Co., Oxnard, CA) format, which reduced assay time to approximately 2 h while maintaining comparable sensitivity (G.H. Campbell et al., personal communication). Lee, Harrison, and Lewis, (64) reduced the amount of MAb required and the assay time to 1 h, excluding preparation of capture MAb-coated plates and overnight incubation, while maintaining sensitivity by using a new peroxidase substrate and a plate shaker. The reduction in assay time may be beneficial in some laboratories; however, the approximate eightfold increase in plate cost of the F.A.S.T. system and the requirement for a plate shaker for both of these methods will limit their use. It should be emphasized that the time during the incubations in the standard ELISA is not wasted, but is usually spent preparing reagents for the next step, triturating mosquitoes for the next day's experiments, or performing routine laboratory duties.

Two groups have described membrane-based sporozoite detection systems developed to eliminate the requirement for microtitre plates and enzyme-labeled MAbs, and to exploit the high protein binding efficacy of membrane-based systems. Petros, Procell, Campbell, and Collins (79) reported a nitrocellulose-based ELISA developed using a *P. inui*-infected *An. dirus* laboratory model. This semiquantitative method had a sensitivity limit of about 200 sporozoites. Long and coworkers used MAb 22:123:14A and a bilayered membrane system to filter out mosquito debris from *P. falciparum*-infected *An. stephensi*. The intensity of reactions was quantified using a portable reflective densitometer and detection of as few as 20 sporozoites per mosquito or 200 sporozoites per pool of 10 mosquitoes was described (G.H. Long, personal communication).

Other Immunological Assays

The circumsporozoite precipitation (CSP) reaction was first described by Vanderberg, Nussenzweig, and Most (105) using *P. berghei* sporozoites in homologous immune mouse serum. The reaction results in the formation of a long threadlike, rapidly increasing precipitate at one end of a sporozoite incubated in immune serum. The CSP reaction was graded following an arbitrary scheme. Chen, Nussenzweig, and Collins (24) and Nardin et al. (75) described the specificity of the CSP antigen for *P. falciparum*, *P. vivax*, and four simian malarias. Nardin et al. (73) reported that the sensitivity of the IFA was five to ten times greater than that of the CSP assay.

Cochrane and coworkers (29) developed a method in which the CS proteins of rodent, simian, or human malaria parasites from mosquitoes could be detected and the molecular weights determined using the Western blot (immunoblot) technique. Sporozoites or dried, infected mosquitoes were triturated, the extracts electrophoresed, transferred to nitrocellulose, and the CS proteins identified by probing with monoclonal antibody followed by ^{125}I-labeled anti-mouse IgG. As few as 100 sporozoites could be detected, which permits the identification and molecular weight determinations of CS proteins of different plasmodial isolates extracted from individual, dried, field-collected mosquitoes.

Other immunological based systems, including the ICA and immunogold techniques, have been used to monitor the development and distribution of CS proteins, primarily in laboratory-infected mosquitoes (52).

Nucleic Acid Methods

A number of nucleic acid probes have been developed for the diagnosis of malaria. This approach is based on the characteristics of the DNA and

RNA of the parasite. These probes, which are strands of nucleotides, will hybridize with preparations of their complementary strands on genes in DNA or the RNA present in the parasite (10).

DNA Probes

Delves et al. (40) evaluated a cloned repetitive DNA sequence (*rep*20) as a diagnostic probe specific for *P. falciparum*-infected *An. stephensi* using a squash blot method. Mosquito head-thoraces squashed directly on nylon filters gave semiqualitative signals, which correlated with the number of oocysts observed in samples of the same batches of mosquitoes examined by dissection. No positive signals were observed with *P. berghei*-infected controls. As few as 1700 sporozoites, equivalent to ca. 34 pg of total DNA, were detected using the ^{32}P-labeled probe. The authors suggest that sensitivity could be improved by using amplification methods, such as polymerase chain reaction (PCR), to replicate the *rep*20 sequences in each sample. However, the added expense associated with PCR would restrict the use of the assay.

The *rep* probe evaluated by Delves and coworkers (40) was cloned from blood stage parasites of a Gambian isolate (HG13) and recognized blood stage DNA of all *P. falciparum* isolates tested to date. It did not cross-hybridize with *P. chabaudi*, *P. berghei*, *P. vivax*, or *P. malariae* DNA. Delves et al. present evidence that sporozoites of the Gambian strain examined have about the same number of sequences. However, they also note that blood-stage DNA from the Papua New Guinea (MAD20), Thailand (K1) and (Tak9) clone (No. 94) cultured isolates tested exhibited a 20-fold range in signal strength, which implies a considerable variation in the number of *rep* sequences among the different parasite strains. A similar variation in the *rep* sequences among sporozoites from different isolates, if it exists, could affect the sensitivity of the assay from isolate to isolate and reduce its usefulness as a quantitative method.

Another *P. falciparum*-specific DNA probe detected sporozoites in laboratory-infected mosquitoes with 2500–5000 parasites (S. Panyim, personal communication in Ref. 59). A DNA probe for *P. berghei* has been used to measure the infectivity of sporozoites (43) and the neutralization of sporozoites by monoclonal antibody (44). The DNA probes for infected erythrocytes capable of detecting approximately 200 parasites (40/μl from 50-μl volume of blood) could be adapted for the detection of infected mosquitoes (10, 63, 121).

Ribosomal RNA (rRNA) Probes

The most abundant cellular macromolecule in malaria parasites is RNA. Theoretically, parasite rRNAs could serve as target sites for specific probes that are 200 to 1000 times more sensitive than a repetitive probe, which accounts for 1% of total DNA. The natural abundance of rRNA and its stability make it an ideal target molecule for the development of probes for studies on the phylogenetic relationship of organisms as well as for quantitative, species-specific diagnostic tools for vectors and parasites (32, 61, 68).

McCutchan et al. (68) reported on *Plasmodium*-specific and species-specific rRNA probes for *P. falciparum* and *P. berghei* blood-stage parasites. In earlier work, Gunderson et al. (56) described rRNA sequence probes that could distinguish between the blood-stage forms and sporozoites of *P. berghei*. Waters and McCutchan (110) described an rRNA probe system for the sensitive and accurate diagnosis of blood-stage *P. falciparum*, *P. vivax*, *P. malariae*, and *P. ovale* parasites. Direct application of treated blood to nylon resulted in the detection of fewer than 10 *P. falciparum* parasites in an overnight exposure using a ^{32}P probe. No cross-reactivity with mosquito rRNA was detected.

The DNA and rRNA probes described were developed to detect blood-stage malaria parasites. If used to screen blood-fed, field-collected mosquitoes for sporozoite nucleic acid, the method would not distinguish between the blood stages of the parasite in blood-fed anophelines and could result in false-positive infection rates. Whether a stage-specific rRNA probe (56) with the desired sensitivity and specificity will be developed for routine use is uncertain. As with the immunological-based IRMA and ELISAs, rRNA probes used to test extracts of whole mosquitoes would indicate the presence of the parasite nucleic acid but not its location. Mosquito dissection and examination of salivary glands would be needed to augment this method for vector incrimination studies.

Discussion

The incidence of malaria continues to increase in many areas of the world. This is attributed to a lack of effective vaccines, mosquito resistance to insecticides, parasite resistance to drugs, movement or inaccessibility of large population groups, and the problems associated with the overall costs and reduced emphasis on antimalarial programs (122, 123). Interruption of vector-human contact is theoretically one of the most effective ways of reducing the incidence of malaria. However, the complex nature of the disease and our inadequate knowledge of the biology of the parasites and vectors, and the dynamics of local malaria transmission have restricted the development of effective regional control strategies. In some areas of the world the primary and/or important secondary vectors are unknown, information on the human plasmodia is unavailable and the required epidemiological studies have not been conducted. The use of the methods described earlier in the chapter will play a vital role in laboratory and field studies designed to develop and evaluate new vaccines, antimalarial drugs, and other control strategies designed to break the vector mosquito-human contact.

Human-use restrictions and logistic constraints have largely eliminated the use of the *in vivo* method for vector incrimination studies. However, feeding of malaria-infected mosquitoes on humans is essential for efficacy testing of malaria vaccines (25, 37, 77) and to obtain basic information on new parasite strains (92).

The dissection of field-collected mosquitoes for vector incrimination and determination of sporozoite and oocyst rates continues to be essential components of malaria epidemiological studies. Dissections also must be used to verify the correlation between the sporozoite rate and the detection of CS protein or parasite nucleic acid, when these methods are used in a new geographic region, with different mosquito species, or with members of a species complex (7, 34, 58, 117). The new technologies described cannot replace dissection, but can augment it superbly.

Modifications that use large pools of mosquitoes to expedite dissections may reduce the epidemiological value of the resulting data (45, 87), and care should be exercised before they are incorporated into routine testing of field-collected specimens. The inability to make a species identification, and the requirements for freshly killed mosquitoes, highly trained technicians, and microscopes with power supplies are disadvantages inherent to the dissection method.

The MAb-based systems have been used extensively in malaria epidemiological studies since their development. Monoclonal antibodies specific for *P. falciparum* (18, 119, 125), *P. malariae* (33), *P. ovale* (84), and the two immunologically distinct isolates of *P. vivax* (92, 118, 125) sporozoites are available for use with the IFA, IHC, IRMA and ELISA. Unfortunately, the *P. malariae* MAb cell line developed by Cochrane, Collins, and Nussenzweig (27) was lost.

The IFA remains the method of choice for confirmation of human malaria sporozoites isolated from the salivary glands of field-collected mosquitoes. The use of fluorescein- and rhodamine-labeled species-specific MAbs can reduce the time and steps required to conduct the assay and the potential for sporozoite loss from the test slide; however, the requirement for a fluorescent microscope remains. Development of an IHC method for sporozoite identification will eliminate this requirement and increase the use of the assay (52). Species identification of salivary gland sporozoites using the IFA or IHC will continue to be an essential component of many malaria studies (91).

Development of assays to detect CS proteins in dried mosquitoes greatly facilitated testing of field-collected specimens. By 1984, an IRMA (125) and an ELISA (18) to detect *P. falciparum* CS protein, based on MAbs that recognized different epitopes, had been reported and greater diversity was expected as more MAbs were developed. Scientists from the Centers for Disease Control, National Institutes of Health, Naval Medical

Research Institute, New York University, and Walter Reed Army Institute of Research met and agreed that a standard ELISA method and MAb would facilitate comparison of data, and the availability of the method as a kit would make it suitable for workers who lacked the resources to develop MAbs. Under the auspices of the World Health Organization, MAbs from four laboratories were evaluated to meet these goals. The MAb and method selected have been incorporated into an ELISA kit, which has been used in 27 countries to test over 250,000 mosquitoes (19, 119, and R.A. Writz et al., unpublished data). Comparative testing and selection of a candidate *P. vivax* MAb has recently been completed (R.A. Writz, unpublished data). These assays will continue to be evaluated and improved, increasing sensitivity and ease of use, while reducing the cost and size of the kits. The use of standard MAbs has greatly facilitated comparison of data from different geographic regions.

Nucleic acid probes for detection of malaria parasites in mosquitoes are still under development and evaluation. The DNA probes are powerful tools and will be used in laboratory studies on sporozoite infectivity, genetics, mixed infections, and taxonomy (81, 107). However, the relatively low sensitivity of the DNA probes described to date, the requirement for expensive, time-consuming, nonquantitative PCR amplification to overcome low sensitivity, and the potential variation in sequence number of repetitive DNA probes limits their routine use as quantitative diagnostic tools.

The *Plasmodium* rRNA probes developed by Waters and McCutchan (110) will be adapted for the detection of sporozoite rRNA and the system evaluated on laboratory-infected and then field-collected mosquitoes. The sensitivity of the assay could be increased by including other species-specific rRNA-directed probes in the hybridization mixture and by raising the specific activity of the probes. The detection of individual sporozoites is theoretically possible and there is tremendous potential for the development of systems for the detection of a variety of parasites in arthropod vectors and members of sibling species complexes using rRNA probes. The rRNA system is the simplest and potentially the most sensitive and least expensive of the nucleic acid diagnostic systems described to date (32, 68, 110).

The conversion of the DNA and RNA probes to a nonradiolabeled detection system, while maintaining sensitivity, will greatly increase their usefulness. McLaughlin, Ruth, Jablonski, Steketee, and Campbell, (69) reported on a 21-base DNA *P. falciparum* blood-stage probe linked to alkaline phosphatase, which was comparable in sensitivity and specificity to the radiolabeled oligomer after a 2-day exposure. An alkaline-phosphastase-linked DNA probe evaluated by Lanar et al. (63) was five times less sensitive than when isotopically labeled (1000 vs. 200 parasites). Other enzymatic and chemiluminescence methods to achieve this goal are under investigation.

The ELISAs and IRMAs are powerful field research tools when used in conjunction with other methods. Perhaps their major advantage is a logistic one, as the assays eliminate the necessity to analyze mosquitoes immediately after collection. Anophelines can be collected and dried rapidly for subsequent analysis. The capability to detect a single infected mosquito in a pool of 20 insects means that two technicians in 1 day could process almost 6000 anophelines for species-specific CS proteins. By dissections, the same two technicians might process 150 mosquitoes in a day (19). Sporozoites could be identified in the salivary glands, but species determinations could not be made unless IFAs were conducted also. This ability to test dried mosquitoes allows investigators to test large numbers of anophelines from areas with very low sporozoite rates, more easily work in remote areas, concurrently study the microepidemiology of malaria in many villages, and monitor the effectiveness of control measures, for example, insecticide, bed-net, and vaccine trials (53, 54, 65).

Despite the potential advantages associated with these new techniques, they reveal little about malaria transmission when used alone. The major constraint when applying these methods occurs in the interpretation of results. In their usual application, the investigator will not actually see the sporozoites in the salivary glands. Because the sporozoite antigen may be found in all parts of the mosquito (52, 66, 89), a positive reaction obtained when assaying the head or thorax does not establish the mosquito as infectious (66, 79, 90). For this reason, investigators have referred to "sporozoite antigen positivity rates" or "CS protein equivalents" and not "sporozoite rates" (33, 116, 125). As nucleic acid probes are evaluated, similar terminology must be used to distinguish DNA/RNA positive mosquitoes from salivary gland sporozoite rates based on microscopic examination.

Numerous field studies have exploited the advantages of the CS protein detection methods (1, 4, 5, 6, 34, 42, 66, 117). However, prior to implementation of these tests, it is essential that their suitability in a particular geographic area be accessed by comparative testing of the assay and dissection, to include species confirmation of salivary gland sporozoites. Only once a reliable correlation is found and salivary gland sporozoites identified can the assays be implemented on a large scale.

These studies are required to insure that the repeat portion of CS protein is reconized by the MAb used in the assay and that the sporozoites, when present, are capable of invading the salivary glands. Several investigators have reported that the CS proteins of the human malarias examined were conserved in the samples tested (111, 126); however, CS protein repeat heterogeneity has been documented in the sporozoites of two simian (28, 46) malarias and *P. vivax* in western Thailand (92). The geographic distribution of this heterogeneity is under investigation. In certain vector–parasite systems, mature sporozoites may be released from oocysts without salivary gland invasion (41, 65, 90).

A CS-like protein present in blood-stage *P. falciparum* and other malarias, detectable with the two-site one antibody IRMA (124), has been reported by Cochrane et al. (30). The amount of CS-like protein appears to vary in different plasmodial species, with mature schizonts having 10 to 1000-fold less than the amount of CS protein in each sporozoite (30).

The application of the ELISAs and IRMAs that has received the most attention has been in the implication of vectors. The ability to test small pools of mosquitoes for CS antigen makes this an excellent approach to use when looking for secondary vectors or searching for the primary vectors in a transmission area where very few, if any, anophelines have been found positive on dissection (109). It must be stressed that vectors cannot be incriminated (vector status established) through the use of these new technologies alone. Studies to incriminate vectors that do not include dissections of wild-caught mosquitoes or feeding suspected vector species on known gametocytemic people must be interpreted as only suspected vectors (1, 23, 38). The identification of suspected vector species permits a focused study to be conducted so that vector status can be established using dissections.

Feeding experiments alone, using suspected vectors on gametocytemic individuals, cannot incriminate a new vector but only establish its susceptibility to infection and ability to produce sporozoites. To be a vector the mosquito must readily feed on humans and must be able to survive in nature at least the length of the parasite's extrinsic incubation period. Anopheline species proven susceptible in the laboratory may then be targeted for sporozoite antigen analyses using wild-caught individuals.

The ELISA, IRMA, and IFA have been used to identify the species of sporozoites in field-collected mosquitoes (6, 23, 38, 42, 66, 92, 117) allowing investigations concerning multiple infections in vectors (17). Sporozoite species identification coupled with relative biting rates to produce relative inoculation rates has enabled investigators to define small area variations in transmission intensity (15). Comparing these relative inoculation rates to parasite prevalence in children has enabled estimates of the relative efficiency of transmission of different malaria species (14). Similarly, measuring malaria incidence with sporozoite antigen and human-biting rates has led to the efficient monitoring of appropriate intervention strategies, for example, those reducing human-mosquito contact such as by untreated or insecticide-treated bed-nets (54, 65, and T.R. Burkot et al., manuscript submitted).

Caution must be used in interpreting results involving both sporozoite antigen rates and measures of the biting rate to provide inoculation rates. Discrepancies between the positivity rate and the true sporozoite rate can be multiplied by errors in measuring the human-biting rate (an error on the log order of magnitude) as well as errors in the proportion of salivary gland sporozoite-positive mosquitoes, which transmit sporozoites when they take a bloodmeal (3, 93). The result can only be expressed as a relative inoculation rate for comparing transmission among different areas or within an area over time.

The use of the assays to quantitate CS antigen has advanced our understanding of the relationship between oocyst infections and sporozoite production (14, 15), between total sporozoite load and the proportion of sporozoites in the salivary glands (4, 66), and between sporozoites in the salivary glands and sporozoite numbers inoculated (3, 4, 37, 93) and development of CS protein in mosquitoes (52). The relationship between the intensity of transmission and the natural development of immunity against the sporozoite stage has been made feasible by the antigen detection systems (16, 42).

Comparing the proportions of the anopheline populations in villages with their respective sporozoite protein rates gives measures in relative susceptibility of different anophelines to malaria infection (13), provided the epidemiology is sufficiently similar among the different villages (55). This approach can also be used to determine vector status of members of a species complex, as exhibited by *An. culicifacies* in India (101).

Defining the fine specificities of the CS protein MAbs now available may give an insight into a "smoke screen" effect of how the parasite might evade the immune system (T.R. Burkot et al., unpublished data). Banks of defined MAbs also permits the screening of infected mosquitoes for clues as to the range of quantitative epitope heterogeneity present in natural populations (118, 119, and T.R. Burkot et al., unpublished data).

Summary

The identification of sporozoite infected mosquitoes is an integral part of many malaria epidemiological studies. Historically, this has been accomplished by dissection of freshly killed mosquitoes and examination of the salivary glands for sporozoites. Dissection is laborious, requires experienced technicians, and does not permit the species identification of the parasite. Development of new biotechnology-based methods for sporozoite detection has significantly improved our ability to conduct such studies.

This is best exemplified by the production of species-specific anti-circumsporozoite protein monoclonal antibodies (MAbs). The use of these MAbs in immunofluorescent antibody assays permits species identification of salivary gland sporozoites from field-collected mosquitoes. Their use in immunohistochemical assays will eliminate the need for a fluorescent microscope and permit tests to be conducted in many more laboratories.

Incorporation of the MAbs into enzyme-linked immunosorbent assays and immunoradiometric assays permits the testing of large numbers of dried mosquitoes and lessens the logistic burden associated with many field studies. The distribution of ELISA kits to scientists without the resources to develop their own assays is one of the most successful examples of the transfer of biotechnology to scientists in developing countries. Prior to the availability of the ELISAs, the problems of dissection and the associated costs discouraged some malaria researchers from conducting field research and made funding such studies more difficult. The ELISAs have allowed many malaria researchers to again focus on field studies, exploiting the capabilities of these new tools in their investigations on vector incrimination and the epidemiology of malaria in new study areas or changing environments. The use of standard MAbs in the ELISAs has greatly facilitated comparison of data from different geographic regions. It is essential to verify that the target epitope of the MAb, present on the sporozoite, is conserved in the study area before these assays are used on field-collected mosquitoes.

The use of nucleic acid probes in malaria research will continue to increase. The rRNA probes offer tremendous potential for the development of diagnostic systems for the quantitative, species-specific detection of both mosquito vectors and malaria parasites. The DNA probes will continue to be valuable laboratory tools. However, these probes must be adapted to nonradioisotopic detection systems before their routine use in field laboratories can be considered.

Acknowledgments. Supported in part by United Nations Development Programme/World Bank/World Health Organization grants to R.A.W. for development and field evaluation of sporozoite ELISAs. Sections of this chapter were written as part of R.A.W.s U.S. Army Reserve active duty training at the Letterman Army Institute of Research. The authors thank R.G. Andre, C.F. Golenda, P.M. Graves, L. Robert, D.R. Roberts, L.W. Roberts, L.C. Rutledge, and R.A. Ward for their suggestions and critical review of this manuscript.

References

1. Baker, E.Z., Beier, J.C., Meek, S.R., and Wirtz, R.A., 1987, Detection and quantitation of *Plasmodium falciparum* and *Plasmodium vivax* infections in Thai-Kampuchean *Anopheles* (Diptera: Culicidae) by enzyme-linked immunosorbent assay, *J. Med. Entomol.* **24**:536–541.
2. Beier, J.C., Asiago, C.M., Onyango, F.K., and Koros, J.K., 1988, ELISA absorbance cut-off method affects malaria sporozoite rate determination in wild Afrotropical *Anopheles*, *Med. Vet. Entomol.* **2**:259–264.
3. Beier, J.C., Onyango, F.K., Koros, J.K., Ramadhan, M., Ogwang, R., Koech, D.K., and Roberts, C.R., 1991, Quantitation of malaria sporozoites transmitted in vitro during salivation by wild Afrotropical *Anopheles*, *Med. Vet. Entomol.* **5**:(in press).

4. Beier, J.C., Onyango, F.K., Ramadhan, M., Koros, J.K., Asiago, C.M., Koech, D.K., and Roberts, C.R., 1991, Quantitation of malaria sporozoites in the salivary glands of wild Afrotropical *Anopheles*, *Med. Vet. Entomol.* **5**:(in press).
5. Beier, J.C., Perkins, P.V., Wirtz, R.A., Whitmire, R.E., Mugambi, M., and Hockmeyer, W.T., 1987, Field evaluation of an enzyme-linked immunosorbent assay (ELISA) for *Plasmodium falciparum* sporozoite detection in anopheline mosquitoes from Kenya, *Am. J. Trop. Med. Hyg.* **36**:459–468.
6. Beier, M.S., Schwartz, I.K., Beier, J.C., Perkins, P.V., Onyango, F., Koros, J.K., Campbell, G.H., Andrysiak, P.M., and Brandling-Bennett, A.D., 1988, Identification of malaria species by ELISA in sporozoite and oocyst infected *Anopheles* from western Kenya, *Am. J. Trop. Med. Hyg.* **39**:323–327.
7. Boudin, C., Robert, V., Verhave, J.P., Carnevale, P. and Meuweissen, J.H.E.T., 1988, La technique ELISA (enzyme-linked immuno-sorbent assay) dans la depistage des moustiques infectes par *Plasmodium falciparum*. I. Evaluation de la fiabilite et de l'efficacite du test. II. Application sur le terrain, *Bull. W.H.O.* **66**:87–97.
8. Boyd, M.F., 1949, Historical review. Boyd, M.F. (ed): in Malariology, vol. 1, W.B. Saunders Company, Philadelphia, pp. 3–25.
9. Bruce-Chwatt, L.J., 1985, Essential Malariology, William Heinemann Medical Books Ltd, London, 452 p.
10. Bruce-Chwatt, L.J., 1987, From Laveran's discovery to DNA probes: New trends in diagnosis of malaria. *Lancet* **2**:1509–1511.
11. Bruce-Chwatt, L.J., 1988, History of malaria from prehistory to eradication. Wernsdorfer, W.H., and McGregor, I. (eds): in Malaria. Principles and Practice of Malariology, vol. 1, Churchill Livingstone, Edinburgh, pp. 1–59.
12. Burkot, T.R., 1988, Non-random host selection by anopheline mosquitoes, *Parasitol. Today* **4**:156–162.
13. Burkot, T.R., Dye, C., and Graves, P.M., 1989, An analysis of some factors affecting the sporozoite rates, human blood indexes and biting rates of the members of the *Anopheles punctulatus* complex in Papua New Guinea, *Am. J. Trop. Med. Hyg.* **40**:229–234.
14. Burkot, T.R., Graves, P.M., Cattani, J.A., Wirtz, R.A., and Gibson, F.D., 1987, The efficiency of sporozoite transmission in the human malaria, *Plasmodium falciparum* and *P. vivax*, *Bull. W.H.O.* **65**:375–380.
15. Burkot, T.R., Graves, P.M., Paru, R., Wirtz, R.A., and Heywood, P., 1988, Human malaria transmission studies in the *Anopheles punctulatus* complex in Papua New Guinea: Sporozoite rates, inoculation rates and sporozoite densities, *Am. J. Trop. Med. Hyg.* **39**:135–144.
16. Burkot, T.R., Graves, P.M., Wirtz, R.A., Brabin, B.J., Battistutta, D., Cattani, J.A., Maizels, R.M., and Alpers, M.P., 1989, Differential antibody responses to *Plasmodium falciparum* and *Plasmodium vivax* circumsporozoite proteins in a human population, *J. Clin. Microbiol.* **27**:1346–1351.
17. Burkot, T.R., Molineaux, L., Graves, P.M., Paru, R., Battistutta, D., Dagoro, H., Barnes, A., Wirtz, R.A., and Garner, P., 1990, The prevalence of naturally acquired multiple infections of *Wuchereria bancrofti* and human malarias in anophelines, *Parasitology* **100**:369–375.

18. Burkot, T.R., Williams, J.L., and Schneider, I., 1984, Identification of *Plasmodium falciparum*-infected mosquitoes by a double antibody enzyme-linked immunosorbent assay, *Am. J. Trop. Med. Hyg.* **33**:783–788.
19. Burkot, T.R., and Wirtz, R.A., 1986, Immunoassays of malaria sporozoites in mosquitoes, *Parasitol. Today* **2**:155–157.
20. Burkot, T.R., Wirtz, R.A., and Lyon, J., 1985, Use of fluorodinitrobenzene to identify monoclonal antibodies which are suitable for conjugation to periodate-oxidized horseradish peroxidase, *J. Immunol. Methods* **84**:25–31.
21. Burkot, T.R., Zavala, F., Gwadz, R.W., Collins, F.H., Nussenzweig, R.S., and Roberts, D., 1984, Identification of malaria-infected mosquitoes by a two site enzyme linked immunosorbent assay, *Am. J. Trop. Med. Hyg.* **33**: 227–231.
22. Carter, R., and Graves, P.M., 1988, Gametocytes, Wernsdorfer, W.H., and McGregor, I. (eds): in Malaria. Principles and Practices in Malariology, vol. 1, Churchhill Livingstone, Edinburgh, pp. 253–306.
23. Carvajal, H., de Herrera, M.A., Quintero, J., Alzate, A., and Herrera, S., 1989, *Anopheles neivai*: A vector of malaria in the Pacific lowlands of Colombia, *Trans. R. Soc. Trop. Med. Hyg.* **83**:609.
24. Chen, D.H., Nussenzweig, R.S., Collins, W.E., 1976, Specificity of the circum-sporozoite precipitation antigen(s) of human and simian malarias, *J. Parasitol.* **62**:636–637.
25. Chulay, J.D., 1989, Development of sporozoite vaccines for malaria, *Trans. R. Soc. Trop. Med. Hyg.* (Suppl) **83**:61–66.
26. Coatney, G.R., Collins, W.E., Contacos, P.G., 1971, The Primate Malarias, U.S. Government Printing Office, District of Columbia, 336 p.
27. Cochrane, A.H., Collins, W.E., and Nussenzweig, R.S., 1984, Monoclonal antibody identifies circumsporozoite protein of *Plasmodium malariae* and detects a common epitope on *Plasmodium brasilianum* sporozoites, *Infect. Immun.* **45**:592–595.
28. Cochrane, A.H., Gwadz, R.W., Barnwell, J.W., Kamboj, K.K., and Nussenzweig, R.S., 1986, Further studies on the antigenic diversity of the circumsporozoite proteins of the *Plasmodium cynomolgi* complex, *Am. J. Trop. Med. Hyg.* **35**:479–487.
29. Cochrane, A.H., Ockenhouse, C.F., and Nussenzweig, R.S., 1984, Identification of circumsporozoite proteins in individual malaria-infected mosquitoes by Western blot analysis, *J. Immunol. Methods* **71**:241–245.
30. Cochrane, A.H., Uni, S., Maracic, M., di Giovanni, L., Aikawa, M., and Nussenzweig, R.S., 1989, A circumsporozoite-like protein is present in micronemes of mature blood stages of malaria parasites, *Exp. Parasitol.* **69**: 351–356.
31. Collins, F.H., Gwadz, R.W., Koontz, L.C., Zavala, F., and Nussenzweig, R.S., 1985, Laboratory assessment of a species-specific radioimmunoassay for the detection of malaria sporozoites in mosquitoes (Diptera: Culicidae), *J. Med. Entomol.* **22**:121–129.
32. Collins, F.H., Mendez, M.A., Rasmussen, P.C., Mehaffey, N.J., Besansky, N.J., and Finnerty, V., 1987, A ribosomal RNA gene probe differentiates member species of the *Anopheles gambiae* complex, *Am. J. Trop. Med. Hyg.* **37**:37–41.

33. Collins, F.H., Procell, P.M., Campbell, G.H., and Collins, W.E., 1988, Monoclonal antibody-based enzyme-linked immunosorbent assay (ELISA) for detection of *Plasmodium malariae* sporozoites in mosquitoes, *Am. J. Trop. Med. Hyg.* **38**:283–288.
34. Collins, F.H., Zavala, F., Graves, P.M., Cochrane, A.H., Gwadz, R.W., and Akoh, J., Nussenzweig, R.S., 1984, First field trial of an immunoradiometric assay for the detection of malaria sporozoites in mosquitoes, *Am. J. Trop. Med. Hyg.* **33**:538–543.
35. Coluzzi, M., 1988, Anopheline mosquitos: Genetic methods for species differentiation. Wernsdorfer, W.H., and McGregor, I. (eds): in Malaria. Principles and Practices in Malariology, vol. 1, Churchhill Livingstone, Edinburgh, pp. 411–430.
36. Corradetti, A., Verolini, R., Sebastiani, A., Proietti, A.M., and Amati, L., 1964, Fluorescent antibody testing with sporozoites of plasmodia, *Bull. W.H.O.* **30**:747–751.
37. Davis, J.R., Murphy, J.R., Clyde, D.F., Baqar, S., Cochrane, A.H., Zavala, F., and Nussenzweig, R.S., 1989, Estimate of *Plasmodium falciparum* sporozoite content of *Anopheles stephensi* used to challenge human volunteers, *Am. J. Trop. Med. Hyg.* **40**:128–130.
38. de Arruda, M., Carvalho, M.B., Nussenzweig, R.S., Maracic, M., Ferreira, A.W., and Cochrane, A.H., 1986, Potential vectors of malaria and their different susceptibility to *Plasmodium falciparum* and *Plasmodium vivax* in northern Brazil by immunoassay, *Am. J. Trop. Med. Hyg.* **35**:873–881.
39. de Arruda, M., Nardin, E.H., Nussenzweig, R.S., and Cochranc, A.H., 1989, Sero-epidemiological studies of malaria in indian tribes and monkeys of the Amazon basin of Brazil. *Am. J. Trop. Med. Hyg.* **41**:379–385.
40. Delves, C.J., Goman, M., Ridley, R.G., Matile, H., Lensen, T.H.W., Ponnudurai, T., and Scaife, J.G., 1989, Identification of *Plasmodium falciparum*-infected mosquitoes using a probe containing repetitive DNA, *Mol. Biochem. Parasitol.* **32**:105–112.
41. Dye, C., 1986, Vectorial capacity: Must we measure all its components? *Parasitol. Today* **2**:203–209.
42. Esposito, F., Lombardi, S., Toure, Y.T., Zavala, F., and Coluzzi, M., 1986, Field observations on the use of antisporozoite monoclonal antibodies for determination of infection rates in malaria vectors, *Parasitologia* **28**:30–37.
43. Ferreira, A., Enea, V., Morimoto, T., and Nussenzweig, V., 1986, Infectivity of *Plasmodium burghei* sporozoites measured with a DNA probe, *Mol. Biochem. Parasitol.* **19**:103–109.
44. Ferreira, A., Morimoto, T., Altszuler, R., and Nussenzweig, V., 1987, Use of a DNA probe to measure the neutralization of *Plasmodium berghei* sporozoites by a monoclonal antibody, *J. Immunol.* **138**:1256–1259.
45. Gabaldon, A., and Ulloa, G., 1978, A quick and easy method to determine the sporozoite index in mosquitoes, *Trans. R. Soc. Trop. Med. Hyg.* **72**: 311–312.
46. Galinski, M.R., Arnot, D.E., Cochrane, A.H., Barnwell, J.W., Nussenzweig, R.S., and Enea, V., 1987, The circumsporozoite gene of the *Plasmodium cynomolgi* complex, *Cell* **48**:311–319.
47. Garnham, P.C.C., 1966, *Malaria Parasites and Other Haemosporidia*, Blackwell, Oxford, 1114 p.

48. Garnham, P.C.C., 1988, Malaria parasites of man: Life-cycles and morphology (excluding ultrastructure), Wernsdorfer, W.H., and McGregor, I. (eds): in Malaria. Principles and Practices in Malariology, vol. 1, Churchhill Livingstone, Edinburgh, pp. 61–96.
49. Garrett-Jones, C., 1964, Prognosis for interruption of malaria transmission through assessment of the mosquito's vectorial capacity, *Nature* **204**:1173–1175.
50. Garrett-Jones, C., and Shidrawi, G.R., 1969, Malaria vectorial capacity of a population of *Anopheles gambiae*. An exercise in epidemiological entomology, *Bull. W.H.O.* **40**:531–545.
51. Gillies, M.T., 1988, Anopheline mosquitoes: Vector behavior and bionomics. Wernsdorfer, W.H. and McGregor, I. (eds): in Malaria. Principles and Practices in Malariology, vol. 1, Churchhill Livingstone, Edinburgh, pp. 453–485.
52. Golenda, C.F., Starkweather, W.H., and Wirtz, R.A., 1990, The distribution of circumsporozoite (CS) protein in *Anopheles stephensi* mosquitoes infected with *Plasmodium falciparum* malaria, *J. Histochem. Cytochem.* **38**:475–481.
53. Graves, P.M., Brabin, B.J., Charlwood, J.D., Burkot, T.R., Ginny, M., Paino, J., Cattani, J.A., Gibson, F.D., and Alpers, M.P., 1987, Reduction in incidence and prevalence of *Plasmodium falciparum* in under 5-year old children by permethrin impregnation of mosquito nets, *Bull. W.H.O.* **65**: 869–877.
54. Graves, P.M., Burkot, T.R., Saul, A. Hayes, R., and Carter, R., 1990, Estimation of anopheline survival rate, vectorial capacity, and mosquito infection probability from vector infection rates in villages near Madang, Papua New Guinea, *J. Appl. Ecol.* **27**:134–147.
55. Greenwood, B.M., 1989, Impact of culture and environmental changes on epidemiology and control of malaria and babesiosis, *Trans. R. Soc. Trop. Med. Hyg.* (Suppl.) **83**:25–29.
56. Gunderson, J.H., Sogin, M.L., Wollett, G., Hollingdale, M., de la Cruz, V.F., Waters, A.P., and McCutchan, T.F., 1987, Structurally distinct, stage-specific ribosomes occur in *Plasmodium*, *Science* **238**:933–937.
57. Harwood, R.F., and James, M.T., 1979, Entomology in Human and Animal Health, New York, Macmillian, 548 p.
58. Hoedojo, Saleha, S., Makimian, R., Campbell, J., Franke, E., Santiyo, K., Gambiro, and Sustriayu, N., 1987, A preliminary study on detection of *Plasmodium falciparum* sporozoites in *Anopheles aconitus*, *Mosquito-Borne Dis. Bull.* **3**:64–66.
59. Holmberg, M., and Wigzell, H., 1987, DNA hybridization assays for detection of malaria sporozoites in mosquitoes, *Parasitol. Today* **3**:380.
60. Ingram, R.L., Otken, L.B., and Jumper, R.J., 1961, Staining of malarial parasites by the fluorescent antibody technique. *Proc. Soc. Exp. Biol. Med.* **106**:52–54.
61. Johnson, A.M., and Baverstock, P.R., 1989, Rapid ribosomal RNA sequencing and the phylogenetic analysis of protists, *Parasitol. Today* **5**: 102–105.
62. Krotoski, W.A., Omar, M.S., and Jumper, J.R., 1974, Immunofluorescent staining of plasmodial oocysts in the mosquito, *J. Parasitol.* **60**:344–347.
63. Lanar, D.E., McLaughlin, G.L., Wirth, D.F., Barker, R.J., Zolg, J.W., and Chulay, J.D., 1989, Comparison of thick films, in vitro culture and DNA

hybridization probes for detecting *Plasmodium falciparum* malaria, *Am. J. Trop. Med. Hyg.* **40**:3–6.

64. Lee, M., Harrison, B.A., and Lewis, G.E., 1990, A rapid sporozoite ELISA using 3,3',5,5'-tetramethylbenzidine as the substrate chromogen, *Am. J. Trop. Med. Hyg.* **42**:314–319.
65. Lindsay, S.W., Snow, R.W., Broomfield, G.L., Janneh, M.S., Wirtz, R.A., and Greenwood, B.M., 1989, Impact of permethrin-treated bednets on malaria transmission by the *Anopheles gambiae* complex in The Gambia, *Med. Vet. Entomol.* **3**:263–271.
66. Lombardi, S., Esposito, F., Zavala, F., Lamizana, L., Rossi, P., Sabatinelli, G., Nussenzweig, R.S., and Coluzzi, M., 1987, Detection and anatomical localization of *Plasmodium falciparum* circumsporozoite protein and sporozoites in the Afrotropical malaria vector *Anopheles gambiae* s.l, *Am. J. Trop. Med. Hyg.* **37**:491–494.
67. Malaria Action Programme, 1987, World malaria situation 1985, *World Health Stat. Q.* **40**:142–170.
68. McCutchan, T.F., de al Cruz, V.F., Lal, A.A., Gunderson, J.H., Elwood, H.J., and Sogin, M.L., 1988, Primary sequences of two small subunit ribosomal RNA genes from *Plasmodium falciparum*, *Mol. Biochem. Parasitol* **28**:63–68.
69. McLaughlin, G.L., Ruth, J.L., Jablonski, E., Steketee, R., and Campbell, G.H., 1987, Use of enzyme-linked synthetic DNA in diagnosis of falciparum malaria, *Lancet* **1**(8535):714–716.
70. Molineaux, L., and Gramiccia, G. 1980. The Garki Project. Research on the Epidemiology and Control of Malaria in the Sudan Savanna of West Africa, World Health Organization, Genera, 311 p.
71. Molineaux, L., Muir, D.A., Spencer, H.C., and Wernsdorfer, W.H., 1988, The Epidemiology of Malaria and Its Measurements. Wernsdorfer, W.H., and McGregor, I. (eds): in Malaria. Principles and Practices of Malariology, vol. 2, Churchhill Livingstone, Edinburgh, pp. 999–1089.
72. Muir, D.A., 1988, Anopheline mosquitoes: Vector reproduction, life-cycle and biotype, Wernsdorfer, W.H., and McGregor, I. (eds): in Malaria. Principles and Practices in Malariology, vol. 1, Churchhill Livingstone, Edinburgh, pp. 431–451.
73. Nardin, E., Gwadz, R.W., and Nussenzweig, R.S., 1979, Characterization of sporozoite surface antigens by indirect immunofluorescence: Detection of stage- and species-specific antimalarial antibodies, *Bull. W.H.O.* **57**(Suppl. 1):211–217.
74. Nardin, E.H., and Nussenzweig, R.S., 1978, Stage-specific antigens on the surface membrane of sporozoites of malaria parasites, *Nature* **274**:55–57.
75. Nardin, E.H., Nussenzweig, R.S., Nussenzweig, V., Harinasuta, K.T., Collins, W.E., Tapschaisri, P., and Chomcharn, Y., 1982, Circumsporozoite (CS) proteins of human malaria parasites *Plasmodium falciparum* and *Plasmodium vivax*, *J. Exp. Med.* **156**:20–30.
76. Nussenzweig, R.S., Montuori, W., Spitalny, and Chen, D., 1973, Antibodies against sporozoites of human and simian malaria produced in rats, *J. Immunol.* **110**:600–601.
77. Nussenzweig, V., and Nussenzweig, R.S., 1986, Development of a sporozoite malaria vaccine, *Am. J. Trop. Med. Hyg.* **35**:678–688.

78. Peters, W., 1960, Studies on the epidemiology of malaria in New Guinea, *Trans. Roy. Soc. Trop. Med. Hyg.* **54**:242–251.
79. Petros, B.L., Procell, P.M., Campbell, G.H., and Collins, F.H., 1989, A nitrocellulose membrane-based ELISA for the detection of *Plasmodium* infections in mosquitoes, *Bull. W.H.O.* **67**:525–533.
80. Ponnudurai, T., Lensen, A.H.W., van Gemert, G.J.A., Bensink, M.P.E., Bolmer, M., and Meuwissen, J.H.E.Th., 1989, Sporozoite load of mosquitoes infected with *Plasmodium falciparum*, *Trans. Roy. Soc. Trop. Med. Hyg.* **83**:67–70.
81. Post, R.J., and Crampton, J.M., 1987, Probing the unknown, *Parasitol. Today* **3**:380–383.
82. Pringle, G., 1965, A count of the sporozoites in an oocyst of *Plasmodium falciparum*, *Trans. R. Soc. Trop. Med. Hyg.* **59**:289–290.
83. Pringle, G., 1966, A quantitative study of naturally acquired malaria infections in *Anopheles gambiae* and *Anopheles funestus* in a highly malarious area of East Africa, *Trans. R. Soc. Trop. Med. Hyg.* **60**:626–632.
84. Procell, P.M., Collins, W.E., and Campbell, G.H., 1988, Circumsporozoite protein of the human malaria parasite *Plasmodium ovale* identified with monoclonal antibodies, *Infect. Immun.* **56**:376–379.
85. Ramsey, J.M., Beaudoin, R.L., Bawden, M.P., and Espinal, C.A., 1981, Taxonomic identification of malaria sporozoites by indirect fluorescent antibody assay, *WHO/MAL81.971*, 7 p.
86. Ramsey, J.M., Beaudoin, R.L., Bawden, M.P., and Espinal, C.A., 1983, Specific identification of *Plasmodium* sporozoites using an indirect fluorescent antibody method, *Trans. Roy. Soc. Trop. Med. Hyg.* **77**:378–381.
87. Ramsey, J.M., Bown, D.N., Aron, J.L., Beaudoin, R.L., and Mendez, J.F., 1986, Field trail in Chiapas, Mexico, of a rapid detection method for malaria in anopheline vectors with low infection rates. *Am. J. Trop. Med. Hyg.* **35**:234–238.
88. Reid, J.A., 1968, Anopheline Mosquitoes of Malaya and Borneo, Government of Malaysia, Kuala Lumpur, 520 p.
89. Robert, V., Verhave, J.P., Ponnudurai, T., Louwe, L., Scholtens, P., and Carnevale, P., 1988, Study of the distribution of circumsporozoite antigen in *Anopheles gambiae* infected with *Plasmodium falciparum*, using the enzymelinked immunosorbent assay, *Trans. R. Soc. Trop. Med. Hyg.* **82**: 289–391.
90. Rosenberg, R., 1985, Inability of *Plasmodium knowlesi* sporozoites to invade *Anopheles freeborni* salivary glands, *Am. J. Trop. Med. Hyg.* **34**:687–691.
91. Rosenberg, R., Andre, R.G., and Somchit, L., 1990, Highly efficient dry season transmission of malaria in Thailand, *Trans. R. Soc. Trop. Med. Hyg.* **84**:22–28.
92. Rosenberg, R., Wirtz, R.A., Lanar, D.E., Sattabongkot, J., Hall, T., Waters, A.P., and Prasittisuk, C., 1989, Circumsporozoite protein heterogeneity in the human malaria parasite *Plasmodium vivax*, *Science* **245**:973–976.
93. Rosenberg, R., Wirtz, R.A., Schneider, I., and Burge, R., 1990, An estimation of the number of malaria sporozoites ejected by a feeding mosquito, *Trans. R. Soc. Trop. Med. Hyg.* **84**:209–212.
94. Russell, P.F., West, L.S., Manwell, R.D., and MacDonald, G., 1963, Practical Malariology, Oxford University Press, London, 2nd ed., 750 p.

95. Saul, A., Graves, P.M., and Kay, B.H., 1990, A cyclical model of disease transmission and its application to determining vectorial capacity from vector infection rates. *J. Appl. Ecol.* **27**:123–133.
96. Service, M., 1976, Mosquito Ecology: Field sampling methods. Applied Science Publishers, London, 583 p.
97. Shute, P.G., and Maryon, M., 1952, A study of human oocysts as an aid to species diagnosis, *Trans. R. Soc. Trop. Med. Hyg.* **46**:275–292.
98. Sinden, R.E., 1984, The biology of *Plasmodium* in the mosquito, *Experientia* **40**:1330–1343.
99. Sodeman, W.A., Jr., and Jeffery, G.M., 1964, Immunofluorescent staining of sporozoites of *Plasmodium gallinaceum*, *J. Parasitol.* **50**:477–478.
100. Sodeman, W.A., Jr., Jeffery, G.M., and Collins, W.E., 1964, Fluorescent antibody studies in experimental malarias. I. Studies on *Plasmodium gallinaceum* and *Plasmodium berghei*, *Proc. First Int. Congr. Parasit.* **1**: 224–230.
101. Sturchler, D., 1989, How much malaria is there worldwide? *Parasitol. Today* **5**:39–40; ibid. **5**:384.
102. Subbarao, S.K., Adak, T., Vasantha, K., Joshi, H., Raghvendra, K., Cochrane, A.H., Nussenzweig, R.A., and Sharma, V.P., 1988. Susceptibility of *Anopheles culicifacies* species A and B to *Plasmodium vivax* and *Plasmodium falciparum* as determined by immunoradiometic assay, *Trans. R. Soc. Trop. Med. Hyg.* **82**:394–397.
103. Tang, V.C.W., Hancock, K., and Maddison, S.E., 1984, Quantitative capacities of glutaraldehyde and sodium *m*-periodate coupled peroxidase-anti-human IgG conjugates in enzyme-linked immunoassays, *J. Immunol. Methods* **70**:91–100.
104. Vanderberg, J.P., and Gwadz, R.W., 1980, The transmission by mosquitoes of plasmodia in the laboratory, Kreier, J.P. (ed): in Malaria, vol. 2, Academic, New York, pp. 154–234.
105. Vanderberg, J.P., Nussenzweig, R., and Most, H. 1969. Protective immunity produced by the injection of X-irradiated sporozoites of *Plasmodium berghei*. V. In vitro effects of immune serum on sporozoites, *Milit. Med.* (Suppl.) **134**:1183–1190.
106. Verhave, J.P., Leewenberg, A.D.E.M., Ponnudurai, T., Meuwissen, J.H.E.Th., and van Druten, J.A.M., 1988, The biotin-streptavidin system in a two-site ELISA for the detection of plasmodial sporozoite antigen in mosquitoes, *Parasite Immunol.* **10**:17–31.
107. Viriyakosol, S., Snounou, G., and Brown, K.N., 1989, The use of a DNA probe for the differentiation of rodent malaria strains and species, *Mol. Biochem. Parasitol.* **32**:93–100.
108. Ward, R.A., 1962, Preservation of mosquitoes for malarial oocyst and sporozoite dissections, *Mosquito News* **22**:306–307.
109. Warren, M., Mason, J., and Hobbs, J., 1975, Natural infections of *Anopheles albimanus* with *Plasmodium* in a small malaria focus, *Am. J. Trop. Med. Hyg.* **24**: 545–546.
110. Waters, A.P., and McCutchan, T., 1989, Rapid, sensitive diagnosis of malaria based on ribosomal RNA, *Lancet* 17 June **8651**:1343–1346.
111. Weber, J.L., and Hockmeyer, W.T., 1985, Structure of the circumsporozoite proteins in 18 strains of *Plasmodium falciparum*, *Mol. Biochem. Parasitol.* **15**:305–316.

112. Wernsdorfer, W.H. 1980. The importance of malaria in the world. Kreier, J.P., (ed): in Malaria, vol. 1, Academic, New York, pp. 1–93.
113. Wharton, R.H., Eyles, D.E., Warren, M., Moorhouse, D.E., and Sandosham, A.A., 1963, Investigations leading to the identification of members of the *Anopheles umbrosus* group as the probable vectors of mouse deer malaria, *Bull. W.H.O.* **29**:357–374.
114. White, G.B., 1989, Malaria, in Geographical Distribution of Arthropod-borne Diseases and their Principal Vectors (*WHO/VBC*/89.967). **1**:7–22. World Health Organization/Division of Vector Biology and Control, Geneva 134 p.
115. Wilkinson, R.N., 1980, Detection of malarial sporozoites by the enzyme linked immunosorbent assay (ELISA), PhD Dissertation, University of Texas Health Science Center at Houston, Texas. 80 p.
116. Wirtz, R.A., Burkot, T.R., Andre, R.G., Rosenberg, R., Collins, W.E., and Roberts, D.R., 1985, Identification of *Plasmodium vivax* sporozoites in mosquitoes using an enzyme-linked immunosorbent assay, *Am. J. Trop. Med. Hyg.* **34**:1048–1054.
117. Wirtz, R.A., Burkot, T.R., Graves, P.M., and Andre, R.G., 1987, Field evaluation of enzyme-linked immunosorbent assays (ELISAs) for *Plasmodium falciparum* and *Plasmodium vivax* sporozoites in mosquitoes (Diptera: Culicidae) from Papua New Guinea, *J. Med. Entomol.* **24**:433–437.
118. Wirtz, R.A., Charoenvit, Y., Burkot, T.R., Esser, K.M., Beaudoin, R.L., Collins, W.E., and Andre, R.G., 1991, Evaluation of monoclonal antibodies against *Plasmodium vivax* sporozoites for ELISA development. *Med. Vet. Entomol.* **5**:(in press).
119. Wirtz, R.A., Zavala, F., Charoenvit, Y., Campbell, G.H., Burkot, T.R., Schneider, I., Esser, K.M., Beaudoin, R.L., and Andre, R.G., 1987, Comparative testing of monoclonal antibodies against *Plasmodium falciparum* sporozoites for ELISA development, *Bull. W.H.O.* **65**:39–45.
120. World Health Organization, 1975, Manual on Practical Entomology in Malaria. World Health Organization, Geneva, 191 p.
121. World Health Organization, 1986, The use of DNA probes for malaria diagnosis: Memorandum from a WHO meeting, *Bull. W.H.O.* **64**:641–652.
122. World Health Organization, 1987, Tropical Disease Research: A global Partnership, Geneva, WHO, 191 p.
123. World Health Organization, 1988, Tropical Disease Research: Science at Work, Geneva, WHO, 64 p.
124. Zavala, F. Cochrane, A.H., Nardin, E.H., Nussenzweig, R.S., and Nussenzweig, V., 1983, Circumsporozoite proteins of malaria parasites contain a single immunodominant region with two or more identical epitopes, *J. Exp. Med.* **157**:1947–1957.
125. Zavala, F., Gwadz, R.W., Collins, F.H., Nussenzweig, R.S. and Nussenzweig, V., 1982, Monoclonal antibodies to circumsporozoite proteins identify the species of malaria parasite in infected mosquitoes, *Nature* **299**:737–738.
126. Zavala, F., Musuda, A., Graves, P.M., Nussenzweig, V., and Nussenzweig, R.S., 1985, Ubiquity of the repetitive epitope of the CS protein in different isolates of human malaria parasites, *J. Immunol.* **135**:2790–2793.

5
Alphavirus Infection in Cultured Tissue Cells

Mary L. Miller and Dennis T. Brown

Introduction

Mosquitoes have been recognized since the early 1900s as vectors of a variety of pathogenic viruses that have plagued humans and domestic animals for centuries. Thorough understanding of the life cycles of these pathogens is essential for developing methods for their control. Epidemiological studies have yielded information on the vector species of many of these disease-causing agents and entomological studies have provided details regarding how arboviruses (arthropod-borne viruses) are cycled in nature through their insect and vertebrate hosts. As a result, eradication measures such as mosquito population control and physical barriers to hematophagous insects have developed, which have proven reasonably effective in certain regions of the world. However, the fact that many vectored phatogens are still responsible for disease outbreaks reaching epidemic proportions and remain a threat to the domestic livestock industry necessitates further research on their control.

In keeping with current biotechnological advances, the interactions between viruses and their animal hosts have been studied intensively at the cellular and molecular levels. Based on the knowledge gained from these investigations, vaccines have been developed that protect against infection by many known viral pathogens. However, these have been produced primarily to protect laboratory workers who must handle these agents routinely and are not generally available for widespread use (134). It must also be considered that prophylactic measures are only effective if administered appropriately and such invasive techniques possess the

Mary L. Miller, Cell Research Institute and Department of Microbiology, The University of Texas at Austin, Austin, Texas 78713, USA.
Dennis T. Brown, Cell Research Institute, BIO 220, The University of Texas at Austin, Austin, Texas 78713, USA.

potential for side effects as serious as the diseases they are meant to prevent. A more effective line of attack would be at the level of virus replication within the vector host. Controlled infection of whole insects allows for analysis of the kinetics of virus replication and transmission mechanisms, but investigation of interactions at the molecular level requires direct manipulation of uniformly grown cells, which is possible only with continuous cell culture.

Two significant breakthroughs, which have accelerated advances in arbovirus research, have been the development of a hemolymph-free medium, which supports growth of arthropod cells in culture (113), and the establishment of continuous mosquito cell lines (43, 129, 170). To date, there are over 100 dipteran species represented by continuous cell lines, many of which are known to be susceptible to one or more arboviruses (70, 89, 91, 137, 199).

Members of five virus taxa are known to be vectored by mosquitoes, representing the togavirus, flavivirus, bunyavirus, rhabdovirus, and reovirus families. This review will focus on the alphaviruses of the Togaviridae, as studies of this genus constitute the greatest body of knowledge to date on arbovirus replication in cultured mosquito cells. In this chapter, we will discuss current contributions and prevalent research directions resulting from examination of infection by these agents in cultured insect and vertebrate cells.

Mosquito Cell Culture

Virologists have provided the primary impetus for developing continuous cell cultures because viruses, as obligate parasites, can only be adequately studied in vitro within cells derived from their hosts. Because knowledge of the physiology and biochemistry of vertebrates was extensive by the time a need for standardized in vitro cell systems was recognized, stable mammalian cell lines were rapidly developed for the study of virus–host interactions. Original medium formulations were based on the composition of blood, with modifications introduced as more information was garnered about the nutritional needs of cells adapted to an in vitro environment. As a direct result of the successful culturing of vertebrate cells, a vast body of literature has evolved that describes the replication of viruses in vertebrate cells and defines the field of molecular virology.

Arboviruses use vertebrate hosts only transiently in their complex life cycles in nature, substantiating the need for studying these agents within cells from invertebrate hosts as well. Far less is understood about the physiology of arthropods in comparison to vertebrate systems, and initial progress in establishing continuous insect cell cultures was tediously slow (44, 90, 91, 199). In the earliest attempts to culture invertebrate cells, investigators used hemolymph as a primary component of the medium.

This approach was based on the logic applied to the successful development of medium for vertebrate cells, which was to provide the nutritional equivalent of blood. The use of hemolymph yielded disappointing results for a variety of reasons. First, untreated hemolymph was discovered to be toxic to cells in culture and required heat inactivation. Also, the use of homologous hemolymph was impractical for the continuous culturing of cells from small insects and the substitution of heterologous hemolymph introduced new variables in addition to being toxic to some cell types (111, 188). A more logical approach seemed to be the analysis of the components of hemolymph and reproduction of its constituent parts in a physiological solution. Such efforts were greatly hindered by the discovery that hemolymph composition varies considerably not only among insect genera and species, but also within an individual insect at different stages of development (111). However, a preoccupation with hemolymph analysis for determining medium formulation set back development of insect culture for several years. An example of how such logic hindered the search for suitable media for invertebrate cell culture was demonstrated in the use of β-alanine. This amino acid was identified as a component of hemolymph in several insect species (210) and has been included in many medium formulations since its initial use (211). It has since been determined that β-alanine hinders cell growth and exerts a detrimental effect on insect cells in culture (109–111). Culture medium suitable for insect cells was eventually developed through an empirical approach, coupled with the insight gained from previous attempts and experience from successful vertebrate cell culture (109, 111, 162, 199). Finally, substitution of fetal calf serum (FCS) for hemolymph yielded the ultimate breakthrough towards progress in establishing continuous insect cell culture (109, 111).

A few of the medium formulations most commonly used for invertebrate cell culture are Mitsuhashi and Maramorosch (M&M) medium, (113) originally designed to support growth of leafhopper cells, Leibovitz's L15 medium (97), and Eagle's minimal essential medium (MEM) (29). The latter two formulations were developed for vertebrate cell culture and were subsequently discovered to be effective in supporting many types of insect cell lines. The addition of tryptose phosphate broth (TPB) and fetal calf serum renders these media partially undefined. Numerous investigators have experimented with serum-free and chemically defined medium recipes in an effort to decrease the number of variables influencing cell growth and also to reduce the costs of maintaining these cultures. Moderate success has been reported on the growth of insect cells in vitro in the absence of TPB and with reduced serum or replacement of serum with lactalbumin hydrolysate (55, 65, 88, 91, 92, 110, 112, 209). The steady progress in this area is attributed to the belief that growth factors in hemolymph, FCS, and lactalbumin hydrolysate have yet to be identified and that once these components are characterized, growth of insect cells in defined, low-cost media will become standard practice (111, 112).

A constant concern in maintaining cell lines in culture is contamination of the cells either by endogenous viruses or extrinsic sources such as microorganisms or cells from another species (56). Bacteria, fungi, and mycoplasma are common invaders that can be controlled through proper handling and the addition of antibiotics. The presence of endogenous viruses in insect cell lines, although less frequent, is well documented in the literature. Viruses have been isolated from apparently uninfected cells that exhibited spontaneous syncytium formation (21, 56, 58, 181), and electron microscopic studies have revealed latent virus infection in a number of cell lines (42, 57). These inapparent infections are often traced to the larvae from which the cells originated or to media additives (63, 79). As many viruses establish a persistent infection with transitory or no cytopathic effect in mosquito cells, the possibility of endogenous infection must always be considered when interpreting data from studies on experimentally virus-infected insect cells.

Although the least common source of contamination, the erroneous mixture of cells of different species has also been reported. The most widely known example of extrinsic contamination involved the *Aedes aegypti* cells of Grace (43) and the *Culiseta inornata* and *Aedes vexans* cell lines established in Sweet's laboratory (188). These three cell lines were identified to be of lepidopteran rather than dipteran origin based on immunological, karyological, and isoenzyme analyses (45, 46). These techniques, in addition to more recently developed protocols, such as mitochondrial DNA restriction mapping and monoclonal antibody marking, have provided the technology for differentiating cell lines not only among different species but within the same species as well (8).

The *Aedes albopictus* cell line established by Singh (170) has since been determined to be free of contamination by extrinsic cells and endogenous virus (41, 45, 46) and many sublines have been cloned from this parent line. These mosquito cell lines are the most widely used in the study of arboviruses and the following review pertains to data derived primarily from experiments involving these cell types, unless otherwise indicated.

Early Events in Alphavirus Infection

Alphaviruses, also known as Group A arboviruses, were the first vectored viruses identified collectively by serological testing. Virions consist of a single strand of positive polarity RNA encased in a virus-encoded capsid protein and enveloped in a host-derived lipid membrane interspersed with viral glycoprotein spikes (159). These viruses comprise the only genus among the Togaviridae known to replicate in both arthropod and vertebrate cells. Alphavirus infection in both cell systems demonstrates equivalent progeny yields and production kinetics (26, 32, 41, 177). Although differences in oligosaccharide and lipid composition are evident, viruses from either source are identical in infectivity and antigenicity (13, 60, 103, 104, 116, 180).

Such a broad host range, spanning major phyla, would imply that these viruses gain access to the host cell's interior through attachment to either a widely ubiquitous cell surface receptor, a variety of receptor types, or possibly no receptor involvement at all. Avian fibroblasts and hamster kidney cells have been shown to adsorb approximately 10^5 Sindbis virus (SV) particles in an evenly distributed array over the cell surface (3). The saturation of a cell surface protein population upon exposure to SV has also been demonstrated by Smith and Tignor (171). These investigators discovered that binding sites on the surface of neuronal cells for an avirulent and neurovirulent strain of SV were unique and that binding sites were more numerous for the latter strain, implicating these putative receptors in the process of establishing virulence. Helenius et al. (54) assigned the Semliki Forest virus (SFV) receptor function to human and mouse major histocompatibility (MHC) antigens. However, Oldstone and co-workers (121) demonstrated successful SFV infection of murine cells that fail to express these antigens, implying that although SFV spike proteins can complex with MHC proteins, this class of antigens serves no apparent role in the infection process. Maassen and Terhorst (105) cross-linked SV to a 90K protein on the surfaces of two lymphoblastic cell lines, one of which lacks complete HLA-A and HLA-B antigens. The binding of antibodies specific for MHC molecules on the surface of the other cell line was not affected by the presence of SV, indicating that the 90K protein is not associated with this class of surface proteins. Virus binding studies such as these underscore the complications inherent in attempts to characterize the phenomenon of virus entry into target cells.

Another approach to understanding the early events in alphavirus infection has been to examine the mechanism by which the viral genome is transferred from the extracellular medium to the host cell interior. It is generally accepted that the lipid bilayer of the virus fuses with a host cell membrane with subsequent release of the viral capsid into the cytoplasm. Data from several studies have yielded conflicting results about the exact route of entry of those virions that are ultimately infectious.

Based on morphological observations at the light and electron microscope levels and on inhibition of virus replication upon pretreatment of cells with lysosomotropic weak bases (53, 191, 192), which are known to raise the pH of acidic intracellular compartments (120), Helenius et al. (52) proposed that SFV gains entry to the vertebrate host cell through receptor-mediated endocytosis. The same laboratory reported a low pH requirement for virus-mediated fusion of host cell membranes (206) and extrapolated these data to further implicate the acidic interior of endosomal vesicles as requisite for triggering release of the virus genome into the cell cytoplasm. However, such interpretation, based largely on circumstantial evidence, must be considered with respect to the following caveats. First, as the authors themselves (52) point out, the amount of virus applied to infect cells for the morphological studies was as much as 1000 times greater than normally used in experimental infections. In addition, subsequent studies on the low pH requirement for membrane fusion have revealed that in vertebrate cells in culture, exposure to acidic pH must be followed by a shift of the extracellular medium to neutral pH to initiate alphavirus-mediated fusion from without (5, 33, 34, 74, 206). This experimentally induced shift in pH is not known to represent any in vivo condition and should be considered a laboratory phenomenon until the mechanism of viral fusion is better understood. Finally, further studies on the effects of lysosomotropic weak bases, such as chloroquine and ammonium chloride, demonstrate that these agents do not prevent penetration of vertebrate cells by alphaviruses. This conclusion was based on experiments that demonstrated that the presence of lysosomotropic weak bases during alphavirus infection did not prevent the detection of newly synthesized virus proteins on the surfaces of mosquito cells or the expression of virus-induced homologous interference (14, 20, 123). These drugs were shown to restrict later events in virus production, including viral RNA synthesis, assembly, and maturation of virus particles, providing an alternative interpretation of previous reports on the inhibitory effects of these agents.

Adding to the complexity of this issue, Omar et al. (122) reported that *Aedes albopictus* cells, in contrast to vertebrate cells, undergo SFV-mediated fusion at low pH without a mandatory return of the medium to neutral pH. These data are also contradictory to findings that *Aedes albopictus* cells require not only a shift up in pH but also a more acidic primary environment than baby hamster kidney (BHK) cells to initiate virus-mediated cell fusion (33). Omar and coworkers attempt to explain this discrepancy by suggesting differences in composition of the media used in the respective laboratories, particularly with regard to cholesterol. This reference to cholesterol is presumably based on reports that fusion of SFV requires the presence of cholesterol in the target membrane (76, 77, 115, 205). Mosquito cells, however, do not synthesize sterols, although they do incorporate them from the medium (16, 114, 168, 200). Edwards and Brown (33) have shown that mosquito cells grown in Eagle's MEM medium will undergo virus-mediated fusion but that the same line of cells cultivated in M&M medium will not fuse by this mechanism at any pH between 4.0 and 7.0. The fact that the latter medium contains an exogenous supply of sterols rules out a lack of cholesterol as an explanation for the absence of fusion and implies that conditions for fusion reside not only within the virus but within the host cell as well. Also, such a stringent requirement for cholesterol fails to account for the ability to infect mosquitoes intrathoracically with virus suspended in saline containing 0.2% bovine serum albumin (BSA) (25) or transovarial and venereal transmission of alphaviruses in nature, particularly in male mosquitoes that never imbibe a bloodmeal and are subsequently never exposed to cholesterol.

The studies that demonstrated a requirement for cholesterol in virus-mediated membrane fusion employed liposomes which contained no proteins. Haywood and Boyer (51) have shown that influenza virus will fuse with liposomes at neutral pH dependent upon their composition. Thus, it must be considered that the cholesterol requirement may be a phenomenon unique to artificial membrane systems and like virus-mediated fusion at low pH, may not be representative of the alphavirus infection process in nature.

The difference in the pH shift-up requirement between vertebrate and invertebrate cells has also been attributed to observations that ATP expenditure accompanies the fusion event in both cell types. Koblet and coworkers (72–74) have proposed that vertebrate cells deplete their ATP supply to maintain internal pH in response to exposure to an acidic extracellular environment and require a shift to neutral conditions for generating energy needed for fusion. Mosquito cells, they suggest, may be more efficient in adapting to fluctuations in extracellular pH and retain the ATP necessary for virus-mediated fusion, reducing the discrepancy between conditions of fusion in the two cell types to a question of energy (82).

The glycoprotein E1 has been shown by several investigators to be the virus surface component responsible for initiating fusion under currently established laboratory conditions (5, 15, 38, 81, 84, 122, 125). Upon experimentally induced exposure to low pH, E1 undergoes a conformational change necessary to initiate fusion (77, 125). A change in trypsin sensitivity has also been detected in the E2 glycoprotein under similar low pH conditions (34, 77, 102), but E2 alone apparently cannot induce cell fusion (22, 83).

The nature of the low pH-induced conformational change of E1 has been examined in detail. Omar and Koblet (125) have demonstrated that exposure to acidic pH induces a significant increase in the hydrophobicity of E1, which probably enhances the interaction between the glycoprotein and the lipid bilayer following initial attachment. Results of studies in which agents that modify thiol and disulfide groups were applied under conditions of virus-mediated cell fusion indicate that a greater number of these groups become exposed during the rearrangement of E1 and that a resulting disulfide–sulfhydride exchange reaction stabilizes the new configuration (124, 126). These findings implicate two regions along the E1 protein as the segments required for mediating fusion. There is a region at amino acid residues 79 through 96, possessing a hydrophobic sequence, which has been suspected to be involved in fusion (207). This piece is included within the segment between positions 61 and 114, containing seven cysteine residues, which appear to play a role in inducing the conformational change of E1 necessary to render it fusogenic (126). It must still be considered that exposure of E1 to a low pH environment under laboratory conditions may only mimic the conditions required in vivo to promote the configuration of the spike protein necessary to mediate fusion.

Recently, the availability of Chinese hamster ovary (CHO) cell lines with temperature-sensitive defects in the ability to acidify endosomes (106, 145, 195) has provided an excellent model system for determining a requirement for a low pH environment to trigger virus-induced membrane fusion. Schmid et al. (161) found that in mutant cells maintained and infected at nonpermissive temperature, internalized SFV E1 does not become exposed to cellular compartments with internal pH $\leq$5.3, as assayed by the pH-dependent trypsin sensitivity of E1 (77). However, these authors failed to examine the ability of alphaviruses to infect these mutant cells productively under conditions in which the phenotype for defective acidification is expressed. Viral RNA synthesis has been shown to be initiated in a CHO mutant cell line found to be severely impaired in the ability to acidify endosomes (J. Edwards and D.T. Brown, unpublished data). These data further stress the demand for reevaluation of the model for receptor-mediated endocytosis as the primary route of entry into cells by alphaviruses and other enveloped viruses.

Replication of the Alphavirus Genome

The alphavirus genome is fully functional as a messenger RNA (187), and almost immediately upon its delivery into the cytosol, host cell-mediated translation of the nonstructural viral proteins is initiated. Four proteins are translated as polypeptides which are proteolytically cleaved to assemble into replication complexes needed for production of additional viral RNA species. Although little is known about this process in invertebrate cells, studies of cultured vertebrate cells have led to the development of a proposed schematic. The replication complex orchestrates the synthesis of (1) full-length negative RNA strands, which, in turn, serve as templates for (2) additional full-length positive strand templates, (3) subgenomic 26S mRNAs from which structural proteins are translated, and (4) full-length positive strand genomes, which are packaged into progeny virions. Such a complex must be capable of a variety of reactions and it is presumed that some, if not all, of the nonstructural proteins play multiple roles in replication (149, 159). Sequencing data and complementation studies of a variety of temperature-sensitive mutants of the heat-resistant strain of SV (SVHR) (10, 182) have allowed for tentative assignment of some of these functions. The collection of mutants determined to be negative for viral RNA synthesis (RNA$^-$) have been assigned to four nonoverlapping groups designated as complementation groups A, B, G and F (9). The genetic lesions in these viruses map to the viral genomic region encoding the nonstructural proteins, nsP1–4 (186).

The protein nsP2 has been shown by in vitro translation experiments to possess an autoproteolytic capability, cleaving the junctions of nsP1–2 and nsP3–4 (27). Several temperature-sensitive mutants whose lesions map to nsP2 become defective in 26S RNA synthesis upon shift up to nonpermissive temperature, suggesting that this protein also functions in initiation of 26S RNA synthesis (75, 151). The nsP2 protein also appears to be involved in the proper functioning of nsP4, which is presumed to be an RNA polymerase (150). This assumption is based on data from cDNA cloning studies of the RNA$^-$ mutant, *ts*118, which contains lesions in both of these nonstructural gene regions. Constructs carrying only one or the other of these defects fail to express fully the phenotype characteristic of *ts*118 when grown at nonpermissive temperatures (48). The temperature-sensitive phenotype of another SV mutant whose lesion maps to nsP4 is the failure to terminate negative RNA strand synthesis late in infection and in the presence of protein synthesis inhibitors. Sawicki et al. (150) have proposed that such aberrant function is the result of impaired ability of nsP4 to preferentially bind minus strands as templates for early replication events. Instead, the defective protein binds positive strands that are subsequently copied into additional minus strands at later times in virus replication when negative strand synthesis would normally have ceased. These observations implicate nsP4 as a regulator of early and late events by functioning at the level of template recognition and binding. Another SV mutant, *ts*17, which is classed in the same complementation group with *ts*24, manifests a similar phenotype of failure to terminate minus strand synthesis at nonpermissive temperature (151, 153, 154). However, the lesion in *ts*17 maps to nsP2 (49), suggesting that this protein may also regulate minus strand synthesis.

Studies of the single member of complementation group B, *ts*11, demonstrate that minus strand RNA synthesis ceases in cells infected with this mutant when shifted from permissive to nonpermissive temperature, whereas 49S plus strand RNA and 26S RNA replication proceeds normally (152). This virus has an altered sequence in the nsP1 region of its genome, which apparently affects the initiation of minus strand synthesis.

Mosquito cell culture has been instrumental in defining another function for nsP1. Viral mutants capable of replicating in methionine-deprived *Aedes albopictus* cells [a prohibitive condition for wild-type virus growth in mosquito cells but not in vertebrate cells (176)] contain lesions in nsP1. This alteration is believed to code for an mRNA methyltransferase with a higher affinity for *S*-adenosylmethionine (ado-met), which is the limiting resource in mosquito cells cultured in the absence of methionine (108). Thus nsP1 may also serve to methylate viral mRNA as a prerequisite to translation.

Hardy and Strauss (50) have determined the temporal sequence of proteolytic processing of SV nonstructural proteins through a series of pulse-chase experiments and immunoprecipitations of the labeled proteins with monospecific polyclonal antibodies. An interesting feature of this proteolytic processing has been exploited to gain further insight on the functioning of the nonstructural proteins. Among the alphaviruses, Sindbis virus, Middleburg virus, and Ross River virus (RRV) contain an in-frame opal termination codon between the genomic regions encoding nsP3 and nsP4 (183–185). In contrast, Semliki Forest virus and O'Nyong-nyong virus retain an arginine codon at this position (183, 190). In those species possessing the nonsense sequence, a readthrough mechanism allows translation of nsP4 and it has been theorized that this function regulates the level of expression of this nonstructural protein (50, 187). Li and Rice (101) replaced the opal codon of SV, through site-directed mutagenesis, with sense codons for amino acids or with amber or ochre termination sequences. These authors found that in chick embryo cells infected with mutants containing sense replacements, nsP34 was still cleaved, albeit at a reduced rate, indicating that the production of nsP4 is not solely regulated by readthrough of the opal codon. It was also observed that the mutants with substituted termination sequences underproduced nsP34, whereas the mutants containing sense codons produced nsP34 in excess. However, an increase in the level of nsP4, which would be expected in cells infected with the latter mutants, was not detected and these investigators suggest that this may be due to a rapid turnover of nsP4. These data conflict with other reports that only small amounts of this protein can be detected in wild-type SV infected cells, using monospecific antibodies and that nsP4 seems to be very stable (50). A possible explanation of these contradictory results is the suggestion that the replication of viral RNA at maximal levels requires very low concentrations of nsP4 and any excess is rapidly removed. Studies of these mutants also support a previous suggestion that nsP34, rather than nsP4 alone, is the functional form of the SV RNA polymerase (50, 183). Finally, these investigators observed different growth kinetics and plaquing properties when infection by these mutants was compared in vertebrate and mosquito cells. These differences were most dramatic in the C7–10 clone of *Aedes albopictus* cells during infection by mutants with amber and ochre stop sequences substituted for the opal codon. These mutants exhibited a temperature-sensitive phenotype not manifested in the vertebrate cell types examined in this study. Such results exemplify the differential roles of host components in vertebrate and invertebrate cells.

Host Cell Involvement in Alphavirus Replication

Although at least one function of the nonstructural proteins has been assigned for alphavirus infection in mosquito cells, little more is known about the location or mechanism of formation of the replication complexes in insect cells. Several lines of evidence implicate one or more host cell factors in viral replication in both vertebrate and invertebrate systems and these components are either not identical or do not serve the same functions. An example of this diversity is demonstrated by the establishment of homologous interference. This virus-related phenomenon is defined as the ability of an established viral infection to interfere with the production of superinfecting identical, or closely related virus (18). As determined from studies in alphavirus-infected vertebrate cells, the mechanism of interference appears to function at the level of transcription of the superinfecting virus RNA. Evidence suggests that a limiting host cell component is consumed or occupied as a result of formation of replication complexes containing this host factor, nonstructural proteins, and positive strand viral RNA. The assembly of these complexes is presumed to be induced by the primary infecting virus. This host component is rendered unavailable for replication of the superinfecting genome (2, 18). This condition is established within 15 min in vertebrate cells infected with SV (69). Homologous interference is also established in invertebrate cells and has been demonstrated during both acute and persistent phases of infection (133). However, the mechanism for this response is different not only among the two cell systems, but among clonal isolates of mosquito cells as well. Two cloned cell lines of *Aedes albopictus* establish a partial interference at 10 h after initial infection, whereas a third clone fails to demonstrate any interference throughout the acute phase of infection (18).

Alphavirus infection in mosquito cells is inhibited by the presence of actinomycin D (156), methionine starvation (176), and enucleation (35). Such alterations do not affect virus production in vertebrate cells. These observations, coupled with evidence that host cell macromolecular synthesis, which is shut down early in infection of vertebrate cells (204), continues at normal levels throughout invertebrate infection, imply that certain labile host functions are required throughout the course of alphavirus infection in insect but not in vertebrate cells, necessitating continual expression of the invertebrate host genome.

Sindbis virions produced in vertebrate cells possess glycoproteins composed of both high mannose sugar moieties and complex oligosaccharides containing galactose, fucose, and sialic acid (11, 165, 166). Mosquito cells do not produce the transferases required for addition of these residues to sugar side chains (12, 13, 60), therefore, glycoproteins on virions matured in these cells contain both oligosaccharides which are processed to high mannose forms and side chains composed of the sequence $Man_3GlcNac_2$ in the locations where vertebrate-produced viruses possess complex sugar structures (60). In vertebrate cells, glycoproteins are modified as they are shuttled through the rough endoplasmic reticulum (RER) and Golgi complex en route to the cell surface (164). The location of these enzymatic processing events in *Aedes albopictus* cells is less well defined. Gillies and Stollar (40) established a functional in vitro translating system from the *Aedes albopictus* clone, LT-C7, which translated the 26S mRNA of SV and vesicular stomatitis virus (VSV) mRNA upon addition of human placental ribonuclease inhibitor as the only exogenous component. In the absence of added intracellular membranes, translation of the subgenomic SV message yielded a large precursor protein that was cleaved in vitro to produce capsid protein and the 100K B polypeptide, which contains PE2 and E1. The G glycoprotein of VSV was glycosylated and inserted into microsomal vesicles when intracellular membranes were added to the translation extract, indicating that mosquito cells possess mechanisms for transmembranal translation and processing that function in a manner similar to equivalent processes in vertebrate cells (39).

It is presumed that the role of the oligosaccharides on alphavirus glycoproteins of either cell origin is to confer the proper protein conformation for additional processing and maturation of infectious virions (60, 71). Experiments with drugs that alter glycosylation of viral proteins reveal additional differences between the host responses in the two systems. Addition of deoxynojirimycin (dNM), *N*-methyl-1-deoxynojirimycin (MdN), or castanospermine to SV-infected vertebrate cells inhibited virion formation and prevented the cleavage of PE2 to E2 but did not prevent the migration of the glycoprotein to the cell surface (107, 157). These drugs inhibit glucosidase I, which cleaves glucose residues from high-mannose asparagine-linked sugar side chains in the RER (148, 163, for review of glycosylation, see 61, 85, 100). The presence of dNM failed to prevent PE2 processing or influence virus yield in SFV-infected *Aedes albopictus* cells (117). Deoxymannojirimycin (dMM), which inhibits the function of Golgi-α-mannosidase I (4) affected virus maturation differently in vertebrate cells. PE2 cleavage did occur but McDowell et al. (107) reported from electron microscopic studies that nucleocapsids preferentially budded through internal membranes rather than at the plasma membrane in dMM-treated, SV-infected vertebrate cells. These authors combined the yield of extracellular virus with titers of intracellular particles released after breaking the cells and found no reduction in overall production in the presence of drug. The significance of a preference for budding at internal sites by virions possessing only high-mannose glycoproteins is interesting because viruses also bud frequently through internal membranes in mosquito cells, in which viral glycoproteins contain sugar moieties more closely resembling high-mannose forms. However, Naim and Koblet (117) failed to detect an increase in intracellular budding in SFV-infected *Aedes albopictus* cells treated with this drug. Two laboratories have reported a similar budding phenomenon in vertebrate cells treated with the ionophore monensin (136), which is believed to block transport of envelope glycoproteins in the Golgi vesicles and inhibits PE2 processing. Johnson and Schlesinger (68) reported that viral oligosaccharides were cleaved to an endo-(β)-acetylglucosaminidase- (endo-H) resistant configuration [indicating that the sugar side chains were processed beyond the high-mannose forms recognized as a substrate for this enzyme (193)] in vertebrate cells treated with 1.0 μ*M* monensin. Griffiths et al. (47) observed that viral glycoproteins remained sensitive to endo-H throughout the infection. These latter investigators added a concentration of 10.0 μ*M* of drug to infected cells and such conflicting observations must be regarded with the caution that monensin is an ionophore known to exhibit a variety of effects on cultured cells.

Alphavirus production is inhibited in both cell systems when infected cells are treated with tunicamycin (TM), which prevents all glycosylation by inhibiting the original oligosaccharide addition reaction in the RER (189, 196). PE2 is not processed to E2, yet it is transported to the plasma membrane in TM-treated vertebrate cells infected with SV (95, 155). However, SFV-infected mosquito cells do process PE2 in the presence of TM (117).

To summarize these data, the presence of glucose residues on viral glycoproteins in vertebrate cells appears to prevent the conformation required for proteolytic cleavage of PE2, although these residues do not hinder transport of the protein to the cell surface. The PE2 precursor is processed in infected invertebrate cells even when glucose moieties are retained on the viral glycoproteins. Inhibitory agents that alter the oligosaccharide sequence after removal of glucose in either cell type do not alter the configuration required for PE2 processing, but the absence of all sugar residues renders the protein unrecognizable by the protease responsible for this cleavage.

Naim and Koblet (117) discovered that in mosquito cells, PE2, in the absence of any glycosylation inhibitors, is sensitive to treatment by endo-H. This indicates that this precursor never acquires a more complex sugar composition and is cleaved before the oligosaccharides are processed to endo-H-resistant forms, implying that PE2 is cleaved before migration to, or early in the Golgi apparatus. Similar observations have been documented by Knipfer and Brown (80) from studies of PE2 processing in vertebrate culture. These investigators showed by pulse-chase experiments that an endo-H-sensitive form of PE2 is cleaved to E2 within 5 min and suggest that this processing event may be of viral origin and independent of cellular protein transport.

Several of the investigators who have studied the effects of glycosylation modulators in vertebrate cells have concluded that the proper processing of viral glycoproteins, although not essential to the transport of these proteins through the cell, is critical to the budding of virus. They assume this maturation event is inhibited by the failure to process PE2 to E2, a step which has long been considered vital to alphavirus formation. However, it is apparent from the data on mosquito cells that glycosylation modulators still inhibit maturation even when E2 is produced. In addition, recent reports of the production of infectious virus particles containing PE2 in the viral membrane (135, 146) demonstrate that PE2 cleavage is not essential to maturation in cultured vertebrate cells. However, it may be required for virulence in vivo (146) and for virion assembly in cultured mosquito cells (J.F. Presley et al., unpublished data). Thus, the importance of the oligosaccharide composition with regard to virus function and maturation requires further examination.

Another approach to understanding the differences in host cell participation between vertebrate and invertebrate cells during alphavirus infection has been through isolation of viral mutants restricted for growth in either cell system. Kowal and Stollar (86) described two SV mutants that were restricted in growth at 34°C in mosquito cells but grew normally in chick fibroblasts at this temperature. Studies on the efficiency of plaquing of RNA from these mutants revealed that the defect in these viruses was at a point in infection beyond adsorption. These mutants were also temperature-sensitive in both cell systems and were found to be RNA^- at the respective nonpermissive temperatures. These authors suggest that activation of the viral RNA polymerase requires binding of a host subunit and the lesion in these viruses affects this binding reaction. The host components in the two cell systems are sufficiently different that the requisite binding of this agent is impaired in vertebrate cells but not in mosquito cells.

A mutant of SV that is restricted in growth only in vertebrate cells has also been identified (28). The mutation in this virus introduces an additional glycosylation site on the PE2 glycoprotein. This mutant, designated $SV_{ap15/21}$, has been assigned to complementation group E, which also includes the temperature-sensitive SV mutant, *ts*20, which contains a defective PE2 sequence that fails to be processed at nonpermissive temperatures (172). Electron micrographs of vertebrate cells infected with either *ts*20 or $SV_{ap15/21}$ reveal an accumulation of nucleocapsids on the cytoplasmic face of the plasma membrane with no evidence of virus budding from the cell. However, in $SV_{ap15/21}$-infected cells, PE2 is processed to E2 and viral glycoproteins are transported to the cell surface, yet virus maturation is still inhibited. These data lend additional support to the developing notion that maturation is not dependent upon the cleavage of PE2. Processing of this viral precursor without subsequent assembly and release of virus has been documented in invertebrate cells (117) and has now been demonstrated in a vertebrate cell system. Durbin and Stollar propose that because of the differences in glycosylation of viral glycoproteins in vertebrate and invertebrate cells, the additional sugar side chain on $SV_{ap15/21}$ does not obstruct maturation of virus in mosquito cells but is prohibitive to virus formation in vertebrate cells.

Stollar's group has isolated a third type of host-restricted mutant (178). Two temperature-sensitive SV mutants that fail to replicate in *Aedes albopictus* cells at 34°C grow to normal titres in five species of intact mosquito following intrathoracic inoculation and incubation within a temperature range of 28° to 34°C. Thus the viral defect that inhibits infection in insect cells in vitro fails to be expressed in whole insects, underscoring the caution in extrapolating data from cell culture systems to processes in the intact organism.

Application of Molecular Genetics to Alphavirus Research

Molecular genetic approaches to understanding virus infection have provided considerable insight into how alphaviruses replicate in host cells. Recombinant DNA technology has been employed to study the expression and transport of the structural proteins of SFV in vertebrate cells in the absence of other viral components (22, 23, 37, 83, 84, 144). These investigators introduced cDNA containing the sequences for the viral structural proteins into the nuclei of host cells via microinjection and calcium phosphate uptake. Rice, Franke, Strauss, and Hruby (141) established successful expression of the SV structural proteins through infection of several vertebrate cell lines with a recombinant vaccinia virus containing the SV sequences. The same virus expression vector was employed to produce SV capsid, E1, and PE2/E2 in *Aedes albopictus* cells (36), demonstrating the successful expression of eukaryotic genetic information in invertebrate cells.

Investigators in the Strauss laboratory have used these techniques for examining the functions of the nontranslated regions of SV. There are four untranslated regions on the alphavirus genome that are highly conserved among all members and are presumed to participate in virus replication. At the 3′ end of the genome adjacent to the polyA tail, there is a conserved sequence of 19 nucleotides that may be a promoter for initiation of synthesis of minus strands (128). At the junction of the genomic regions that encode the nonstructural and structural proteins lies another conserved sequence composed of 21 nucleotides that contains the initiation site for the subgenomic message. A stem-and-loop structure is conserved at the extreme 5′ end of the genome, which is postulated to function as the promoter for initiation of synthesis of positive strands (127). The fourth conserved region consists of 51 nucleotides located within the gene for nsP1. Although no function has been identified for this sequence, defective interfering particles that lack this segment show reduced replication efficiency (187).

Kuhn, Hong, and Strauss (87) produced a battery of SV mutants with site-specific alterations within the 3′ nontranslated region of the genome, most of which mapped within the 19-nucleotide-conserved sequence. These investigators found that growth was hindered for almost all of the mutants and the impairment was more severe in mosquito cells than in vertebrate cells in most cases. However, growth parameters of a few of the mutants exceeded those of wild-type virus in both cell systems. The conclusions drawn from this study indicate that the entire 3′ nontranslated region is essential for efficient virus replication, although some variability of the conformation of the region is tolerated. Also, the differential host responses implicate the interaction of host components during replication and suggest that alphavirus genomes that are found in nature represent a compromise between sequences that allow for optimal replication in vertebrate and invertebrate hosts.

Niesters et al. (119) used the same genetic approach to examine the function of the 51-nucleotide-conserved sequence contained within the nsP1 coding sequence of the SV genome. This group produced 25 mutants with site-specific lesions within this region, which is known to be capable of forming two hairpin structures. Most of the mutations were silent and did not alter any amino acids but did change the linear sequence and the stability of the hairpin structures. Almost all of the silent mutants grew more slowly in mosquito cells than in chicken cells and produced lower titres. Two of the mutants produced virus more efficiently than did the wild-type virus in mosquito cells, prompting the same interpretation, that the sequence found in this region represents a compromise, facilitating successful cycling of this virus through animal and insect hosts. Alterations in the efficiency of viral replication in cells infected with these mutants indicate that components encoded by either the virus or the host cell bind to this hairpin region in a sequence-specific fashion that promotes viral RNA replication.

Alphavirus Morphogenesis and Cytopathic Response

The most distinguishing feature of alphavirus replication in vertebrate and invertebrate cells involves viral morphogenesis and cytopathic response. Hallmarks of the infection in vertebrate cells are the production of nucleocapsids in the cytoplasm and maturation of virions by budding through the plasma membrane, with subsequent cell destruction and death (1, 96, 139, 204). Studies of alphavirus infection in the original heterogeneous populations of Singh's *Aedes albopictus* line indicate that these cells lapse into a persistently infected state after an acute phase of virus production without obvious cytopathic effect (26, 130, 140, 175). Ultrastructural examination of viral infection in these mixed populations reveals a variety of mechanisms for virus maturation in these cells. Raghow et al. (138, 139) examined the morphogenesis of two alphaviruses, Ross River virus and SFV and concluded that maturation of virus by budding through the plasma membrane was the primary route for production of infectious progeny. A study of SV infection by Stollar, Harrap, Thomas, and Sarver (179) provided evidence that, in addition to acquiring membranes at the cell surface, virions also matured intracellularly by budding through membrane-bounded vesicles within infected cells. These investigators proposed that these internally matured viruses are released by reverse phagocytosis, based on observations that these virus-laden vesicles were often located proximal to the cell surface and were occasionally seen with membranes that appeared to be contiguous with the plasma membrane.

Many clones have been derived from Singh's original *Aedes albopictus* population which show various degrees of cytopathic effect upon infection by alphaviruses. Tooker and Kennedy (197) examined 115 clonal isolates and discovered that the degree of cytopathology correlated directly with virus yield, viral RNA synthesis, and shutdown of host functions, whereas Sarver and Stollar (147) failed to detect such a direct relationship in the clones isolated in their laboratory. These latter investigators did observe an increase in viral RNA synthesis in cells that demonstrated cytopathic effect (CPE) and determined that this response was variable within a given cloned cell line with respect to media conditions and temperature (179). Tatem and Stollar (194) showed that the phenotype for CPE dominates in cell fusion studies between CPE+ and CPE− cells.

Two clonal isolates have been examined at the electron microscope level and reported in the literature. Simizu and Maeda (169) describe the ultrastructural features of Western equine encephalitis virus (WEE) infection in C6/36 cells (62) but do not illustrate temporal morphogenesis and offer little interpretation of the mechanism of virus release from these cells. Gliedman et al. (41) detailed the time sequence of SV infection in cells, which they refer to as *Aedes albopictus* cells, that represent a subcloned cell line later designated u4.4. These authors observed that virus maturation appears to occur almost exclusively within membrane-bounded structures inside the cells and infectious progeny are apparently released by reverse phagocytosis. No significant amount of budding of virions through the plasma membrane was observed in these cells.

Three subcloned cell lines, each of which exhibit a degree of cytopathology directly related to the amount of virus they produce, (under infection conditions of incubation at 28°C, in MEM medium containing 10% FCS) have been extensively studied at the ultrastructural level to define differences in morphogenesis of SV that correlate with variations in CPE during infection (M.L. Miller and D.T. Brown, unpublished data). These three cell lines, consisting of the u4.4 and C6/36 lines previously mentioned and another subclone, C7–10 (194) respond uniquely with respect to such virus-associated phenomena as homologous interference (18), actinomycin D treatment (17), and production of and response to an antiviral factor (AVF) (19). Such variations suggest that these cultures may contain cells that have undergone some degree of differentiation and represent different cell types which exist in the whole mosquito. SV morphogenesis in these three subcloned lines was examined ultrastructurally at various time points throughout the acute phase of infection until 5 days postinfection.

Features of the infection in u4.4 cells are similar to those reported by Gliedman et al. (41) with the exception that virus production was apparent in only a small number of cells despite the fact that extracellular yields of virus from these cultures ranged from 10^8 to 10^9 plaque-forming units (PFU)/ml of medium. Also, vesicular structures containing membranous strands were observed in mock-infected as well as in infected u4.4 cells, implying that these structures are not unique to the presence of an alphavirus, as was alluded to by these authors. The morphogenetic features of SV infection were found to be similar in C6/36 and C7–10 cells although the latter cells appeared qualitatively to contain more nucleocapsids and virus particles, which correlates with the tendency for these cells to release slightly higher titres of virus than C6/36 cells. In both cell types, virions were observed budding through the plasma membrane and through internal membranes into vesicles, with ultimate release of the contents through exocytosis (Fig. 5.1). Nucleocapsids were detected in the cytoplasm and embedded in amorphous, electron-dense matrices, which appeared to be the only structures unique to the presence of virus (Figs. 5.2, 5.3).

These studies indicate that among cell clones derived from a single parental *Aedes albopictus* population, the host response varies significantly and some cell types are better adapted to restrict the process of virus replication and thus avoid the deleterious effects of a cytopathic response.

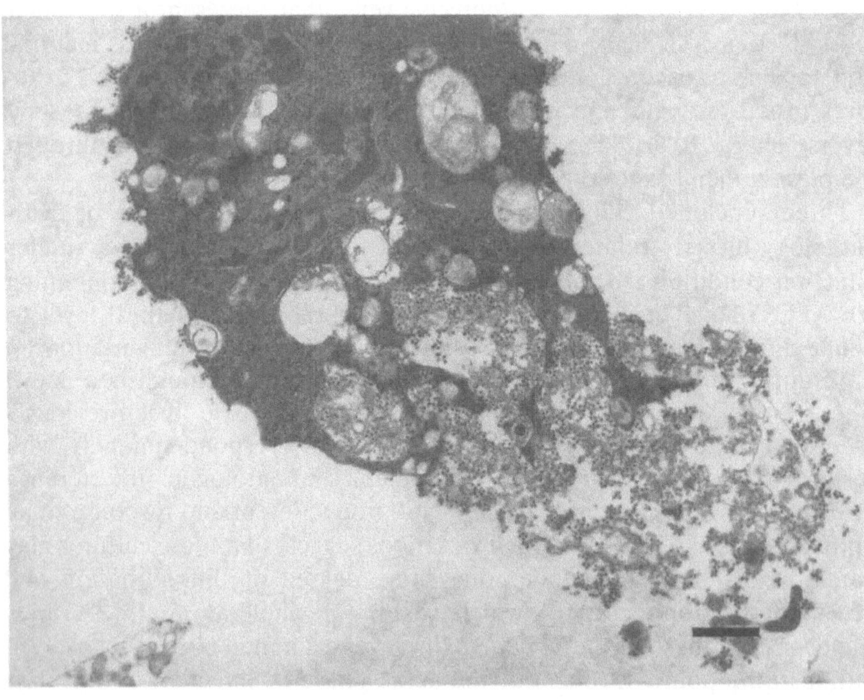

FIGURE 5.1. Exocytosis of Sindbis virus from a C7–10 mosquito cell. Nucleocapsids bud through the membranes of intracellular vesicles and accumulate as mature particles. The membranes of the vesicles fuse with one another and the plasma membrane, opening channels through which the virions are released from the cell. Scale bar = 1 μM.

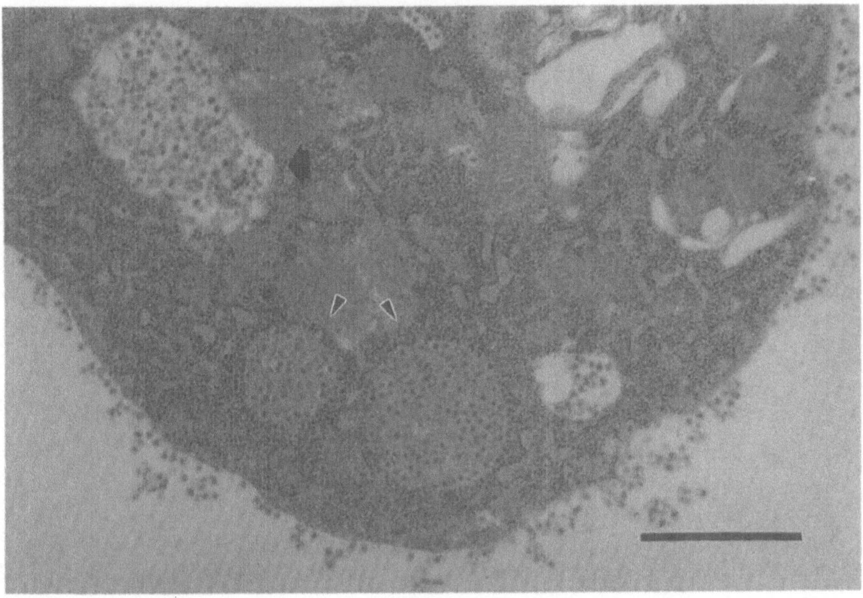

FIGURE 5.2. C7–10 mosquito cell at 36 h postinfection. Nucleocapsids are embedded in an amorphous, electron-dense matrix in the cytoplasm (arrowheads) and budding virions are evident at numerous sites along the cell surface. Enveloped particles accumulate in internal vesicles (wide arrow) and are ultimately released from the cell by exocytosis. Scale bar = 1 μ*M*.

Such differences may reflect similar variations among certain tissues in the whole insect with respect to whether they are resistant or susceptible to alphavirus infection. The earliest electron microscope studies on alphavirus infection in intact mosquitoes failed to show evidence of any cytopathological response to the presence of virus (93, 201, 208). Weaver, Scott, Lorenz, Lerdthusnee, Romoser (202) have since reported cytopathological lesions in the midgut of the mosquito, *Culiseta melanura* in response to oral infection with eastern equine encephalomyelitis virus (EEE). The observation that certain cell types show cytopathology upon infection with alphaviruses in both in vitro and in vivo systems may provide insight into the mechanisms that restrict the host range of many viruses to one or at most, very few insect species.

Persistent Infection by Alphaviruses in Mosquito Cells

Alphavirus infection in mosquito cell culture progresses from an acute phase, which lasts several days after virus is introduced and is characterized by the release of high titres of infectious particles, to a persistently infected

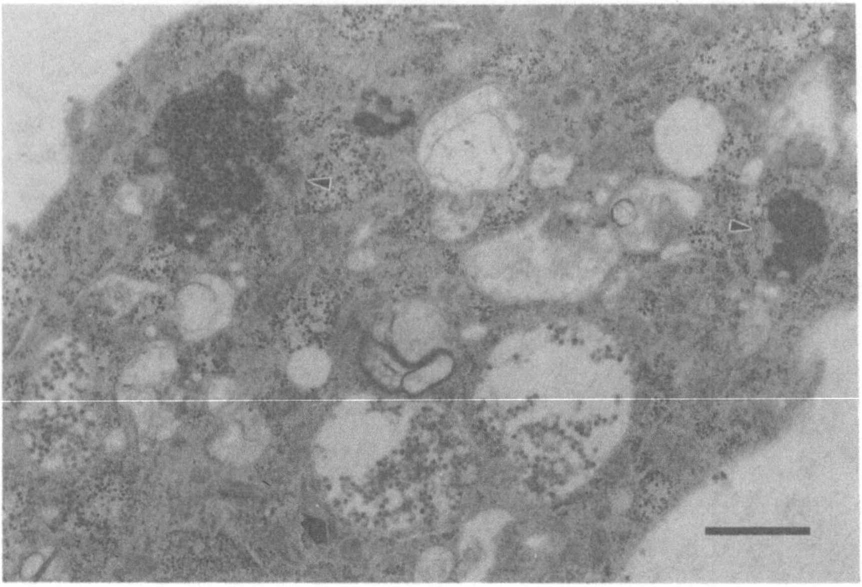

FIGURE 5.3. C7–10 mosquito cell at five days postinfection. Nucleocapsids are localized in amorphous, electron-dense regions (arrowheads) and are interspersed throughout the cytoplasm in greater numbers than observed at earlier infection points. This cell contains vesicles filled with mature virus particles (wide arrow) and shows fewer nucleocapsids budding through the plasma membrane. Scale bar = 1 μM.

or chronic state of infection. During this latter phase, viral protein and RNA synthesis shut down and virus production becomes limited to approximately 2% of the cell population (24, 66, 130, 140, 142). The persistent state is also defined by the feature that, regardless of the amount of cytopathic effect a given cell line exhibits during the acute infection, the cells become indistinguishable from uninfected cell populations (Fig. 5.4). The establishment of the persistent state has been the topic of considerable investigation and several phenomena have been associated with its development. These include small plaque variants, homologous interference, antiviral activity, and defective interfering (DI) particles (for review, see 6).

Small plaque variants can be detected in the media of infected mosquito cells within a few days of inoculation with a virus and dominate the extracellular milieu by 8 to 9 days postinfection (24, 31, 167). The role of these variants in establishing the persistently infected state is not clear although the presence of these mutants does appear to affect the establishment of homologous interference. In *Aedes aegypti* cells adapted to growth at 15°C, titres of SV released from these cells failed to drop to levels

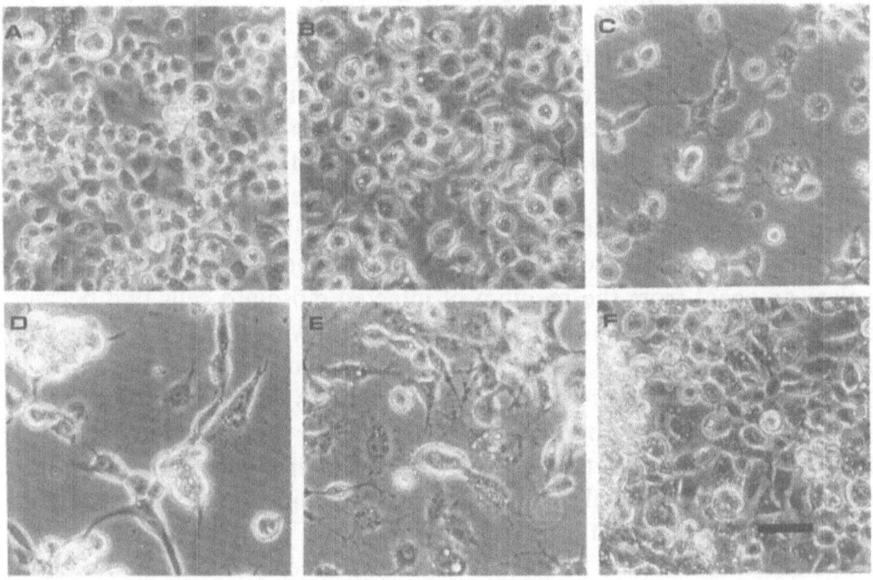

FIGURE 5.4. Cytopathic response and recovery from acute infection in C7–10 cells. A, Mock-infected C7–10 cells at day 0 of infection. B–F, C7–10 cells at days 1 through 5 of Sindbis virus infection. Cells demonstrate the most severe CPE at day 3 (D) and recover completely by day 5 (F). Scale bar = 10 μ*M*.

characteristic of the persistent state over a 130-day test period, and plaque morphology remained constant as well. These cells did not exhibit the ability to exclude the superinfecting homologous virus except under certain conditions when the preadapted cultures were preinoculated with a small plaque-forming variant of SV (132).

Eaton (30) demonstrated that uncloned *Aedes albopictus* cells infected with SV become refractory to infection by all alphaviruses at approximately 3 days postinfection but remain susceptible to a separate family of viruses (Bunyaviridae). Heterologous interference to alphaviruses persists for 8 days after which infection can be initiated but yields of the superinfecting virus are significantly reduced and only 8% to 10% of the persistently infected population shows capability of supporting heterologous virus replication. Eaton determined that both heterologous and homologous interference were established within 1 h following infection in these cells and that the population remained resistant to homologous superinfection indefinitely. Condreay and Brown (18) examined the establishment of homologous interference in the three subcloned *Aedes albopictus* cell lines u4.4, C6/36, and C7–10. These investigators observed that the latter two cell populations demonstrated this phenomenon by 10 h postinfection, which was manifested by complete interference against superinfecting homologous virus in C7–10 cells by 24 h postinfection and incomplete interference at the same time point in C6/36 cells. The third cloned population, u4.4, failed to exhibited interference at any time during the acute or early persistent stages of infection. This study was initially carried out to compare the establishment of homologous interference to the antiviral activity also associated with the transition of alphavirus-infected cells from the acute to the persistently infected state. The production of an antiviral compound in cells infected with SV was first documented by Riedel and Brown (143). These authors were able to isolate an agent from the medium of infected mosquito cells that became detectable at 48 to 72 h postinfection. This agent was found to be virus- and cell-specific, which are characteristics of a similar substance produced in SFV-infected *Aedes albopictus* cells (118). It was determined that in u4.4 cells, replication of a superinfecting virus genome was inhibited only when antiviral activity was detected. This type of interference requires a 48 h pretreatment of the cells with medium containing the agent, does not require initial infection, and does not occur in C7–10 cells. These investigators concluded that the inhibitory mechanism of homologous interference differs from the mechanism of antiviral activity. Further studies on the antiviral agent have revealed that this protein specifically inhibits synthesis of all viral RNA species in a temporal fashion, providing additional evidence that host cell participation in viral replication is variable among mosquito cell types (19).

One phenomenon implicated in the establishment of persistent infection in mosquito cells is the generation of defective interfering particles. These viral agents are defined as truncated genomic sequences that accumulate after repeated passage of virus in cultured cells. These mutants are distinguished by their ability to specifically interfere with replication of infectious virions in cells containing homologous or closely related viruses. These abbreviated RNA strands outcompete full-length genomes for access to the limited sites available for replication in the cell and are overproduced relative to other viral RNA sequences. DI particles have been well characterized in vertebrate cell infections (for review, see 59, 158, 160). Recombinant DNA applications have transformed these truncated viral sequences into valuable tools for localizing the genomic regions necessary for replication and encapsidation of viral RNA (99, 198, 203). These particles have also been employed in the delivery of foreign genomic sequences into target cells (98).

It is unclear whether DI particles function in establishing persistent infection in invertebrate cells. The presence of abbreviated genomes in alphavirus-infected mosquito cells has been documented as early as 24 h postinfection (173, 197) but particles are not detectable in the medium, suggesting that the defective RNAs fail to be encapsidated. Other investigators have found virus particles which are smaller than normal virions (7) and DI particles released into the medium (31, 78), but the appearance of these agents does not correlate with the establishment of persistence. Also, DI particles produced in chicken or hamster cells fail to be expressed in *Aedes albopictus* cells (67). Steacie & Eaton (174) have reported that certain DI particles generated in mosquito cells do not replicate in vertebrate cells. These studies indicate that DI particles may serve some virus-modulating role in certain types of invertebrate cells but function by a mechanism different than that demonstrated in vertebrate cell infections.

Conclusion

The availability of mosquito cell cultures has greatly facilitated the study of how pathogenic viruses multiply in insect tissues without apparent injury to the vector host. Insect cell lines have also proven useful for the isolation and characterization of viruses from natural sources and for differentiation between arboviruses and nonvectored viruses (64, 70, 94). Through continuous cultivation of viruses in mosquito cells, changes in the properties of viruses can be monitored, large quantities of virus can be produced, and attenuated virus strains can be established for vaccine production (131, 134).

At the cellular and molecular level, many questions remain unanswered with regard to how viruses replicate in insect cells. How do viruses gain access to the cell's interior? Where do replication complexes form and what host factors are involved in viral protein translation? What effect does glycosylation have on the processing of viral proteins into mature infectious virions? Why do certain cell types exhibit dramatic CPE, whereas other cell types demonstrate none? What are the mechanisms for establishing the persistently infected state?

A great deal of information is available regarding alphavirus infection in vertebrate cells in culture although there is still much to be learned. Features of infection within these cells, such as viral entry, replication of the viral genome, and processing of viral glycoproteins, have been examined extensively and have provided insight on both viral and cellular processes. Recombinant DNA technology has allowed for a better understanding of the mechanisms for viral replication and for studies of individual viral proteins as models for cellular protein processing mechanisms. Identification of the host cell factors that participate in alphavirus replication and assembly will further enhance understanding of virus infection in cultured vertebrate cells.

Molecular genetic applications and studies of cell mutants with phenotypes restrictive for virus infection are valuable technological tools for defining host cell involvement in insect culture as well. These techniques need to be applied to invertebrate cell systems to understand the mechanisms of cytopathic response and persistence. Also, matching of cloned mosquito cell lines with corresponding cell types in the adult insect is necessary to characterize the features of a cell that render it susceptible to virus infection. Once the factors that restrict or enhance virus infection in various mosquito cell types are defined, new methods for eradication of vectored viral pathogens can be developed to eliminate these agents as health hazards worldwide.

References

1. Acheson, N.H., and Tamm, I., 1967, Replication of Semliki Forest virus: An electron microscopic study, *Virology* **32**:128–143.
2. Adams, R., and Brown, D.T., 1985, BHK cells expressing Sindbis virus-induced homologous interference allow the translation of nonstructural genes of superinfecting virus, *J. Virol.* **54**:351–357.
3. Birdwell, C.R., and Strauss, J.H., 1974, Distribution of the receptor sites for Sindbis virus on the surface of chicken and BHK cells, *J. Virol.* **14**: 672–678.
4. Bischoff, J., and Kornfeld, R., 1984, The effect of 1-deoxymannojirimycin on rat liver α-mannosidases, *Biochem. Biophys. Res. Commun.* **125**:324–331.
5. Boggs, W.M., Hahn, C.S., Strauss, E.G., and Strauss, J.H., 1989, Low pH-dependent Sindbis virus-induced fusion of BHK cells: Differences between strains correlate with amino acid changes in the E1 glycoprotein, *Virology* **169**:485–488.
6. Brown, D.T., and Condreay, L.D., 1986, Replication of alphaviruses in mosquito cells, in The Togaviridae and Flaviviridae, Schlesinger, S., and Schlesinger, M.J. (eds): Plenum Press, New York, pp. 171–207.
7. Brown, D.T., and Gliedman, J., 1973, Morphological variants of Sindbis virus obtained from infected mosquito tissue culture cells, *J. Virol.* **12**:1534–1539.
8. Brown, S.E., and Knudson, D.L., 1987, Characterization and identification of arthropod cell lines, Yunker, C.E. (ed): in Arboviruses in Arthropod Cells in vitro, Vol. I, CRC Press, Inc., Boca Raton, Florida, pp. 53–65.
9. Burge, B.W., and Pfefferkorn, E.R., 1966, Complementation between temperature-sensitive mutants of Sindbis virus, *Virology* **30**:214–223.
10. Burge, B.W., and Pfefferkorn, E.R., 1966, Isolation and characterization of conditional-lethal mutants of Sindbis virus, *Virology* **30**:204–213.
11. Burke, D.J., and Keegstra, K., 1979, Carbohydrate structure of Sindbis virus glycoprotein E2 from virus grown in hamster and chicken cells, *J. Virol.* **29**: 546–554.
12. Butters, T.D., and Hughes, R.C., 1981, Isolation and characterization of mosquito cell membrane glycoproteins, *Biochim. Biophys. Acta.* **640**:655–671.
13. Butters, T.D., Hughes, R.C., and Vischer, P., 1981, Steps in the biosynthesis of mosquito cell membrane glycoproteins and the effects of tunicamycin, *Biochim. Biophys. Acta.* **640**:672–686.
14. Cassell, S., Edwards, J., and Brown, D.T., 1984, Effects of lysosomotropic weak bases on infection of BHK-21 cells by Sindbis virus, *J. Virol.* **52**: 857–864.

15. Chanas, A.C., Gould, E.A., Clegg, J.C.S., and Varma, M.G.R., 1982, Monoclonal antibodies to Sindbis virus glycoprotein E1 can neutralize, enhance infectivity, and independently inhibit haemagglutination or haemolysis, *J. Gen. Virol.* **58**:37–49.
16. Clayton, R.B., 1964, The utilization of sterols by insects, *J. Lipid Res.* **5**: 3–19.
17. Condreay, L.D., Adams, R.H., Edwards, J., and Brown, D.T., 1988, Effect of Actinonycin D and cycloheximide on replication of Sindbis virus in *Aedes albopictus* (mosquito) cells, *J. Virol.* **62**:2629–2635.
18. Condreay, L.D., and Brown, D.T., 1986, Exclusion of superinfecting homologous virus by Sindbis virus-infected *Aedes albopictus* (mosquito) cells, *J. Virol.* **58**:81–86.
19. Condreay, L.D., and Brown, D.T., 1988, Suppression of RNA synthesis by a specific antiviral activity in Sindbis virus-infected *Aedes albopictus* cells, *J. Virol.* **62**:346–348.
20. Coombs, K., Mann, E., Edwards, J., and Brown, D.T., 1981, Effects of chloroquine and cytochalasin B on the infection of cells by Sindbis virus and vesicular stomatitis virus, *J. Virol.* **37**:1060–1065.
21. Cunningham, A., Buckley, S.M., Casals, J., and Webb, S.R., 1975, Isolation of chikungunya virus contaminating an *Aedes albopictus* cell line, *J. Gen. Virol.* **27**:97–100.
22. Cutler, D.F., and Garoff, H., 1986, Mutants of the membrane-binding region of Semliki Forest virus E2 protein. I. Cell surface transport and fusogenic activity, *J. Cell Biol.* **102**:889–901.
23. Cutler, D.F., Melancon, P., and Garoff, H., 1986, Mutants of the membrane-binding region of Semliki Forest virus E2 protein. II. Topology and membrane binding, *J. Cell Biol.* **102**:902–910.
24. Davey, M.W., and Dalgarno, L., 1974, Semliki Forest virus replication in cultured *Aedes albopictus* cells: Studies on the establishment of persistence, *J. Gen. Virol.* **24**:453–463.
25. Davey, M.W., Mahon, R.J., and Gibbs, A.J., 1979, Togavirus interference in *Culex annulirostris* mosquitoes, *J. Gen. Virol.* **42**:641–643.
26. Davey, M.W., Dennett, D.P., and Dalgarno, L., 1973, The growth of two togaviruses in cultured mosquito and vertebrate cells, *J. Gen. Virol.* **20**: 225–232.
27. Ding, M., and Schlesinger, M.J., 1989, Evidence that Sindbis virus nsP2 is an autoprotease which processes the virus nonstructural polyprotein, *Virology* **171**:280–284.
28. Durbin, R.K., and Stollar, V., 1984, A mutant of Sindbis virus with a host-dependent defect in maturation associated with hyperglycosylation of E2, *Virology* **135**:331–344.
29. Eagle, H., 1959, Amino acid metabolism in mammalian cell cultures, *Science* **130**:432–437.
30. Eaton, B.T., 1979, Heterologous interference in *Aedes albopictus* cells infected with alphaviruses, *J. Virol.* **30**:45–55.
31. Eaton, B.T., 1981, Viral interference and persistence in Sindbis virus infected *Aedes albopictus* cells, *Can. J. Microbiol.* **27**:563–567.
32. Eaton, B.T., and Regnery, R.L., 1975, Polysomal RNA in Semliki Forest virus infected *Aedes albopictus* cells, *J. Gen. Virol.* **29**:35–49.

33. Edwards, J., and Brown, D.T., 1986, Sindbis virus-mediated fusion from without is a two-step event, *J. Gen. Virol.* **67**:377–380.
34. Edwards, J., Mann, E., and Brown, D.T., 1983, Conformational changes in Sindbis virus envelope proteins accompanying exposure to low pH, *J. Virol.* **45**:1090–1097.
35. Erwin, C., and Brown, D.T., 1983, Requirement of cell nucleus for Sindbis virus replication in cultured *Aedes albopictus* cells, *J. Virol.* **45**:792–799.
36. Franke, C.A., and Hruby, D.E., 1985, Expression of recombinant vaccinia virus-derived alphavirus proteins in mosquito cells, *J. Gen. Virol.* **66**:2761–2765.
37. Garoff, H., Kondor-Koch, C., Petterson, R., and Burke, B., 1983, Expression of Semliki Forest virus proteins from cloned complementary DNA. II. The membrane-spanning glycoprotein E2 is transported to the cell surface without its normal cytoplasmic domain, *J. Cell Biol.* **97**:652–658.
38. Garoff, H., Kondor-Koch, C., and Riedel, H., 1982, Structure and assembly of alpha viruses, *Curr. Top. Microbiol. Immunol.* **99**:1–50.
39. Garoff, H., Simons, K., and Dobberstein, B., 1978, Assembly of the Semliki Forest virus membrane glycoproteins in the membrane of the endoplasmic reticulum in vitro, *J. Mol. Biol.* **124**:587–600.
40. Gillies, S., and Stollar, V., 1981, Translation of vesicular stomatitis and Sindbis virus mRNAs in cell-free extracts of *Aedes albopictus* cells, *J. Biol. Chem.* **256**:13188–13192.
41. Gliedman, J.B., Smith, J.F., and Brown, D.T., 1975, Morphogenesis of Sindbis virus in cultured *Aedes albopictus* cells, *J. Virol.* **16**:913–926.
42. Gorziglia, M., Botero, L., Gil, F., and Esparza, J., 1980, Preliminary characterization of virus-like particles in a mosquito (*Aedes pseudocutellaris*) cell line (Mos. 61), *Intervirology* **13**:232–240.
43. Grace, T.D.C., 1966, Establishment of a line of mosquito (*Aedes aegypti* L.) cells grown in vitro, *Nature* **211**:366–367.
44. Grace, T.D.C., 1982, Development of insect cell culture, Maramorosch, K., and Mitsuhashi, J. (eds): in Invertebrate Cell Culture Applications, Academic Press, Inc., New York, pp. 1–8.
45. Greene, A.E., and Charney, J., 1971, Characterization and identification of insect cell cultures, *Curr. Top. Microbiol. Immunol.* **55**:51–61.
46. Greene, A.F., Charney, J., Nichols, W.W., and Coriell, L.L., 1972, Species identity of insect cell lines, *In Vitro* **7**:313–322.
47. Griffiths, G., Quinn, P., and Warren, G., 1983, Dissection of the Golgi complex. I. Monensin inhibits the transport of viral membrane proteins from medial to trans Golgi cisternae in baby hamster kidney cells infected with Semliki Forest virus, *J. Cell Biol.* **96**:835–850.
48. Hahn, S., Grakoui, A., Rice, C.M., Strauss, E.G., and Strauss, J.H., 1989, Mapping of RNA^- temperature-sensitive mutants of Sindbis virus: Complementation group F mutants have lesions in nsP4, *J. Virol.* **63**:1194–1202.
49. Hahn, Y.S., Strauss, E.G., and Strauss, J.H., 1989, Mapping of RNA^- temperature-sensitive mutants of Sindbis virus: Assignment of complementation groups A, B, and G to nonstructural proteins, *J. Virol.* **63**:3142–3150.
50. Hardy, W.R., and Strauss, J.H., 1988, Processing the nonstructural polyproteins of Sindbis virus: Study of the kinetics in vivo by using monospecific antibodies, *J. Virol.* **62**:998–1007.

51. Haywood, A.M., and Boyer, B.P., 1985, Fusion of influenza virus membranes with liposomes at pH 7.5, *Proc. Natl. Acad. Sci. USA.* **82**:4611–4617.
52. Helenius, A., Kartenbeck, J., Simons, K., and Fries, F., 1980, On the entry of Semliki Forest virus into BHK-21 cells, *J. Cell Biol.* **84**:404–420.
53. Helenius, A., Marsh, M., and White, J., 1982, Inhibition of Semliki Forest virus penetration by lysosomotropic weak bases, *J. Gen. Virol.* **58**:47–61.
54. Helenius, A., Morrin, B., Fries, E., Simons, K., Robinson, P., Schirrmacher, V., Terhorst, C., and Strominger, J.L., 1978, Human (HLA-A and HLA-B) and murine (H-2K and H-2D) histocompatibility antigens are cell surface receptors for Semliki Forest virus, *Proc. Nat. Acad. Sci. USA.* **75**:3846–3850.
55. Hink, W.F., and Bezanson, D.R., 1985, Invertebrate cell culture media and cell lines, Kurstak, E. (ed): in Techniques in the Life Sciences, C1. Techniques in Setting Up and Maintenance of Tissue and Cell Cultures, Vol. C111, Elsevier Scientific Publishers, Ltd., New York, pp. 1–30.
56. Hirumi, H., 1976, Viral, microbial, and extrinsic cell contamination of insect cell cultures, Maramorosch, K. (ed): in Invertebrate Tissue Culture. Research Applications, Academic Press, Inc., New York, pp. 233–268.
57. Hirumi, H., Hirumi, K., and Speyer, G., 1976, Further studies on the latent viruses isolated from Singh's *Aedes albopictus* cell line, Kurstak, E., and Maramorosch, K. (eds): in Invertebrate Tissue Culture. Applications in Medicine, Biology, and Agriculture, Academic Press, New York, pp. 69–76.
58. Hirumi, H., Hirumi, K., Speyer, G., Yunker, C.E., Thomas, L.A., Cory, J., and Sweet, B.H., 1976, Viral contamination of a mosquito cell line, *Aedes albopictus*, associated with syncytium formation, *In Vitro* **12**:83–97.
59. Holland, J.J., Kennedy, S.I.T., Semler, B.L., Jones, C.L., Roux, L., and Grabau, E.A., 1980, Defective interfering RNA viruses and host-cell response, Frankel-Conrat, H., and Wagner, R.R. (eds): in Comprehensive Virology, Vol. 16, Plenum Press, New York, pp. 137–192.
60. Hsieh, P., Robbins, P.W., 1984, Regulation of asparagine-linked oligosaccharide processing. Oligosaccharide processing in *Aedes albopictus* mosquito cells, *J. Biol. Chem.* **259**:2375–2382.
61. Hubbard, S.C., Ivatt, R.J., 1981, Synthesis and processing of asparagine-linked oligosaccharides, *Annu. Rev. Biochem.* **50**:555–583.
62. Igarashi, A., 1978, Isolation of a Singh's *Aedes albopictus* cell clone sensitive to Dengue and Chikungunya viruses, *J. Gen. Virol.* **40**:531–544.
63. Igarashi, A., 1979, A mutant of chikungunya virus isolated from a line of Singh's *Aedes albopictus* cells by plaque formation on virus-sensitive cloned cells obtained from another Singh's *Aedes albopictus* cell line, *Virology* **98**: 385–392.
64. Igarashi, A., 1987, Application of *Aedes albopictus* clone C6/36 cells to the isolation of mosquito-borne togaviruses in Japan, Indonesia, and Thailand, Yunker, C.E. (ed): in Arboviruses in Arthropod Cells in vitro, Vol. I, CRC Press, Inc., Boca Raton, Florida, pp. 103–114.
65. Igarashi, A., 1988, Adaptation of *Aedes albopictus* clone C6/36 cells to serum free growth medium, Kuroda, Y., Kurstak, E., and Maramorosch, K. (eds): in Invertebrate and Fish Tissue Culture, Japan Scientific Societies Press, Tokyo, p. 28.
66. Igarashi, A., Koo, R., and Stollar, V., 1977, Evolution and properties of *Aedes albopictus* cell cultures persistently infected with Sindbis virus, *Virology* **82**:69–83.

67. Igarashi, A., and Stollar, V., 1976, Failure of defective interfering particles of Sindbis virus produced in BHK or chicken cells to affect viral replication in *Aedes albopictus* cells, *J. Virol.* **19**:393–408.
68. Johnson, D.C., and Schlesinger, M.J., 1980, Vesicular stomatitis virus and Sindbis virus glycoprotein transport to the cell surface is inhibited by ionophores, *Virology* **103**:407–424.
69. Johnston, R.E., Wan, K., and Bose, H.R., Jr., 1974, Homologous interference induced by Sindbis virus, *J. Virol.* **14**:1076–1082.
70. Jozan, M., 1987, Of arboviruses, arthropods and arthropod cell cultures: History and expectations, Yunker, C.E. (ed): in Arboviruses in Arthropod Cells in vitro, Vol. I, CRC Press, Inc., Boca Raton, Florida, pp. 3–22.
71. Kaluza, G., Rott, R., Schwarz, R.T., 1980, Carbohydrate-induced conformational changes of Semliki Forest virus glycoproteins determine antigenicity, *Virology* **102**:286–299.
72. Kempf, C., Kohler, U., Michel, M.R., and Koblet, H., 1987, Semliki Forest virus-induced polykaryocyte formation is an ATP-dependent event, *Arch. Virol.* **95**:111–122.
73. Kempf, C., Michel, M.R., Kohler, U., and Koblet, H., 1987, A novel method for the detection of early events in cell-cell fusion of Semliki Forest virus infected cells growing in monolayer cultures, *Arch. Virol.* **95**:283–289.
74. Kempf, C., Michel, M.R., Kohler, U., and Koblet, H., 1988, Exposure of Semliki Forest virus-infected baby hamster kidney cells to low pH leads to a proton influx and a rapid depletion of intracellular ATP which in turn prevents cell-cell fusion, *Arch. Virol.* **99**:111–115.
75. Keränen, S., and Kääriäinen, L., 1979, Functional defects of RNA negative *ts* mutants of Sindbis and Semliki Forest viruses, *J. Virol.* **32**:19–29.
76. Kielian, M., and Helenius, A., 1984, Role of cholesterol in fusion of Semliki Forest virus with membranes, *J. Virol.* **52**:281–283.
77. Kielian, M., and Helenius, A., 1985, pH-induced alterations in the fusogenic spike protein of Semliki Forest virus, *J. Cell Biol.* **101**:2284–2291.
78. King, C.-C., King, M.W., Garry, R.F., Wan, K.M.-M., Ulug, E.T., and Waite, M.R.F., 1979, Effect of incubation time on the generation of defective-interfering particles during undiluted serial passage of Sindbis virus in *Aedes albopictus* and chick cells. *Virology* **96**:229–238.
79. Kitamura, S., Imai, T., and Grace, T.D.C., 1973, Adaptation of two mosquito cell lines to medium free of calf serum, *J. Med. Entomol.* **10**: 488–489.
80. Knipfer, M.E., and Brown, D.T., 1989, Intracellular transport and processing of Sindbis virus glycoproteins, *Virology* **170**:117–122.
81. Koblet, H., Kempf, C., Kohler, U., and Omar, A., 1985, Conformational changes at pH 6 on the cell surface of Semliki Forest virus-infected *Aedes albopictus* cells, *Virology* **143**:334–336.
82. Koblet, H., Omar, A., Kohler, U., and Kempf, C., 1988, Investigation of cell-cell fusion in Semliki Forest virus (SFV) infected C6/36 (mosquito) cells, Kuroda, Y., Kurstak, E., and Maramorosch, K. (eds): in Invertebrate and Fish Tissue Culture, Japan Scientific Societies Press, pp. 140–143.
83. Kondor-Koch, C., Burke, B., and Garoff, H., 1983, Expression of Semliki Forest virus proteins from cloned complementary DNA. I. The fusion activity of the spike glycoprotein, *J. Cell Biol.* **97**:644–651.

84. Kondor-Koch, C., Riedel, H., Soderberg, K., and Garoff, H., 1982, Expression of the structural proteins of Semliki Forest virus from cloned cDNA microinjected into the nucleus of baby hamster kidney cells, *Proc. Natl. Acad. Sci. USA*. **79**:4525–4529.
85. Kornfeld, R., and Kornfeld, S., 1985, Assembly of asparagine-linked oligosaccharides, *Annu. Rev. Biochem.* **54**:631–664.
86. Kowal, K.J., and Stollar, V., 1981, Temperature-sensitive host-dependent mutants of Sindbis virus, *Virology* **114**:140–148.
87. Kuhn, R., Hong, Z., and Strauss, J.H., 1990, Mutagenesis of the 3′ non-translated region of Sindbis virus RNA: Requirement of the 3′ terminal 19 nucleotide conserved region for virus replication, *J. Virol* **64**:1465–1476.
88. Kuno, G., 1983, Cultivation of mosquito cell lines in serum-free media and their effects on dengue virus replication, *In Vitro* **19**:707–713.
89. Kurstak, E., Tijssen, P., and Kurstak, C., 1987, In vitro immunoenzymatic detection and screening of arthropod-borne togavirus antigens and antibodies, Yunker, C.E. (ed): in Arboviruses in Arthropod Cells in vitro, Vol. I, CRC Press, Inc., Boca Raton, Florida, pp. 67–75.
90. Kurtti, T.J., and Munderloh, U.G., 1984, Mosquito cell culture, *Adv. Cell Cult.* **3**:259–302.
91. Kurtti, T.J., and Munderloh, U.G., 1989, Advances in the definition of culture media for mosquito cells, Mitsuhashi, J. (ed): in Invertebrate Cell System Applications, Vol. I, CRC Press, Inc., Boca Raton, Florida.
92. Landureau, J.C., and Lenar-Rousseaux, J.J., 1988, New culture media for insect cells, Kuroda, Y., Kurstak, E., and Maramorosch, K. (eds): in Invertebrate and Fish Tissue Culture, Japan Scientific Societies Press, Tokyo, pp. 23–27.
93. Larsen, J.R., and Ashley, R.F., 1971, Demonstration of Venezuelan equine encephalitis virus in tissues of *Aedes aegypti*, *Am. J. Trop. Med. Hyg.* **20**: 754–760.
94. Leake, C.J., and Varma, M.G.R., 1987, Application of *Aedes pseudocutellaris* (AP-61) cells to arbovirus isolation and identification, Yunker, C.E. (ed): in Arboviruses in Arthropod Cells in vitro, Vol. I, CRC Press, Inc., Boca Raton, Florida, pp. 79–86.
95. Leavitt, R., Schlesinger, S., and Kornfeld, S., 1977, Tunicamycin inhibits glycosylation and multiplication of Sindbis and vesicular stomatitis viruses, *J. Virol.* **21**:375–385.
96. Lehane, M.J., and Leake, C.J., 1982, A kinetic and ultrastructural comparison of alphavirus infection of cultured mosquito and vertebrate cells, *J. Trop. Med. Hyg.* **85**:229–238.
97. Leibovitz, A., 1963, The growth and maintenance of tissue-cell cultures in free gas exchange with the atmosphere, *Am. J. Hyg.* **78**:173–180.
98. Levis, R., Huang, H., and Schlesinger, S., 1987, Engineered defective interfering RNAs of Sindbis virus express bacterial chloramphenicol acetyltransferase in avian cells, *Proc. Natl. Acad. Sci. USA*. **84**:4811–4815.
99. Levis, R., Weiss, B.G., Tsiang, M., Huang, H., and Schlesinger, S., 1986, Deletion mapping of Sindbis virus DI RNAs derived from cDNAs defines the sequences essential for replication and packaging, *Cell* **44**:137–145.
100. Li, E., Tabas, I., and Kornfeld, S., 1978, The synthesis of complex-type oligosaccharides. I. Structure of the lipid-linked oligosaccharide precursor of

the complex-type oligosaccharides of the vesicular stomatitis virus G protein, *J. Biol. Chem.* **253**:7762–7770.
101. Li, G., and Rice, C.M., 1989, Mutagenesis of the in-frame opal termination codon preceding nsP4 of Sindbis virus: Studies of translational readthrough and its effect on virus replication, *J. Virol.* **63**:1326–1337.
102. Lobigs, M., and Garoff, H., 1990, Fusion function of the Semliki Forest virus spike is activated by proteolytic cleavage of the envelope glycoprotein, *J. Virol.* **64**:1233–1240.
103. Luukkonen, A., Kääriäinen, L., and Renkonen, O., 1976, Phospholipids of Semliki Forest virus grown in cultured mosquito cells, *Biochim. Biophys. Acta.* **450**:109–120.
104. Luukkonen, A., von Bonsdorff, C.-H., and Renkonen, O., 1977, Characterization of Semliki Forest virus grown in mosquito cells. Comparison with the virus from hamster cells, *Virology* **78**:331–335.
105. Maassen, J.A., and Terhorst, C., 1981, Identification of a cell-surface protein involved in the binding site of Sindbis virus on human lymphoblastoic cell lines using a hetero bifunctional cross-linker, *Eur. J. Biochem.* **115**:153–158.
106. Marnell, M.H., Mathis, L.S., Stookey, M., Shia, S.-P., Stowe, D.K., and Draper, R.K., 1984, A Chinese hamster ovary cell mutant with a heat-sensitive conditional-lethal defect in vacuolar function, *J. Cell Biol.* **99**: 1907–1916.
107. McDowell, W., Romero, P.A., and Datema, R., Schwarz, R.T., 1987, Glucose trimming and mannose trimming affect different phases of the maturation of Sindbis virus in infected BHK cells, *Virology* **161**:37–44.
108. Mi, S., Durbin, R., Huang, H.V., Rice, C.M., and Stollar, V., 1989, Association of the Sindbis virus RNA methyltransferase activity with the nonstructural protein nsP1, *Virology* **170**:385–391.
109. Mitsuhashi, J., 1982, Determination of essential amino acids for insect cell lines, Mitsuhashi, J., and Maramorosch, K. (eds): in Invertebrate Cell Culture Applications, Academic Press, Inc., New York, pp. 9–51.
110. Mitsuhashi, J., 1988, Simplification of media and utilization of sugars by insect cells in cultures, Kuroda, Y., Kurstak, E., and Maramorosch, K. (eds): in Invertebrate and Fish Tissue Culture, Japan Scientific Societies Press, Tokyo, pp. 15–18.
111. Mitsuhashi, J., 1989, Nutritional requirements of insect cells in vitro, Mitsuhashi, J. (ed): in Invertebrate Cell System Applications, Vol. I, CRC Press, Inc., Boca Raton, Florida, pp. 3–20.
112. Mitsuhashi, J., and Goodwin, R.H., 1989, The serum-free culture of insect cells in vitro, Mitsuhashi, J. (ed): in Invertebrate Cell System Applications, Vol. I, CRC Press, Inc., Boca Raton, Florida, pp. 31–43.
113. Mitsuhashi, J., and Maramorosch, K., 1964, Leafhopper tissue culture: Embryonic, nymphal and imaginal tissues from aseptic insects, *Contrib. Boyce Thompson Inst.* **22**:435–460.
114. Mitsuhashi, J., Nakasone, S., and Horie, Y., 1983, Sterol-free eukaryotic cells from continuous cell lines of insects, *Cell Biol. Intl. Rep.* **7**:1057–1062.
115. Mooney, J.J., Dalrymple, J.M., Alving, C.R., and Russell, P.K., 1975, Interaction of Sindbis virus with liposomal model membranes, *J. Virol.* **15**: 225–231.

116. Moore, N.F., Barenholz, Y., and Wagner, R.R., 1976, Microviscosity of togavirus membranes studied by fluorescence depolarization: Influence of envelope proteins and the host cell, *J. Virol.* **19**:126–135.
117. Naim, H.Y., and Koblet, H., 1988, Investigation of the role of glycans for the biological activity of Semliki Forest virus grown in *Aedes albopictus* cells using inhibitors of asparagine-linked oligosaccharides trimming, *Arch. Virol.* **102**: 73–89.
118. Newton, S.E., and Dalgarno, L., 1983, Antiviral activity released from *Aedes albopictus* persistently infected with Semliki Forest virus, *J. Virol.* **47**:652–655.
119. Niesters, H.G.M., and Strauss, J.H., 1990, Mutagenesis of the conserved 51 nucleotide region of Sindbis virus, *J. Virol.* **64**:1639–1647.
120. Ohkuma, S., and Poole, B., 1978, Fluorescence probe measurement of the intralysosomal pH in living cells and the perturbation of pH by various agents, *Proc. Natl. Acad. Sci. USA.* **75**:3327–3331.
121. Oldstone, M.B.A., Tishon, A., Dutko, F.J., Kennedy, S.I.T., Holland, J.J., and Lampert, P.W., 1980, Does the major histocompatibility complex serve as a specific receptor for Semliki Forest virus? *J. Virol.* **34**:256–265.
122. Omar, A., Flaviano, A., Kohler, U., and Koblet, H., 1986, Fusion of Semliki Forest infected *Aedes albopictus* cells at low pH is a fusion from within, *Arch. Virol.* **89**:145–159.
123. Omar, A., Flaviano, A., Reigel, F., Kohler, U., and Koblet, H., 1989, Syncytium formation and inhibition in Semliki-Forest-virus-infected *Aedes albopictus* cells at low pH, Mitsuhashi, J. (ed): in Invertebrate Cell System Applications, Vol. II, CRC Press, Inc., Boca Raton, Florida, pp. 147–150.
124. Omar, A., Kempf, C., Kohler, U., and Koblet, H., 1985, Involvement of thiol groups in the fusion process of *Aedes albopictus* cells infected with Semliki Forest virus (SFV), *Experientia* **41**:536 (Abstr.).
125. Omar, A., and Koblet, H., 1988, Semliki Forest virus particles containing only the E1 envelope glycoprotein are infectious and can induce cell-cell fusion, *Virology* **166**:17–23.
126. Omar, A., and Koblet, H., 1989, Application of mosquito cell culture and toga virus for studying the mechanism of membrane fusion, Mitsuhashi, J. (ed): in Invertebrate Cell System Applications, Vol. II, CRC Press, Inc., Boca Raton, Florida, pp. 151–155.
127. Ou, J.-H., Strauss, E.G., and Strauss, J.H., 1983, The 5′ terminal sequences of the genomic RNAs of several alphaviruses, *J. Mol. Biol.* **168**:1–15.
128. Ou, J.-H., Trent, D.W., and Strauss, J.H., 1982, The 3′-non-coding regions of alphavirus RNAs contain repeating sequences, *J. Mol. Biol.* **156**:719–730.
129. Peleg, J., 1968, Growth of arboviruses in monolayers from subcultured mosquito embryo cells, *Virology* **35**:617–619.
130. Peleg, J., 1969, Inapparent persistent virus infection in continuously grown *Aedes aegypti* mosquito cells, *J. Gen. Virol.* **5**:463–471.
131. Peleg, J., 1971, Growth of arboviruses in arthropod cell cultures: Applications. I. Attenuation of Semliki Forest (SF) virus in continuously cultured *Aedes aegypti* mosquito cells (Peleg) as a step in production of vaccines, *Curr. Top. Microbiol. Immunol.* **55**:155–161.

132. Peleg, J., and Pecht, M., 1978, Adaptation of an *Aedes aegypti* mosquito cell line to growth at 15°C and its response to infection by Sindbis virus, *J. Gen. Virol.* **38**:231–239.
133. Peleg, J., Stollar, V., 1974, Homologous interference in *Aedes aegypti* cell cultures infected with Sindbis virus, *Arch. Ges. Virusforsch.* **45**:309–318.
134. Peters, C.J., and Dalrymple, J.M., 1990, Alphaviruses, Fields, B.N., and Knipe, D.M. (eds): in Virology, Vol. I, Raven Press, Ltd., New York, pp. 713–761.
135. Presley, J.F., and Brown, D.T., 1989, The proteolytic cleavage of PE2 to envelope glycoprotein E2 is not strictly required for the maturation of Sindbis virus, *J. Virol.* **63**:1975–1980.
136. Pressman, B.C., and Fahim, M., 1982, Pharmacology and toxicology of the monovalent carboxylic ionophores, *Ann. Rev. Pharm. Toxicol.* **22**: 851–856.
137. Pudney, M., Leake, C.J., and Buckley, S.M., 1982, Replication of arboviruses in arthropod in vitro systems: An overview, Maramorosch, K., and Mitsuhashi, J. (eds): in Invertebrate Cell Culture Applications, Academic Press, Inc., New York, pp. 159–194.
138. Raghow, R.S., Davey, M.W., and Dalgarno, L., 1973, The growth of Semliki Forest virus in cultured mosquito cells: Ultrastructural observations, *Arch. Ges. Virusforsch.* **43**:165–168.
139. Raghow, R.S., Grace, T.D.C., Filshie, B.K., Bartley, W., and Dalgarno, L., 1973, Ross River virus replication in cultured mosquito and mammalian cells: Virus growth and correlated ultrastructural changes, *J. Gen. Virol.* **21**: 109–122.
140. Rehacek, J., 1968, The growth of arboviruses in mosquito cells in vitro, *Acta Virol.* **12**:241–246.
141. Rice, C.M., Franke, C.A., Strauss, J.H., and Hruby, D.F., 1985, Expression of Sindbis virus structural proteins via recombinant vaccinia virus: Synthesis, processing, and incorporation into mature Sindbis virions, *J. Virol.* **56**: 227–239.
142. Riedel, B., and Brown, D.T., 1977, Role of extracellular virus in the maintenance of the persistent infection induced in *Aedes albopictus* (mosquito) cells by Sindbis virus, *J. Virol.* **23**:554–561.
143. Riedel, B., and Brown, D.T., 1979, Novel antiviral activity found in the media of Sindbis virus-persistently infected mosquito (*Aedes albopictus*) cell cultures, *J. Virol.* **29**:51–60.
144. Riedel, H., 1985, Different membrane anchors allow the Semliki Forest virus spike subunit E2 to reach the cell surface, *J. Virol.* **54**:224–228.
145. Robbins, A.R., Peng, S.S., and Marshall, J.L., 1983, Mutant Chinese hamster ovary cells pleiotropically defective in receptor-mediated endocytosis, *J. Cell Biol.* **96**:1064–1071.
146. Russell, D.L., Dalrymple, J.M., and Johnston, R.E., 1989, Sindbis virus mutations which coordinately affect glycoprotein processing, penetration, and virulence in mice, *J. Virol.* **63**:1619–1629.
147. Sarver, N., and Stollar, V., 1977, Sindbis virus-induced cytopathic effect in clones of *Aedes albopictus* (Singh) cells, *Virology* **80**:390–400.
148. Saunier, B., Kilker, R.D., Tkacz, J.S., Quaroni, A., and Herscovics, A., 1982, Inhibition of *N*-linked complex oligosaccharide formation by 1-deoxy-

nojirimycin, an inhibitor of processing glucosidases, *J. Biol. Chem.* **257**: 14155–14161.
149. Sawicki, D., and Sawicki, S., 1987, Alphavirus plus strand and minus strand RNA synthesis, Brinton, M.A., and Rueckert, R.R. (eds): in Positive Strand RNA Viruses, Alan R. Liss, Inc., New York, pp. 251–260.
150. Sawicki, D.L., Barkhimer, D.B., Sawicki, S.G., Rice, C.M., and Schlesinger, S., 1990, Temperature sensitive shut off of alphavirus minus strand RNA synthesis maps to a nonstructural protein, nsP4, *Virology* **174**:43–52.
151. Sawicki, D.L., and Sawicki, S.G., 1985, Functional analysis of the A complementation group mutants of Sindbis HR virus, *Virology* **144**:20–34.
152. Sawicki, D.L., Sawicki, S.G., Keränen, S., and Kääriäinen, L., 1981, Specific Sindbis virus coded function for minus-strand RNA synthesis, *J. Virol.* **39**: 348–358.
153. Sawicki, S.G., and Sawicki, D.L., 1986, The effect of loss of regulation of minus-strand RNA synthesis on Sindbis virus replication, *Virology* **151**: 339–349.
154. Sawicki, S.G., Sawicki, D.L., Kääriäinen, L., and Keränen, S., 1981, A Sindbis virus mutant temperature-sensitive in the regulation of minus-strand synthesis, *Virology* **115**:161–172.
155. Scheefers, H., Scheefers-Borchel, U., Edwards, J., and Brown, D.T., 1980, Distribution of virus structural proteins and protein-protein interactions in plasma membrane of baby hamster kidney cells infected with Sindbis or vesicular stomatitis virus, *Proc. Nat. Acad. Sci. USA.* **77**:7277–7281.
156. Scheefers-Borchel, U., Scheefers, H., Edwards, J., and Brown, D.T., 1981, Sindbis virus maturation in cultured mosquito cells is sensitive to Actinomycin D, *Virology* **110**:292–301.
157. Schlesinger, S., Koyama, A.H., Malfer, C., Gee, S.L., and Schlesinger, M.J., 1985, The effects of inhibitors of glucosidase I on the formation of Sindbis virus, *Virus Res.* **2**:139–149.
158. Schlesinger, S., Levis, R., Weiss, B.G., Tsiang, M., and Huang, H., 1987, Replication and packaging sequences in defective interfering RNAs of Sindbis virus, Brinton, M.A., and Rueckert, R.R. (eds): in Positive Strand RNA Viruses, Alan R. Liss, Inc., New York, pp. 241–250.
159. Schlesinger, S., Schlesinger, M.J., 1990, Replication of Togaviridae and Flaviviridae, Knipe, D.M., and Fields, B.N. (eds): in Virology, Vol. I, Raven Press, Ltd., New York, pp. 697–711.
160. Schlesinger, S., and Weiss, B.G., 1986, Defective RNAs of alphaviruses, Schlesinger, S., and Schlesinger, M.J. (eds): in The Togaviridae and Flaviviridae, Plenum Press, New York, pp. 149–170.
161. Schmid, S., Fuchs, R., Kielian, M., Helenius, A., and Mellman, I., 1989, Acidification of endosome subpopulations in wild-type Chinese hamster ovary cells and temperature-sensitive acidification-defective mutants, *J. Cell Biol.* **108**:1291–1300.
162. Schneider, I., 1987, Preparation and maintenance of arthropod cell cultures: Diptera, with emphasis on mosquitoes, Yunker, C.E. (ed): in Arboviruses in Arthropod Cells in vitro, Vol. I, CRC Press, Inc., Boca Raton, Florida, pp. 25–34.
163. Schwarz, R.T., and Datema, R., 1984, Inhibitors of trimming: New tools in glycoprotein research, *Trends Biochem. Sci.* **9**:32–34.

164. Sefton, B.M., 1977, Immediate glycosylation of Sindbis virus membrane proteins, *Cell* **10**:659–668.
165. Sefton, B.M., and Burge, B.W., 1973, Biosynthesis of Sindbis virus carbohydrates, *J. Virol.* **12**:1366–1374.
166. Sefton, B.M., and Keegstra, K., 1974, Glycoproteins of Sindbis virus: Preliminary characterization of the oligosaccharides, *J. Virol.* **14**:522–530.
167. Shenk, T.E., Koshelnyk, K.A., and Stollar, V., 1974, Temperature-sensitive virus from *Aedes albopictus* cells chronically infected with Sindbis virus, *J. Virol.* **13**:439–447.
168. Silberkang, M., Havel, C.M., Friend, D.S., McCarthy, B.J., and Watson, J.A., 1983, Isoprene synthesis in isolated embryonic *Drosophila* cells. I. Sterol-deficient eukaryotic cells, *J. Biol. Chem.* **258**:8503–8511.
169. Simizu, B., and Maeda, S., 1981, Growth patterns of temperature-sensitive mutants of Western Equine Encephalitis virus in cultured *Aedes albopictus* (mosquito) cells, *J. Gen. Virol.* **56**:349–361.
170. Singh, K.R.P., 1967, Cell cultures derived from larvae of *Aedes albopictus* (Skuse) and *Aedes aegypti* (L.). *Curr. Sci.* **36**:506–508.
171. Smith, A.L., and Tignor, G.H., 1980, Host cell receptors for two strains of Sindbis virus, *Arch. Virol.* **66**:11–26.
172. Smith, J.F., and Brown, D.T., 1977, Envelopment of Sindbis virus: Synthesis and organization of proteins in cells infected with wild type and maturation defective mutants, *J. Virol.* **22**:662–678.
173. Stalder, J., Reigel, F., and Koblet, H., 1983, Defective viral RNAs in *Aedes albopictus* C6/36 cells persistently infected with Semliki Forest virus, *Virology* **129**:247–254.
174. Steacie, A.D., and Eaton, B.T., 1984, Properties of defective interfering particles of Sindbis virus generated in vertebrate and mosquito cells, *J. Gen. Virol.* **65**:333–341.
175. Stevens, T.M., 1970, Arbovirus replication in mosquito cell lines (Singh) grown in monolayer or suspension culture, *Proc. Soc. Exp. Biol. Med.* **134**: 356–361.
176. Stollar, V., 1978, Inhibition of Sindbis virus replication in *Aedes albopictus* cells deprived of methionine, *Virology* **91**:504–507.
177. Stollar, V., 1980, Togaviruses in cultured arthropod cells, Schlesinger, R.W. (ed): in The Togaviruses, Academic Press, New York, pp. 584–622.
178. Stollar, V., and Hardy, J.L., 1984, Host dependent mutants of Sindbis virus whose growth is restricted in cultured *Aedes albopictus* cells produce normal yields of virus in intact mosquitoes, *Virology* **134**:177–183.
179. Stollar, V., Harrap, K., Thomas, V., and Sarver, N., 1979, Observations related to cytopathic effect in *Aedes albopictus* cells infected with Sindbis virus, Kurstak, E. (ed): in Arctic and Tropical Arboviruses, Academic Press, Inc., New York, pp. 277–296.
180. Stollar, V., Stollar, B.D., Koo, R., Harrap, K.A., and Schlesinger, R.W., 1976, Sialic acid contents of Sindbis virus from vertebrate and mosquito cells, *Virology* **69**:104–115.
181. Stollar, V., and Thomas, V.L., 1975, An agent in the *Aedes aegypti* cell line (Peleg) which causes fusion of *Aedes albopictus* cells. *Virology* **64**:367–377.
182. Strauss, E.G., Lenches, E.M., and Strauss, J.H., 1976, Mutants of Sindbis virus. I. Isolation and partial characterization of 89 new temperature-sensitive mutants, *Virology* **74**:154–168.

183. Strauss, E.G., Levinson, R., Rice, C.M., Dalrymple, J., and Strauss, J.H., 1988, Nonstructural proteins nsP3 and nsP4 of Ross River and O'Nyong-nyong viruses: Sequence and comparison with those of other alphaviruses, *Virology* **164**:265–274.
184. Strauss, E.G., and Rice, C.M., and Strauss, J.H., 1983, Sequence coding for the alphavirus nonstructural proteins is interrupted by an opal termination codon, *Proc. Natl. Acad. Sci. USA.* **80**:5271–5275.
185. Strauss, E.G., Rice, C.M., and Strauss, J.H., 1984, Complete nucleotide sequence of the genomic RNA of Sindbis virus, *Virology* **133**:92–110.
186. Strauss, E.G., and Strauss, J.H., 1980, Mutants of alphaviruses: Genetics and physiology, Schlesinger, R.W. (ed): in The Togaviruses, Academic Press, Inc., New York, pp. 393–426.
187. Strauss, E.G., and Strauss, J.H., 1986, Structure and replication of the alphavirus genome, Schlesinger, S., and Schlesinger, M.J. (eds): in The Togaviridae and Flaviviridae, Plenum Press, New York, pp. 35–90.
188. Sweet, B.H., and McHale, J.S., 1970, Characterization of cell lines derived from *Culiseta inornata* and *Aedes vexans* mosquitoes, *Exp. Cell Res.* **61**: 51–63.
189. Takatsuki, A., Kohno, K., and Tamura, G., 1975, Inhibition of biosynthesis of polyisoprenol sugars in chick embryo microsomes by tunicamycin, *Agric. Biol. Chem.* **39**:2089–2091.
190. Takkinen, K., 1986, Complete nucleotide sequence of the nonstructural protein genes of Semliki Forest virus, *Nucleic Acids Res.* **14**:5667–5682.
191. Talbot, P.J., and Vance, D.E., 1980, Evidence that Sindbis virus infects BHK-21 cells via a lysosomal route, *Can. J. Biochem.* **58**:1131–1137.
192. Talbot, P.J., and Vance, D.E., 1982, Biochemical studies on the entry of Sindbis virus into BHK-21 cells and the effect of NH_4Cl, *Virology* **118**: 451–455.
193. Tarentino, A.L., and Maley, F., 1974, Purification and properties of an endo-(β)-acetylglucosaminidase from *Streptomyces griseus*, *J. Biol. Chem.* **249**: 811–817.
194. Tatem, J., and Stollar, V., 1986, Dominance of the CPE (+) phenotype in hybrid *Aedes albopictus* cells infected with Sindbis virus, *Virus Res.* **5**:121–130.
195. Timchak, L.M., Kruse,. F., Marnell, M.H., and Draper, R.K., 1986, A thermosensitive lesion in a Chinese hamster cell mutant causing differential effects of the acidification of endosomes and lysosomes, *J. Biol. Chem.* **261**: 14154–14159.
196. Tkacz, J.S., and Lampen, J.O., 1975, Tunicamycin inhibition of polyisoprenol *N*-acetylglucosaminyl pyrophosphate formation in calf liver microsomes, *Biochem. Biophys. Res. Commun.* **65**:248–257.
197. Tooker, P., and Kennedy, S.I.T., 1981, Semliki Forest virus multiplication in clones of *Aedes albopictus* cells, *J. Virol.* **37**:589–600.
198. Tsiang, M., Weiss, B.G., and Schlesinger, S., 1988, Effects of 5′-terminal modifications on the biological activity of defective interfering RNAs of Sindbis virus, *J. Virol.* **62**:47–53.
199. Vaughn, J.L., 1985, Insect tissue culture: Techniques and development, Kurstak, E. (ed): in Techniques in the Life Sciences. C1. Techniques in Setting Up and Maintenance of Tissue and Cell Cultures, Vol. C108, Elsevier Scientific Publishers, Ltd., New York, pp. 1–35.

200. Vaughn, J.L., Louloudes, S.J., and Dougherty, K., 1971, The uptake of free and serum-bound sterols by insect cells in vitro, *Curr. Top. Microbiol. Immunol.* **55**:92–97.
201. Weaver, S.C., 1986, Electron microscopic analysis of infection patterns for Venezuelan equine encephalomyelitis virus in the vector mosquito, *Culex (Melanoconian) taeniopus*, *Am. J. Trop. Med. Hyg.* **35**:624–631.
202. Weaver, S.C., Scott, T.W., Lorenz, L.H., Lerdthusnee, K., and Romoser, W.S., 1988, Togavirus-associated pathologic changes in the midgut of a natural mosquito vector, *J. Virol.* **62**:2083–2090.
203. Weiss, B., Nitschko, H., Ghattas, I., Wright, R., and Schlesinger, S., 1989, Evidence for specificity in the encapsidation of Sindbis virus RNAs, *J. Virol.* **63**:5310–5318.
204. Wengler, G., 1980, Effects of alphavirus on host cell macromolecular synthesis, Schlesinger, R.W. (ed): in The Togaviruses, Academic Press, Inc., New York, pp. 459–471.
205. White, J., and Helenius, A., 1980, pH-dependent fusion between the Semliki Forest virus membrane and liposomes, *Proc. Natl. Acad. Sci. USA.* **77**:3273–3277.
206. White, J., Kartenbeck, J., and Helenius, A., 1980, Fusion of Semliki Forest virus with the plasma membrane can be induced by low pH, *J. Cell Biol.* **87**: 264–272.
207. White, J., Kielian, M., and Helenius, A., 1983, Membrane fusion proteins of enveloped animal viruses, *Q. Rev. Biophys.* **16**:151–195.
208. Whitfield, S.G., Murphy, A., and Sudia, W.D., 1971, Eastern equine encephalomyelitis virus: An electron microscopic study of *Aedes triseriatus* (Say) salivary gland infection, *Virology* **43**:110–122.
209. Wilkie, G.E.I., Stockdale, H., and Pirt, S.V., 1980, Chemically defined media for production of insect cells and viruses in vitro, *Dev. Biol. Stand.* **46**: 29–37.
210. Wyatt, G.R., Loughheed, T.C., and Wyatt, S.S., 1956, The chemistry of insect hemolymph. Organic components of the hemolymph of the silkworm, *Bombyx mori*, and two other species, *J. Gen. Physiol.* **39**:853–868.
211. Wyatt, S.S., 1956, Culture in vitro of tissue from the silkworm, *Bombyx mori* L., *J. Gen. Physiol.* **39**:841–852.

6
Advances in Triatomine Bug Ecology in Relation to Chagas' Disease

Toby V. Barrett

Introduction

The bugs of the reduviid subfamily Triatominae require repeated bloodmeals over several months in order to reach maturity, and are independent of individual host animals between meals. It is thus not surprising that they are intermediate hosts and vectors of protozoan blood and tissue parasites: *Hepatozoon* spp. of reptiles (1, 8, 116), and *Trypanosoma conorhini*, *Trypanosoma rangeli* and *Trypanosoma cruzi* of their mammalian hosts (37, 83) (Triatominae are not known to transmit any parasites of birds or amphibians). Unlike many trypanosomes, *T. rangeli** and *T. cruzi** are found in many mammals of different orders, in keeping with the lack of host specificity of most of their triatomine vectors. Humans are susceptible to both *T. rangeli* and *T. cruzi*, but only the latter is a serious pathogen, and the medical importance of Triatominae is due principally to their role as vectors of *T. cruzi*, the etiological agent of Chagas' disease. Humans may become infected by direct (25, 42, 84, 115) or indirect (11, 168) contact with enzootic cycles of transmission, but the main reason for the very high prevalence (90, 137) of human trypanosomiasis in many parts of Latin America is the presence of breeding colonies of Triatominae in houses in which people and domestic mammals serve as reservoirs of the parasite (12, 90, 112).

It is now thought that *T. cruzi* does not occur naturally outside the Western Hemisphere (83). *T. cruzi* occupies most (83, 90, 132) of the range of the Triatominae in the Americas, which is approximately between latitudes 40°N (*Triatoma protracta*) and 46°S (*Triatoma infestans*) (89,

Toby V. Barrett, Departamento de Ciências da Saúde, Instituto Nacional de Pesquisas da Amazônia, Caixa Postal 478, 69083 Manaus-AM, Brazil.

* There are no Triatominae with these specific names.

119). Natural infection with *T. cruzi* has been reported even in triatomines not primarily associated with mammals (19), and it is prudent to assume that all species are potential vectors.

The literature on Triatominae is large, and much of it is published in sources that are not readily accessible. Fortunately, various reviews relating to the ecology of Triatominae are available (16–18, 31, 90, 114, 133, 137, 145, 159, 166, 167, 169, 171), and a recent bibliography on Chagas' disease contains many relevant entries (129). The species have usually been grouped according to the degree to which they are associated with humans, and the anthropocentric and teleological concept that triatomines are evolving towards greater adaptation to the domestic environment, with species that colonize peridomestic structures representing an intermediate stage in this process, may appear to be firmly established. In fact, with the exception of resistance to organochlorine insecticides in some populations of *Rhodnius prolixus* (107), there is very little evidence that colonies in houses are genetically different from wild populations of the same species.

The systematic arrangement used here follows Lent and Wygodzinsky's taxonomic monograph of the Triatominae (89). Species not recognized in that work, either described since 1979 or considered to be junior synonyms, will occasionally be mentioned, but no judgement as to the systematic status of these populations is intended here. More detailed information on geographical distribution can be found in the Reference list (32, 38, 56–58, 81, 89, 119–124, 149). Lent and Wygodzinsky (89) also provide notes on the biology of the species, with particular reference to habitat. I have attempted to update this information. Silvatic refers here only to forest or woodland. Elsewhere the term has been used indiscriminately for nonsynanthropic populations, obscuring the fact that many triatomines, particularly of the tribe Triatomini, are primarily saxicolous inhabitants of rocky areas in arid and semiarid environments.

Habits and Habitats

The Tribe Alberproseniini

The smallest (5 mm long) triatomine, *Alberprosenia goyovargasi* has been collected only in Zulia State, Venezuela, in tropical xerophytic woodland between sea level and 400 m. Specimens were associated with snakes and lizards in galleries excavated by passalid beetles in tree trunks. In the laboratory it will feed on reptiles, chickens, and people, and appears to have a rapid life cycle for a triatomine, a second instar nymph having been reared to adult in 44 days. It is not known to transmit *Trypanosoma cruzi* in nature but has been found infected with another flagellate, possibly *Blastocrithidia* (31).

The Tribe Cavernicolini

The tribe is restricted to tropical America. Most reports of *Cavernicola pilosa* are from hollow trees (33, 39, 123), although it was first found in caves in Panama (4). *Cavernicola lenti* (10) is known only from a hollow tree in the Brazilian state of Amazonas, and the type locality of this species is therefore surrounded by the known distribution of *C. pilosa.* Both species are associated with bats, and *C. pilosa* is unusually specialized for a triatomine in that it refuses to feed on other animals in the laboratory (33), whereas *C. lenti* can be reared on mice (10). Both species are vectors of *Trypanosoma cruzi marinkellei*, a parasite of phyllostomatid bats (10, 45).

The Tribe Bolboderini

The Bolboderini include four genera of small (10 mm long) dorsoventrally flattened triatomines from silvatic habitats in tropical America. The species are poorly collected and appear not to have been established in laboratory colonies. The compression of the body can be related to life in narrow spaces under tree bark, between folded dead leaves, and at the bases of bromeliad epiphytes. In those species for which the eggs are known these are glued to the substrate, as in several other arboreal triatomines. *Bolbodera scabrosa* is restricted to Cuba, where it has been reported from nests of the rodent *Capromys* (89, 123). *Belminus costaricensis* (89, 123) from Mexico (89) and Costa Rica has been found in bromeliad epiphytes (89, 110) and in nests of termites and bees, as well as on a sloth (160). *Belminus herreri* (99, 103, 152) is found under loose bark on forest trees: *Anacardium* spp. in Panama and *Hymenolobium* spp. in the Brazilian Amazon. It is thought to feed on lizards. Few specimens have been dissected and in Manaus we have found infections with *Machadoella* spp. (a schizogregarine). *Belminus peruvianus* (80, 89) is known only from the upper Marañon Valley in Peru, a relatively dry environment for the tribe. Nymphs and adults were found under the bark of a large tree near chickens and an opossum, as well as in the bedrooms of adobe houses with *Panstrongylus herreri.* In the laboratory, first and second instar nymphs fed only on reptiles and on hemolymph and midgut contents of triatomines, whereas older nymphs and adults would feed on chickens and, less readily, on humans. All specimens examined were negative for trypanosomes, although *T. cruzi* was frequent in the associated *Panstrongylus herreri.* The biology of *Belminus rugulosus* (89), from Colombia and Venezuela, is unknown.

Parabelminus carioca from the Atlantic coastal forest in Rio de Janeiro was discovered in a nest of *Didelphis* in a palm, and specimens were found infected with *T. cruzi* (77). A later report (105) also associates this species with opossums, this time in a hollow tree. *Parabelminus yurupucu* (8, 89) occurs further north, in the Atlantic forest of Bahia State, where it inhabits bromeliad epiphytes. Although frequently associated with infected *Triatoma tibiamaculata* in this habitat, 31 specimens dissected were all negative for *T. cruzi*. Although adults and nymphs have been fed on anesthetized laboratory mice, a single fresh bloodmeal in a specimen from the field contained nucleated erythrocytes. Reptiles and tree frogs are common in the bromeliads, birds' nests are rarer. The known distribution of *Parabelminus* is restricted to eastern Brazil; a report from Bolivia does not appear to have been confirmed. In other areas, analogous habitats are occupied by the closely related (89) genus *Microtriatoma*.

Microtriatoma trinidadensis (29, 38, 89, 103, 152) is a wide ranging species associated with epiphytic bromeliads. There are also reports of specimens from under tree bark, in a palm, and (as *M. mansosotoi*) (31) from a bat refuge. Specimens from opossum nests have been found infected with *T. cruzi* (105). In the Amazon forest I suspect that the majority of *M. trinidadensis* live among fallen leaves trapped above ground by entanglements of lianas, although few specimens have been collected from this habitat, from which it is often difficult to sample. Hairs found among the dead leaves indicate that opossums and other mammals use these sites, but the presence of pale fluid in the midgut of many nymphs suggests that insect hemolymph may be a more important food source for *M. trinidadensis*. Bugs collected from this habitat are often associated with detrivorous caterpillars, which consolidate the leaf litter with their silk. An adult *M. trinidadensis* placed together with one of these caterpillars made determined attacks with its extended rostrum on the region just behind the head capsule of the (much larger) caterpillar, which was rocking the anterior half of its body from side to side in what appeared to be a defensive maneuver. When the bug succeeded in making contact, the swaying movements ceased abruptly; the same bug had previously refused to feed on man. *Microtriatoma borbai* (89) has been collected in bromeliads in association with opossums and rodents in Southern Brazil. One specimen was found to be infected with *T. cruzi*, although in the laboratory the bugs refused to feed on mammals. Further study is required, but the above observations suggest that the Bolboderini may be primarily micropredators on arthropods.

The Tribe Rhodniini

The genus *Psammolestes* (6, 20, 30) contains three species, all closely associated with birds' nests in scrubland or open country with scattered small trees. The main hosts are those members of the family Furnariidae that build nest with sticks, particularly *Phacellodomus* spp. and *Anumbius annumbi*. *Psammolestes arthuri* from Venezuela and Western Colombia (39) is isolated from the Brazilian *P. tertius* by the Amazon rainforest. The latter species closely resembles (89) *P. correodes*, from Argentina, Bolivia, and Paraguay. *Psammolestes* spp. have occasionally been found infected with *T. cruzi* (19), probably aquired from secondary mammalian inhabitants of the birds nests, but are not known to be of any importance in the transmission of the parasite.

In the genus *Rhodnius*, 12 species, ranging from Southern Mexico to Southern Brazil, are at present recognized (89). *R. dalessandroi*, *R. nasutus*, *R. neglectus*, and *R. robustus* are morphologically close to each other and to *R. prolixus*, and preliminary work on population genetics suggests that the status of some of the populations included in these species may in future require reconsideration (9).

R. prolixus is abundant in houses in Southern Mexico, Guatemala, El Salvador, and Honduras, infrequent, in Costa Rica and Nicaragua, and possibly absent from Panama (123), where the main domestic vector is *R. pallescens*. *R. prolixus* is the principal domestic vector of *T. cruzi* in Venezuela, where it occurs throughout most of the country (32, 35, 73). *R. prolixus* is a common domestic species in Colombia, where it occurs between 20 and 2600 m (38). In Venezuela and Colombia *R. prolixus* occurs in the wild, particularly in palms (92) but also in birds nests (67), and there are even reports of this species from animal burrows (38). Domestic infestations by *R. prolixus* may be extremely heavy, particularly in houses with thatch roofs (68). In El Porvenir (Colombia) *R. prolixus* was found to be abundant in *Scheelea* palms, and adults frequently flew into houses, but only in one house were a few nymphs found (39). In Venezuela palms are thought to be an important source of *R. prolixus*, which gives rise to domestic colonies (73).

Colonies derived from domestic and silvatic populations of *R. prolixus* from Honduras, Venezuela, and Colombia, along with material labeled as *R. robustus* from Peru were found to be fully interfertile in laboratory crosses (9). Most reports of *R. robustus* are from areas of tropical rainforest in and around the Amazon region. In Brazil, north of the Amazon River, bugs classified as this species have been found in palms (*Attalea* spp., *Jessenia bataua*, *Mauritia carana*), and adults infected with *T. cruzi* frequently fly into houses around Manaus. In Venezuela (88, 156) the species has been found in palms, principally *Attalea* (= *Scheelea*), and also in bromeliads.

R. neglectus, from Central and Southern Brazil occurs in palms (*Acrocomia sclerocarpa*, *Orbignya oleifera*) and is widespread in chicken houses in the state of Minas Gerais (21, 23, 61). Occasional nymphs have been found in houses following eradication of *Triatoma infestans*. *R. nasutus* represents the population from the arid Northeast of Brazil, where it is found in palms (113) and birds nests. Peridomestic colonies of this species occur in chicken houses in Ceara State (2, 26). Uncharacterized populations of the *R. prolixus* complex occur in palms (*Orbignya phalerata*) in Northern Brazil south of the Amazon River (9).

Rhodnius pictipes is a silvatic species found in and around the Amazon Basin, with one record from Central America (Belize) (89). It inhabits palms where it may occur together with *R. prolixus* or *R. robustus* (101), but it is also found in bromeliad epiphytes and has been reported from a bird nest (108). Adults infected with *T. cruzi* frequently fly into houses near Manaus and Belem (101) in Brazil, and small colonies including nymphs have been found in houses in Pará (10) and Piauí States in that country. In Peru, *R. pictipes* is reported to infest houses in an area of San Martin province (G. Calderón, personal communication).

Rhodnius pallescens is a Central American (123) species, which, like the somewhat similar (89) *R. pictipes*, is associated particularly with palms (163). In Panama it is the principal domestic triatomine and is most frequent in houses with palm thatch roofs, in which *Rattus rattus* acts as an important domestic host (66). The species has also been reported from birds nests (36) and tree holes (38), and has been found in limited numbers in extradomiciliary sites in Colombia (38).

Rhodnius ecuadoriensis, colonizes in houses, chicken houses, and guinea pig pens in areas of xerophytic vegetation on the Pacific and Amazonian slopes of the Andes in Ecuador and Northern Peru. It has been found on trees (*Schinus molle*) in association with *Didelphis* and *Belminus peruvianus*, in palms near Guayaquil, and among cacti. *R. ecuadoriensis* is possibly more closely related to *R. pictipes* and *R. pallescens* than to other species (31, 82, 89) and G. Calderón, personal communication).

Rhodnius neivai is found only in dry or very dry areas in Venezuela (Lara, Falcón, Zulia) and in the Magdalena Valley in Colombia. Nymphs were found once in a dead tree and once in a *Copernicia* palm; the species is not known to colonize in houses (31, 34).

Rhodnius paraensis is known only from the type locality near Belem in Brazil. It was found in a nest of the rodent *Echimys chrysurus* in the forest canopy (103).

Rhodnius domesticus occurs in the Atlantic rainforest and transitional vegetation from Bahia to Santa Catarina (13, 85). In the wild this species is found in epiphytic bromeliads, particularly *Aechmea multiflora* (13). It is not known to colonize in houses. *R. domesticus* inhabits the southeastern extreme of the range of the genus, and the finding of a specimen infected with *T. rangeli* in Bahia (13), along with the recent isolation of *T. rangeli* from a spiny rat in Santa Catarina (M. Steindel, personal communication), extends the known range of this parasite considerably.

Reports of *Rhodnius brethesi* from areas other than the Orinoco basin and northern tributaries of the upper and middle Rio Negro, where it is associated with the palm *Leopoldinia piassaba* are doubtful. This species readily attacks humans and has been blamed for the appearence of cutaneous lesions at the site of the bites (96). One case of mixed infeetion with *T. cruzi* and *T. rangeli* in a man engaged in collecting the fibers of *L. piassaba* is known, and other piasaba collectors were found to have positive serology for *T. cruzi* (55), but the role of *R. brethesi* as a vector of Chagas' disease to humans remains to be studied. The results of a more recent collection of *R. brethesi* from *L. piassaba* suggests that the bugs in that sample were feeding mainly on lizards (B. Mascarenhas, unpublished thesis).

Rhodnius dallesandroi has been reported from the palm *Jessenia polycarpa* in Meta, Colombia, but the taxonomic status of this species of *Rhodnius* is not well established (89).

The Tribe Triatomini

The Triatomini include six genera from throughout the range of the subfamily. The large genus *Triatoma* has been tentatively divided into species groups based on morphological characters. This arrangement (89) will be followed here, since there are good correlations with habitat and distribution.

The Genus *Linshcosteus*

The genus is known only from India, where *L. costalis* occurs together with *L. confumus* under boulders and rocks. The biology of *L. carnifex*, *L. chota*, and *L. kali* is unknown, and the genus has no known public health importance. Together with the eight members of the *Triatoma rubrofasciata* complex, these are the only Triatominae so far known from the Eastern Hemisphere (71, 89, 124).

The Genus *Dipetalogaster*

The only species in a genus of very restricted distribution, *D. maxima*, in common with many other members of the tribe Triatomini, is saxicolous. It is restricted to rocky outcrops in the desert environment of southernmost Baja California in Mexico (93, 123, 127) and is most abundant where the rocks have been fractured. It has been found infected with *T. cruzi* and will readily feed on mammals, but its main natural host seems to be the large herbivorous lizard *Sauromalus australis*. It is the largest known triatomine, and in recent years has been much used for xenodiagnosis on patients suspected of having *T. cruzi* infections because of the advantages in logistics and safety of the unfed first instar nymphs for this procedure.

The Genus *Paratriatoma*

The monotypic genus *Paratriatoma* is restricted to the United States of America and Mexico, and in nature has been found only in *Neotoma* nests (123). Although *P. hirsuta* has not been reported as a natural host of *T. cruzi* (123), it is of public health importance due to hypersensitivity to bites. A literature review (120) with reports on geographical variation, distribution, and hybridization studies is available for this genus, as is a discussion (89) of its systematic position within the tribe Triatomini and possible relationships with the ecologically similar *Triatoma protracta* complex.

The Genus *Eratyrus*

Eratyrus cuspidatus occurs from Mexico to Peru and parts of Venezuela (123). The species has been cited as peridomestic in association with goats, but an original source (117) refers only to a few adults found in a goat yard, with the observation that the true habitat of the species is probably silvatic. The occurrence of *Eratyrus* in palms is probably also accidental. Nymphs of *E. cuspidatus* were found associated with bats in an abandoned observation tower in primary forest in Panama (64).

E. mucronatus is a silvatic species occurring east of the Andes from Bolivia to Trinidad (89). In the Brazilian Amazon *E. mucronatus* inhabits the interior of large living hollow trees, and if these are entered at ground level, then hungry fourth and fifth instar nymphs will usually approach the collector from above, after 15–30 min. These hollow trees often have an opening at canopy level and it is common to find adults and nymphs at the bases of hollow branches containing porcupine quills, rodent nests, or shelters of *Potos flavus* (Procyonidae). Externally, the tree forks are used as resting places by sloths and monkeys, and there are usually small colonies of bats in the hollow trunk. Porcupine blood has been identified in the gut contents of *E. mucronatus*, and nymphs are also micropredators on the hemolymph of invertebrates (Amblypygi) (103). The long head, long antennae, and the habit of nymphs in camouflaging themselves with dust are presumably adaptations to the environment inside the trees, but small nymphs may also be found externally, under loose bark, a habitat shared with *Belminus herreri*. Despite the large size of the habitat, the number of *E. mucronatus* collected from individual trees does not usually exceed a dozen specimens. In the laboratory, colonies can be maintained on mouse blood, and the bugs will readily feed on humans. Both species of *Eratyrus* have been found infected with *T. cruzi*, but in our experience trypanosome infections are relatively rare in *E. mucronatus*, which does however often carry heavy infections by an undescribed species of *Machadoella* (Schizogregarinidae) in the hindgut and malpighian tubules. The two species of *Eratyrus* are very similar morphologically and may be sympatric in northern and western Venezuela (89), so the genus would be an interesting subject for a study on population genetics. To the published distribution of *E. mucronatus*, the Brazilian states of Rondonia (Samuel hydroelectric project) and Roraima (Maraca Island) can be added from our records.

The Genus *Panstrongylus*

This genus contains 13 species from South and Central America. Five species forming a distinct cladistic group on adult morphology (89) are found in the less humid southern and eastern parts of the range of the genus; *P. guentheri* (31), from Argentina, Bolivia, and Paraguay, is said to be frequent in woodpiles and may be associated with birds nests. *P. diasi*, *P. lutzi*, *P. lenti*, and *P. tupynambai* from Brazil south of the Amazon region are known only from adult specimens accidentally associated with humans (89). *P. diasi* has also been reported from Bolivia and *P. tupynambai* from Uruguay (89).

Another group of three, apparently closely related, species inhabits more humid regions in the northern and western parts of the range of the genus. *P. humeralis* has been taken at light in Panama (151). *P. lignarius* is found in the Amazon Region of Brazil and neighboring countries, and is morphologically and chromatically very close (89) to the Peruvian *P. herreri*, with which it hybridizes in the laboratory. *P. lignarius* has been found in mammal nests in the forest canopy (103). First and fifth instar nymphs have been found on tree trunks, and mosquito collectors have been attacked by this species on canopy platforms (41), suggesting that nymphs will disperse in search of food. Unfed first instar nymphs were found in the crown of a *Mauritia carana* palm used by monkeys as a resting place in the forests near Manaus. In the laboratory *P. lignarius* can be reared on rodent blood, provided the eggs are kept in contact with a moist surface. *P. herreri* may be parapatric with *P. lignarius*, because it occurs in rainforest areas between the Marañon and Huallaga rivers in Peru, at altitudes between 400 and 1500 m (31). This species colonizes houses and peridomestic structures (80), and in the laboratory no special precautions are required with the eggs.

P. chinai and *P. howardi* have been reported from Ecuador, and the former species also occurs in Peru. *P. chinai* inhabits rocky areas up to 2500 m on both sides of the Andes, in regions with median isotherms of 17° to 25°C. This species colonizes in chicken houses and in human inhabitations with wooden walls. It is considered to be the principal domestic vector of Chagas' disease in the Peruvian Department of Piura. Fifty-six specimens were found under tree trunks, which served as benches in a rural school, where they fed on the pupils in daytime (54). The wild habitat of *P. chinai* is unknown, as is that of *P. howardi*, known only from specimens found in houses in Ecuador (Manabi). Specimens from Peru, provided by Dr. G. Calderón, show a greater range of morphological and chromatic variation than is indicated by descriptions of *P. chinai* and *P. howardi* (89), but the geographical basis of this variability has not been studied.

P. rufotuberculatus is a silvatic species inhabiting tropical rainforest from Mexico (Chiapas) to Bolivia and northern Brazil. This species has been found in great numbers in cane and mud-walled houses in coastal Ecuador and in 38% of houses examined near Cuzco (Peru) (31). *P. rufotuberculatus* has been collected from a hollow tree, in association with *Desmodus* bats, and is a vector of *T. cruzi* (31, 38, 40, 117, 123).

Panstrongylus geniculatus occupies most of the range of the genus, from Nicaragua and Trinidad to Argentina, and is the only triatomine other than

Cavernicola pilosa to occur in both the Atlantic and Amazonian forests of Brazil. It also occurs in the intervening semiarid regions but requires a humid microclimate, which is often provided by armadillo burrows (15, 104). In the Amazon forest *P. geniculatus* is found in armadillo burrows even among dead leaves at the entrance, and in live hollow trees below ground level. It is easiest to collect from within fallen hollow trunks and branches inhabited by ground-dwelling rodents. Reports of *P. geniculatus* from the crowns of palm trees probably represent accidental finds of dispersing adults; in the Amazon forest this species appears to be ecologically separated from *P. lignarius* by vertical stratification. In the laboratory *P. geniculatus* will feed on humans, and is readily reared on rodents provided a humid atmosphere is maintained in the containers. Adult females have been observed to feed on anesthetized mice for several hours, depositing large quantities of excreta as the bloodmeal is concentrated. *P. geniculatus* commonly flies into houses and, unless in a state of complete inanition (as is often the case) these specimens are usually found to be infected with *T. cruzi*. On three occasions in Manaus freshly fed female *P. geniculatus* were found in sleeping quarters under circumstances which suggested that they had fed on people after entering the house.

Panstrongylus megistus is a silvatic species in the southern (more humid) part of the Brazilian Atlantic rainforest, where it is found in bromeliad epiphytes, tree holes, and other habitats. Beyond the limit of the South Atlantic Polar Front the species breeds in humid mud-walled houses and chicken houses and has rarely been found in silvatic habitats. Before the spread of *Triatoma infestans*, *P. megistus* was the principal domestic vector of *T. cruzi* in the areas of Brazil most highly endemic for Chagas' disease (11, 12, 15, 24, 44, 56–61).

The *Triatoma protracta* Group

Except for *Triatoma nitida*, which extends into Costa Rica, these species are confined to the U.S.A. and Mexico. The group is divided into two complexes (89).

In the *protracta* complex, *T. neotomae*, *T. peninsularis*, *T. protracta*, and *T. sinaloensis* have been found in the wild only in association with woodrat (125) (*Neotoma* spp.) lodges (89, 123). *T. protracta* is of public health importance due to hypersensitivity reactions to bites from adults that fly into houses (94), and has also been found infected with *T. cruzi*. *T. nitida*, which is possibly conspecific (89, 123) with *T. neotomae*, occurs from Yucatan to Costa Rica and is known from a few specimens including nymphs found in domestic and peridomestic situations in areas free from *Triatoma dimidiata* and *Rhodnius prolixus* (74). The Mexican *T. barberi* colonizes in and around houses and feeds on man (123). The natural habitat of this species is unknown, but may be arboreal as eggs adhere to the substrate (89). There is no information on the biology of *T. incrassata* (123).

In the *lecticularia* complex, *T. indictiva* is known mainly from specimens taken at light but has also been found in *Neotoma* nests (123). *T. lecticularia* and *T. sanguisuga* are found in *Neotoma* nests but are not restricted to this habitat. *T. lecticularia* colonizes *Neotoma* nests in open country, and hollow trees in forest regions, as well as breeding in domestic and peridomestic situations, and will attack people. Specimens of *T. sanguisuga* infected with *T. cruzi* have been found in dead or drying trees hollow or riddled with insect tunnels, in hollow roots in association with armadillos (*Dasypus novemcintus*) and up to 20 ft above ground in dead trees with opossums (*Didelphis virginiana*) and racoons (*Pyocyon lotor*) (123). In New Orleans adults of *T. sanguisuga* were found in a house and under a kennel where a dog died of acute chagasic myocarditis (164). The species is frequently found in houses even in urban situations, but is not known to colonize there. One population (*T. sanguisuga ambigua*) is reported from under loose bark and under dead leaf stocks of palmetto, in associations with lizards and toads (123).

The *Triatoma rubrofasciata* Group

The *Triatoma phyllosoma* complex consists of six large Mexican species and includes a number of populations that colonize in and around houses. In a region of tropical deciduous and subdeciduous forest, domestic colonies of *T. mazzottii* were confined to that part of the dwelling used as storage space for corn and shelter for domestic animals. The species was also found infesting small caves used as shelter by the local peasants, where adults were observed in cracks and on the walls, and nymphs camouflaged with dust on the floor. Specimens were found infected with *T. cruzi* and may have been feeding on bats and rodents in the caves (118). Previous reports describe domestic infestations by adults and nymphs of this species and of *T. pallidipennis* as frequent, and they have been found in association with armadillos and *Neotoma* spp. (123). *T. phyllosoma* is abundant in peridomestic situations, and in the wild appears to be a saxicolous species associated with lizards and mammals (123). *T. longipennis* colonizes around houses and is possibly also cavernicolous, in association with bats (89). There is no information on the biology of *T. mexicana* and *T. picturata* (89).

Triatoma dimidiata has morphological affinities with the members of the *phyllosoma* complex, but extends beyond Mexico as far as Peru (89). It is an important domestic vector of Chagas' disease and has been the subject of recent reviews (168, 170) containing numerous bibliographical references, which will not be repeated here. Although domestic populations occur in some regions where houses are infested by *Rhodnius prolixus*, *T. dimidiata* tends to predominate in the cooler areas and the relative abundance of the two species is often correlated with altitude. Populations in houses are usually densest near ground level, and houses with mud floors are particularly liable to heavy infestations. *T. dimidiata* is an urban pest in the city of Guayaquil but in most areas there appears to be no clear boundary between domestic, peridomestic, and silvatic populations, with bugs from the woodland being introduced into the domestic area with firewood, and household bugs feeding on opossums and other mammals in the peridomestic area and also in the space under houses with raised wooden floors (172). Under these circumstances a continuous input of enzootic *T. cruzi* into the domestic environment is highly probable. In the wild the principal habitat of the species appears to be tree holes, in association with *Didelphis* and other mammals. Other reports refer to armadillo burrows (38), palms in Panama, rocks in Yucatan, stone walls in Guatemala, and to an association with a snake. Cavernicolous populations with characteristic morphological adaptations are known from Guatemala and Belize (89).

The *Triatoma recurva* complex includes two species from Southwest U.S.A. and parts of Mexico. *T. recurva* (123, 128) is saxicolous and has also been reported from nests of the rodents *Spermophilus* and (rarely) *Neotoma*, in arid environments similar to those occupied by the allopatric *Dipetalogaster maxima*. It will feed on reptiles in the laboratory and is said to prefer them in the field. *T. recurva* has been found infected with *T. cruzi* and is of medical importance due to bite reactions. *T. gerstaekeri* (123) has been found in nests of the woodrat *Neotoma micropus*, and also in shelters of *Didelphis*, rodent burrows, peridomestic situations, and feeding on a snake. It has been reported infected with *T. cruzi* and adults have been found in houses, but it does not colonize there.

The *Triatoma flavida* complex contains three species. *T. obscura* is restricted to Jamaica and little information is available on its biology. It has been caught biting people, and in the wild may be associated with limestone caves or hollow trees (123). *T. flavida* and *T. bruneri* are restricted to Cuba. The resurrection of *T. bruneri* as a valid species (87) was not available until after field observations on the biology of Cuban Triatomines (109) in 1981, so some confusion remains regarding the biology of these two species. The Cuban members of the complex include populations that infest the entrances of caves in the western part of the island. Humans and pigs are attacked by day and night in the caves, which are also used by dogs, bats, and rodents of the genus *Capromys*. Following agricultural modifications in regions of abundant vegetation, infestation of houses by adults of a noncavernicolous population was reported. People were attacked at night, but there was no evidence of establishment of domiciliary colonies. Bugs from the cave populations were dissected and were all negative for trypanosomes.

Apart from *Triatoma rubrofasciata*, which is tropicopolitan, the species of the *Triatoma rubrofasciata* complex are restricted to Asia and North

Queensland in Australia (106, 124). Nothing is known of the ecology of *T. amicitiae*, represented by a single specimen from Sri Lanka, *T. leopoldi*, from Australia and Indonesia, *T. pugasi*, from Java, or *T. sinica*, from Nankin in China (124). *T. migrans* occurs from India to Papua New Guinea; a specimen from Sarawak was reported from rotten heartwood of a felled tree (89). The closely related (89) *T. bouvieri* has been reported from the Nicobar Islands, the Phillipines, and South Vietnam. From the distribution of these species, they are likley to be mainly silvatic inhabitants of tropical rainforest, and may be vectors of trypanosomes of Asian primates (161). *T. cavernicola* was collected in a limestone cave in Malaya inhabited by monks, who were attacked by the insects (52).

Triatoma rubrofasciata is a synanthropic species whose wild habitat is unknown. It is widespread in India but elsewhere is mainly confined to port cities, which suggests that it was spread by international sea trade from India to the New World (124), although one reviewer (137) favors a Neotropical origin for this species. It is frequently associated with *Rattus rattus*, among which it transmits *Trypanosoma conorhini* (83). *T. rubrofasciata* has been found infected with *Trypanosoma cruzi* in the Americas and colonizes in human dwellings (28, 103) but is not considered to be an important vector of Chagas' disease. In Asia, species of the *rubrofasciata* complex may possibly be responsible for occasional transmission of monkey trypanosomes to people (161).

The *Triatoma spinolai* complex is restricted to Argentina and Chile. *T. breyeri* is native to dry areas in Central Argentina, where it has been found in large numbers in the brushwood used for goat enclosures, in association with rodents (31). *T. eratyrusiformis* is a morphologically variable group of populations from Argentina, and some authors recognize two species (31). *T. eratyrusiformis* sensu strictu, is a saxicolous population from xeric environments, found in nests of *Microcavia australis*. It does not colonize in houses but will attack people who enter its habitat and is frequently found infected with *T. cruzi*. *T. ninioi* is also saxicolous in association with cavimorph rodents but is restricted to areas near watercourses and requires high (70%) relative humidity to develop in laboratory colonies (31). *T. spinolai* is a saxicolous species restricted to arid and semiarid areas of Chile. On rocky shores the species has been reported to attack sea birds and sea lions (C.J. Schofield, personal communication), and inland it is common in stone walls where it feeds on reptiles and mammals. One specimen was found infected with hemogregarines (1), and the species is found naturally infected with *T. cruzi*. People are attacked even in daylight when they enter the bugs' habitat but the species does not colonize in houses (89). Females are invariably micropterous, whereas males may be macropterous, brachypterous, or micropterus. Wingedness in males appears to be genetically determined, with male offspring following their parental phenotype. In coastal populations bordering the Atacama Desert, winged males have not been recorded, nor have they emerged in laboratory colonies established from these areas (143).

Most of the remaining species of *Triatoma* are included in the *infestans* subgroup of the *rubrofasciata* group. Of the three complexes assigned to this subgroup, the *infestans* complex is the largest, and includes the majority of species from South America, to which it is restricted. Many of the species are inhabitants of the less humid areas, where they tend to be either saxicolous, in association with reptiles and rodents, or to colonize in birds nests. Several of these species also colonize analogous synanthropic habitats, and some are important household pests.

Of the saxicolous species, *T. arthurneivai* (22) from Central and Southern Brazil is a vector of a hemogregarine of the lizard *Tropidurus torquatus* (116). Rock cavies and other rodents also occur in the habitat of this species but *T. arthurneivai* has not been found infected with *T. cruzi*. It will colonize in stone walls but only adults have been reported from houses. *Triatoma brasiliensis* from northeast Brazil occupies similar habitats in the wild and one population associated with lizards was also found to be heavily infected with hemogregarines (11). Other populations do however colonize in houses, and in the drier parts of Ceara State *T. brasiliensis* is considered to be the main vector of Chagas' disease. In a study of peridomestic habitats, *T. brasiliensis* was found in goat corrals, but only in those with stone bases to the fence. *T. brasiliensis* infected with *T. cruzi* were found among rocks used by free-ranging goats as nocturnal resting places, and the species has also been found in chicken houses and in piles of wood and tiles in the peridomestic environment (2). Specimens from the rocky habitats presumably represent a ready source for the rapid recolonization of sprayed houses, although saxicolous populations do exist in regions where this species is not a domestic pest (11). *Triatoma costalimai* is found in outcrops of calcareous rocks in Central Brazil. These rocks are inhabited by cavimorph rodents, and *T. costalimai* has been found infected with *T. cruzi*. Bloodmeal analysis of one sample suggested however that the bugs were feeding principally on reptiles. Adults occasionally fly into houses but do not colonize there (70, 140). *Triatoma lenti* is a saxicolous species from Bahia in Brazil and has been reported from goat corrals (146). *T. petrochii* is sympatric with *T. brasiliensis* and has been found together with this species in rocks inhabited by cavies (53). *T. patagonica* is widespread in Argentina under stones and tree trunks, often associated with cavies. It will colonize peridomestic stone walls, has been found infected with *T. cruzi*, and readily attacks people both in the open and indoors, although it is not known to colonize in houses (31). *T. rubrovaria*, from Argentina, Uruguay, and Southern Brazil is associated with reptiles and amphibians in rocky areas. In the laboratory the species will feed on birds and mammals as well as on invertebrate hemolymph (89). It has been found infected with *T. cruzi* and hemogregarines, and is not known to colonize in houses. *Triatoma infestans* has previously (153, 159) been refered to as a saxicolous species in Chile and Bolivia, but it is only recently that reports have become available of collections of this species from what is thought to be its primary habitat among stones near Cochabamba (51) and Sucre (J.P. Dujardin, personal communication) in Bolivia. *T. infestans* is highly synanthropic, and throughout most of its range from Ecuador to Southern Argentina it is not normally found outside the domestic environment. It is a very dangerous vector of *T. cruzi* and when introduced into new areas may cause outbreaks of acute Chagas' disease (11, 12, 91). Wild populations from Cochabamba were not distinguishable by isoenzyme markers from domestic populations, and it may be argued that domestic populations are invading wild ecotopes in this area (51), but the evidence is equally compatible with the hypothesis that the species is preadapted to conditions in houses and that no evolutionary changes were necessary for it to take advantage of the new habitat provided by humans.

Of the species of the *infestans* complex associated with birds nests, *Triatoma delpontei* from Argentina, Paraguay, and Uruguay has adhesive eggs and is particularly associated with nests of *Myopsitta monacha*. It has also been reported from nests of *Phacellodomus* in Uruguay and may occasionally be found in association with rodents at the base of trees with bird nests. Bird nests may be taken over by mammals and *T. delpontei* has been found infected with *T. cruzi*. Fertile hybirds can be obtained in the laboratory between female *T. delpontei* and the sympatric *T. platensis*, but in nature the two species appear to be separated by ecological and other barriers. *T. delpontei* has not been reported from synanthropic situations and is therefore ecologically separated from the introduced *T. infestans* (31, 89, 159). *T. platensis* also has adhesive eggs and is found in nests of birds of the family Furnariidae, rarely in those of *Myopsitta*. It occasionally occurs in primitive chickens houses, where it may hybridize with *Triatoma infestans* (31, 89, 159). *T. sordida* is widespread in central South America and in the wild has been collected from a variety of habitats, particularly birds nests, tree holes, and under bark. Peridomestically, it occurs mostly in chicken houses, under the bark of fence posts, and in other wooden structures. In houses it does not appear to compete successfully with *Triatoma infestans* or *Panstrongylus megistus*, the main domestic triatomines in its area of distribution. Peridomestic populations of *T. sordida* can however be important in maintaining an enzootic cycle of *T. cruzi* transmission among rats and domestic animals, which may subsequently introduce the parasite into populations of *T. infestans* inside houses (12, 21, 60). A population from birds nests in semidesert zones of north and central Argentina is recognized as a distinct species (*T. garciabesi*) by some authors (31).

Triatoma maculata and *T. pseudomaculata* are morphologically (89) and ecologically similar species occurring respectively north and south of the Amazon rainforest. *T. maculata* (39, 157) has been collected in large numbers in the semiarid lowlands of Venezuela, particularly in association with peridomestic chickens, although there is some overflow into houses.

In the wild the species occurs under tree bark, in birds' nests, and occasionally in bromeliads and in palms (especially *Scheelea* spp.) in association with *Rhodnius* spp., the latter invariably with higher trypanosome infection rates. Avian blood predominated in the samples analyzed, even from inside houses, and 20% of a silvatic sample were positive for reptilian blood. In Colombia *T. maculata* has been reported from *Scheelea* palms, and from a hollow *Mauritia* palm with bats. In the Brazilian State of Roraima investigators at a field station complained of attacks by nymphs and adults of this species, and the focus of the infestation was traced to nests of grey-breasted martins and palm tanagers in the roofs of the buildings. *Triatoma pseudomaculata* from central and northeast Brazil is also associated with chickens around houses, but tends to be found in lower numbers, possibly because of competition by *Triatoma sordida*. In the arid northeast, in areas free from *T. sordida*, it is a more common peridomestic species (2). In the wild it has been found in tree holes and under bark and in termite nests on trees, where it is often associated with reptiles, a finding supported by the results of precipitin tests on bloodmeals (V. Py-Daniel, personal communication). It has also been reported from palms (26). *Triatoma guasayana* is ecologically intermediate between the saxicolous and ornithophilic species of the *infestans* complex in that it colonizes both under stones and in birds nests. As with *T. sordida*, *T. maculata*, and *T. pseudomaculata*, the eggs are laid loose. The species occurs in Argentina, Bolivia, and Paraguay under tree bark, under stones with toads, under fallen logs with lizards and in chicken houses, but also feeds on mammals as it has been found naturally infected with *T. cruzi*. In houses it may replace *T. infestans* after control of that species (31, 89).

Of the species of the *infestans* complex, only *T. vitticeps* and *T. tibiamaculata* extend to the more humid coastal regions of eastern Brazil. *T. tibiamaculata* is a silvatic species found in epiphytic bromeliads, particularly *Aechmea multiflora*, in remnants of the Atlantic rainforest and transitional vegetation, from Pernambuco (149) to Santa Catarina States. Opossums (*Didelphis* spp.) commonly use these bromeliads as shelter, and *T. tibiamaculata* is frequently infected with *T. cruzi*. *T. tibiamaculata* shares its bromeliad habitat with *Rhodnius domesticus*, but has never been found infected with *Trypanosoma rangeli* (8, 13). *Triatoma vitticeps* is known only from southeast Brazil. It is widespread in the state of Espirito Santo, where nymphs have been collected in houses, although with one exception only adults were infected with *T. cruzi* (25). *T. vitticeps* has been reported in association with rock cavies and opossums (89).

Nymphs of *Triatoma melanocephala* have been collected once from terrestrial bromeliads in semiarid open country in eastern Brazil. The nymphs were associated with hairs of *Didelphis albiventris* and were infected with *T. cruzi* (12). The species is otherwise known only from adults that have flown into houses. Little information is available on the remaining species of the *infestans* complex, all from Brazil. *T. wygodzinskyi*, from Minas Gerais, appears to be closely related to *T. arthurneivai*. The natural habitat of *T. matogrossensis*, from Mato Grosso, is unknown. *T. williami* (158) occurs in houses in Goias and Mato Grosso. *T. deanei* may represent a hybrid between *T. williami* and *T. infestans*. Adults, and fifth-instar nymphs attributed to this species, are known only from specimens found in houses (89).

The *Triatoma circummaculata* complex consists of the two species which previously comprised the genus *Neotriatoma* Pinto, and both are saxicolous. *T. circummaculata*, from southern Brazil and Uruguay, occurs under rocks and in stone walls together with *T. rubrovaria*, and has been found infected with *T. cruzi*. Argentinian records of *T. circummaculata* are now believed to refer to *T. limai*, which occurs in rocks inhabited by rodents in Cordoba Province (31, 89).

The three species of the *Triatoma dispar* complex occur in areas of mesic forest in central and northwestern South America. *T. dispar*, known from Costa Rica, Ecuador, and Panama (89) and more recently from Colombia (5), is an arboreal species for which monkeys may be an important host. Nymphs have been found in tree forks occupied by the sloth *Choloepus hoffmani*, and specimens have been caught attempting to feed on humans on tree platforms (7, 64–66). *T. venosa* also occurs in Colombia and Costa Rica, between 1600 and 2000 m above sea level in the former country. Its hosts and habits are unknown, but it has been found infected with *T. cruzi* (89). *T. carrioni* is found between 1000 and 2650 m in Ecuador and Peru, in tree holes inhabited by wild mammals (80, 89).

The remaining species of *Triatoma* have yet to be placed in the above arrangement of species complexes. The recently described *T. brailovskyi* (95) is known only from adults taken at light in premontane areas of Mexico (31). *T. hegneri* has been described as phenetically isolated (89) or as closely related to *Triatoma dimidiata* (123). It is an insular species from Cozumel (Quintana Roo), Mexico. *T. hegneri* is reported to be saxicolous and cavernicolous, associated with *Didelphis*, and has been found infected with *T. cruzi*. Specimens including nymphs have been collected in peri-domestic situations (74, 123). *T. nigromaculata* is found in tree holes in association with birds and didelphids in Venezuela (31). The biology of *T. ryckmani* is unknown, but there is indirect evidence associating it with arboreal bromeliads in Guatemala and Honduras (123). *T. rubida* is associated with *Neotoma* nests in the U.S.A. and Mexico, and has been found infected with *T. cruzi*. It will bite man, and hypersensitive reactions to the bug's saliva may be severe in susceptible persons. An insular population (*T. rubida jaegeri*) is saxicolous, and associated with fish-eating bats in boulders a few feet above sea level (123). *T. guazu* is known only from a single specimen from Paraguay (89). *T. oliverai* from southern Brazil was found in shelters of the rodent *Cavia apera* (89). *T. matsunoi* is a recently described species from La Libertad Department in Peru. Specimens were collected on human bait in caves at 1890 m above sea level in an area of low (231 mm–522 mm) annual rainfall and moderate (13°C–18°C) temperatures. The bugs fed on mice in the laboratory (54 a).

Dispersal

Triatomines may disperse by flight, by walking, or by being passively transported. With the exception of *T. spinolai*, all adult Triatominae are macropterous. *Parabelminus yurupucu* and *Microtriatoma trinidadensis* will readily take to the wing in daylight, in what appears to be an escape reaction, but in most species flight activity is nocturnal. The use of strategically placed chicken houses and marked bugs to study patterns of colonization in South Brazil has been explored in a series of papers by Forattini (60, 61), and similar studies with *R. prolixus* in Venezuela have been reviewed elsewhere (35, 68, 114). Flight ranges of several hundred meters have been recorded, and Schofield and colleagues (86, 141) have calculated that flight, as a factor in the colonization of houses by *T. infestans*, is important at a distance of up to 200 m from the source.

Flight activity tends to be seasonal but it is difficult to separate the direct effects of meteorological factors from the effects of seasonal variation in population structure and host availability. Reduced nutritional status is certainly a stimulus to dispersal by flight (see below). Even in the relatively constant climate or Manaus, triatomines (principally *P. geniculatus*, *R. robustus*, and *R. pictipes*) that have flown into houses tend to be delivered to our laboratory irregularly, several specimens appearing within a few days following months without a record. In the Amazon region the probable source of silvatic bugs that have flown into houses can usually be identified nearby, and in the case of palms it may be practical to remove or treat them where zoonotic Chagas' disease is considered to be a danger (101). It should be noted that terms such as *light-attracted*, although widely used, are teleological and misleading when applied to bugs that have flown into houses, as the processes leading to the arrestment of triatomines in illuminated areas have not been analyzed.

Engorged first instar nymphs of *T. sordida* have been detected in the plumage of sparrows captured in flight in a few meters from the roost (62), and in Venezuela eggs and first instar nymphs of *R. prolixus* have been found in the wing feathers of nestlings of the wood ibis *Mycteria americana* (68). *Rhodnius* eggs are cemented to the substrate, and the transport of *Rhodnius prolixus* over long distances by migratory birds is an attractive hypothesis that deserves study (169). Dispersal by humans is undoubtedly one of the principal factors accounting for the present distribution of synanthropic species, and the history of their spread continues to be studied and related to human migratory movements (11, 15, 46, 47, 56, 79, 137, 147, 148, 150, 169). *T. infestans* has accompanied ships (79), railways (150), mule trains, wars, forced migrations, and postal services, and has also been spread deliberately through ignorance or malice (79). A recent work finds a relation between the coffee boom in São Paulo, and the establishment of *T. infestans* in Brazil at the beginning of the century (148). West of the Andes, *T. infestans* carried by people crossed the barrier of the Atacama desert from Chile to Peru around 1880 (79). The risk of this species crossing the Amazon rainforest to Roraima in north Brazil has recently been increased by the traffic of light aircraft carrying gold miners from northeast Brazil, and it is fortunate in this respect that *T. infestans* is being controlled in Brazil south of the Amazon (48, 154). *T. infestans* formerly spread as far noth as the pre-Amazonian State of Maranhão and in northern Goias reached a latitude of approximately 5°30′S in the Tocantins Valley (149).

Natural Enemies and Symbionts

The literature on the parasites, predadors, and symbionts of Triatominae up to 1978 has been reviewed in a fairly comprehensive anotated bibliography (8). Since then a further bibliography has been published (126), and De Santis and others have added to the list of microhymenopteran parasitoids of triatomine eggs (43). Schaub has studied the host–parasite relations of *Blastocrithidia triatomae* (131) and the effect of *T. cruzi* infection on *T. infestans* (130). Most reviewers agree that natural enemies play little part in regulating domestic triatomine populations, and the results of field trials of biological control have not been encouraging (114). The hypothesis that DDT may facilitate the establishment of domestic triatomine populations by eliminating natural enemies (11) has not been cited elsewhere, possibly because of conflicting reports on the effect of this insecticide on *T. infestans* (11, 78). Hemogregarines in Triatominae continue to be referred to as *Hepatozoon triatomae*, although several additional species are involved (8), and the most complete study (116) of the life cycle of a triatomine-transmitted hemogregarine was probably based on a distinct, unnamed species (8). Heavy infections of *Eratyrus mucronatus* by a gregarine of the genus *Machadoella* are frequent and may contribute to the low prevalence of *T. cruzi* in this species, but a detailed study is lacking.

Population Dynamics

Work on the population ecology of domestic triatomines is beset with practical and ethical difficulties associated with long-term studies in infested houses. These difficulties have been overcome to some extent by using as experimental models chicken houses designed so that they can be readily dismantled and rebuilt at regular intervals (76), and by the development and evaluation of passive sampling methods (69, 165). A comparison of reviews published in 1981 and 1985 shows that this is an area in which significant advances were made (114, 136, 171), although both of the 1985 reviews indicated that much remained to be done. The general picture that emerges is that triatomines are K-strategists with a low intrinsic rate of natural increase whose populations are limited by food availability (111) through density-dependent irritability of the hosts. Schofield and colleagues (134–136, 144) have proposed on the basis of experimental evidence, that as bug density increases relative to a fixed availability of hosts, this provokes an increase in host grooming behavior that leads to an interruption of feeding and a reduced nutritional status of the bugs, and consequently to a reduced rate of recruitment to the adult stage, reduced fecundity, and increased dispersal. Space is not normally limiting (139) and little evidence has been found for density-dependent mortality (75, 76). Although reduced fecundity and increased dispersal acting in a density-dependent manner should limit population size directly, Rabinovitch (114) has noted that a reduced rate of recruitment unaccompanied by increased mortality affects the time taken to reach a given population, rather than its final size. In practice a longer development time and need for an increased number of feeds will expose individual nymphs to an increased risk of mortality, particularly if the host is insectivorous or if host defense reactions include killing the bugs (128). Irritability at high bug densities may also cause the hosts to abandon the habitat.

The development time from egg to adult for *T. infestans* in central Brazil in about 6 months (134), which is relatively short in comparison with other species of *Triatoma* (171). In the Argentine Chaco, development rates and oviposition of *T. infestans* were correlated with mean minimum temperatures and were severely constrained during the winter. In regions with a pronounced cold season, year to year population stability in *T. infestans* appears to be maintained by compensatory development and recruitment during the warmer months (76). The effect of temperature on seasonal variation in vector population density and age (or stage) structure, along with the inhibitory effect of low temperature on the development of the infective metacyclic forms of *T. cruzi*, may explain observations of seasonality in the incidence of cases of acute Chagas' disease (44, 76, 114). In eastern Brazil, population density of domestic *Panstrongylus megistus* was related to household seropositivity to *T. cruzi* (112).

The Domiciliary Habitat

House design varies regionally in areas with endemic Chagas' disease, depending on local tradition and availability of building materials. Ecologically important features are revealed by structural modifications that successfully reduce infestation. Thus replacement of beaten earth floors with cement, or palm thatch with metal, has been effective in the control of *T. dimidiata* (172) and *R. prolixus* (68), respectively. Plastering walls can reduce available refuges to a point at which space becomes limiting (139). Engineering in relation to domestic triatomines has been reviewed by Schofield and White (142).

Host defensive behavior as a factor regulating triatomine populations evidently depends not only on the intensity of infestation (see above), but also on the threshold of sensitivity of the host and effectiveness of the host reaction. Dias and colleagues (46, 47) conclude from field studies that poverty and desperate living conditions prevalent in endemic areas of Chagas' disease result in a scale of subjective priorities that relegate the presence of domestic triatomines to the status of a comparatively minor nuisance, from the point of view of the inhabitants. Where social and economic conditions are better, tolerance is reduced to a point at which domestic populations fail to become established or are rapidly eliminated (46).

The peridomestic habitats of triatomines often are little more than extensions of contiguous natural ecotopes, the principal difference being that greater host availability may result in higher bug populations. Thus saxicolous species are found in stone walls, and species inhabiting birds nests are found in primitive chicken houses built of sticks. In areas where the domestic species has no wild population, peridomestic colonies may be extensions of the domestic population. This is the case with *P. megistus* in the mud-walled chicken houses in eastern Bahia, Brazil. In western Bahia, *T. infestans* colonized peridomestic structures where these were mud-brick extensions of the houses, but did not become established in wooden structures occupied by *T. sordida* (11). The analogies between domestic habitats and the wild habitats of domestic species are less clear, which makes it more difficult to predict which additional species are most likely to exploit the domestic environment. The ability to occupy a variety of different habitats in the wild is a feature of *P. megistus* and *T. dimidiata*, but it is not immediately clear why *T. infestans* should have become a more successful domestic pest than other saxicolous species, or why *R. prolixus* is more troublesome than other palm-tree-inhabiting species of the genus *Rhodnius*.

Final Considerations

Information on the habits and habitats of Triatominae continues slowly to accumulate, but many species including such conspicuous bugs as *Panstrongylus diasi* and *P. lutzi* are still known only from adult specimens that have flown into houses. Inconspicuous bugs, such as the Bolboderini, are poorly collected even in South America and it may be premature to declare this tribe absent from Africa and Asia. A useful methodological advance has been the development of a tracking device that allows triatomine habitats to be identified by following the hosts to their resting places (104), but this does not yet appear to have been widely used.

Palms are evidently important habitats for Triatominae, particularly for several species or populations of the genus *Rhodnius*. Names of palms in the entomological literature include many synonyms as their classification involves numerous ill-defined genera and species (27, 72, 162). The mode of leaf abscission appears to be an important character correlated with the suitability of palms as habitats for triatomines and their hosts, palms in which the petiole of the dead leaf fractures some distance from the trunk to leave a series of old leaf bases being most commonly infested. Thus in the forest north of Manaus, *Rhodnius robustus* was found in *Mauritia carana*, *Jessenia bataua*, and *Attalea* spp., palms of three different subfamilies but which share this feature.

Stands of the babaçu palm *Orbignya phalerata* are estimated to occupy an area of nearly 200,000 km^2 in Brazil, where they are concentrated in the southern portion of the Amazon Basin (97). These palms are inhabited by *Rhodnius pictipes* and populations close to *R. prolixus*, and owe their dominance of the landscape to a cryptic underground germination that allows the young palms to survive cutting and burning. Thus in the southern Amazon forest human settlement has actually increased the available habitat of palm-tree-inhabiting *Rhodnius* populations (97, 98). At the same time, clearance of the primary forest removes a barrier to the dispersal of domiciliary triatomines by flight, and on a larger scale increased aridity caused by deforestation may extend the area climatically suitable for *T. infestans*. Rural houses in south Para State commonly have mud walls that appear suitable for colonization by triatomines and the area has direct road links with central Brazil. The southern Amazon region can therefore be regarded as vulnerable to the establishment of domestic triatomines introduced from the south, and the possibility that local populations of *Rhodnius* may find conditions suitable for the establishment of domestic colonies cannot be excluded. Landscape degradation due to ecologically unsound agricultural practices may favor the domestic vectors of Chagas' disease, as resulting impoverishment of rural communities is reflected in standards of housing and education (138). Elsewhere human population growth exposes increasing numbers of people to silvatic triatomines (42), although autochthonous cases of Chagas' disease in areas without domiciliary bugs are still relatively rare.

The large literature on identification of hosts by serological tests on bloodmeals has not been reviewed here, partly because many workers found it unnecessary to mention any kind of controls or precautions against cross-contamination of samples, even when reporting unusually high rates of multiple mixed feeds or improbable host associations.

Progress made in recent years on the population ecology of domestic triatomines has been mentioned above, but a glance at any recent symposium proceedings on Chagas' disease will show that the main emphasis has been on the biochemistry and immunology of the trypanosome parasites rather than on vector ecology. Several papers include information on the prevalence of different biochemically characterized strains of *T. cruzi* in different vectors (3, 12, 100, 102, 155), but the number of samples analyzed is still small in relation to the number of vector species and populations, and much remains to be done on the ecological aspects of different vector–parasite systems using wild rather than laboratory strains of triatomines and trypanosomes. Techniques, such as enzyme electrophoresis (49–51, 63) and analysis of cuticular hydrocarbons, could usefully be applied more widely to the characterization of morphologically similar vector populations, to define populations geographically and detect clines or hybrid zones.

The frequent use of dogmatic negative statements as in this chapter is of course hazardous, but will have been worthwhile if it stimulates the divulgence of any important unpublished or obscurely published information that I may have missed, or encourages efforts to identify the habitats of the many species for which these are unknown.

Acknowledgments. I gratefully acknowledge the help received from colleagues who provided reprints, publications, and unpublished information. Jose Camilo Hurtado Guerrero helped transform the handwritten draft into a form ready for the typist, and other past and present students of the INPA postgraduate entomology course have provided the stimulus to try to keep up with literature on triatomine ecology. Original work on Amazonian Triatominae was supported in part by the research agreement ELETRONORTE/INPA. This review was written during the tenure of CNPq grant 301382 from the Brazilian National Research Council.

References

1. Aguilera, X., Miles, M.A., and Apt, W., 1986, *Triatoma spinolai* in Chile: A new host for *Hepatozoon triatomae*. *Trans. R. Soc. Trop. Med. Hyg.* **80**: 492–493.
2. Alencar, J.E., 1987, Historia Natural da Doença de Chagas no Estado do Ceará. Imprensa Universitaria da Universidade Federal do Ceará, Fortaleza, 341 p.
3. Apt, W., Aguilera, X., Arribada, A., Gomez, Z., Miles, M.A.M., and Widmer, G., 1987, Epidemiology of Chagas' disease in northern Chile: Isozyme profiles of *Trypanosoma cruzi* from sylvatic and domestic transmission cycles and their association with cardiopathy, *Am. J. Trop. Med. Hyg.* **37**:302–307.
4. Barber, H.G., 1937, A new bat-cave bug from Panama (Hempitera—Heteroptera: Reduviidae), *Proc. Entomol. Soc. Washington* **39**:60–63.

5. Barreto, M., and Barreto, P., 1984, *Triatoma dispar* (Hemiptera: Reduviidae), a new record for Colombia. *J. Med. Entomol.* **21**:750.
6. Barreto, M., Barreto, P., and D'Alessandro, A., 1984, *Psammolestes arthuri* (Hemiptera: Reduviidae) and its parasite *Telenomus capito* (Hymenoptera: Scelionidae) in Colombia, *J. Med. Entomol.* **21**:703–705.
7. Barreto, P., Barreto, M., and Hurtado, C., 1988, Nuevos hallazgos en Colombia de *Panstrongylus geniculatus* (Latreille, 1811) y *Triatoma dispar* Lent, 1950 (Hemiptera: Reduviidae), *Colombia Méd.* **19**:64–67.
8. Barrett, T.V., 1979, The ecology of triatomine bugs (Hemiptera: Reduviidae) and their hosts in relation to the transmission of *Trypanosoma cruzi* Chagas, 1909 in the State of Bahia, Brazil, PhD Thesis, London University, British Lending Library reference D 29306/80.
9. Barrett, T.V., 1988, Current research on amazonian Triatominae, *Mem. Inst. Oswaldo Cruz* **83**(Suppl. 1):441–447.
10. Barrett, T.V., and Arias, J.R., 1985, A new Triatomine host of *Trypanosoma* from the Central Amazon of Brazil: *Carvenicola lenti* n. sp. (Hemiptera, Reduviidae, Triatominae), *Mem. Inst. Oswaldo Cruz* **80**:91–96.
11. Barrett, T.V., Hoff, R., Mott, K.E., Guedes, F., and Sherlock, I.A., 1979, An outbreak of acute Chagas' disease in the São Francisco Valley region of Bahia, Brazil: Triatomine vectors and animal reservoirs of *Trypanosoma cruzi*, *Trans. R. Soc. Trop. Med. Hyg.* **73**:703–709.
12. Barrett, T.V., Hoff, R.H., Mott, K.E., Miles, M.A., Godfrey, D.G., Teixeira, R., Souza, J.A.A., and Sherlock, I.A., 1980, Epidemiological aspects of three *Trypanosoma cruzi* zymodemes in Bahia State, Brazil, *Trans. R. Soc. Trop. Med. Hyg.* **74**:84–90.
13. Barrett, T.V., and Oliveira, T.S., 1977, A trypansome, indistinguishable from *Trypanosoma rangeli*, in the haemolymph of *Rhodnius domesticus* from Brazil, *Trans. R. Soc. Trop. Med. Hyg.* **71**:445–446.
14. Barretto, M.P., 1967, Estudos sôbre reservatórios e vectores silvestres do *Trypanosoma cruzi*. XXI: Observações sôbre a ecologia do *Panstrongylus geniculatus* (Latreille, 1811) (Hemiptera, Reduviidae), *Rev. Brasileira Biol.* **27**:337–348.
15. Barretto, M.P., 1967, Estudos sôbre reservatórios e vectores silvestres do *Trypanosoma cruzi*. XXII. Modificações dos focos naturais da tripanossomose Americana e suas consequências, *Rev. Soc. Brasileira Med. Trop.* **1**:167–173.
16. Barretto, M.P., 1968, Transmissores do *Trypanosoma cruzi*: Os triatomíneos, Cançado, J.R. (ed): in Doença de Chagas. Universidade Federal de Minas Gerais, Belo Horizonte, *Imprensa Oficial do Estado de Minas Gerais*, pp. 189–224.
17. Barretto, M.P., 1976, Ecologia de triatomineos e transmissão do *Trypanosoma cruzi*, com especial referência ao Brasil, *Rev. Soc. Brasileira Med. Trop.* **10**:339–354.
18. Barretto, M.P., 1979, Epidemiologia, Brener, Z., and Andrade, Z.A. (eds): in Trypanosoma cruzi e Doença de Chagas, Guanabara Koogan, Rio de Janeiro, pp. 89–151.
19. Barretto, M.P., and Albuquerque, R.D.R., 1969, Estudos sôbre reservatórios e vectores silvestres do *Trypanosoma cruzi*. XXXIII. Infecção experimental e natural do *Psammolestes tertius* Lent & Jurberg, 1965 pelo *T. cruzi*, *Rev. Inst. Med. Trop. S. Paulo* **11**:165–168.

20. Barretto, M.P., and Carvalheiro, J.R., 1967, Estudos sôbre reservatórios silvestres do *Trypanosoma cruzi*. XVIII. Observações sôbre a ecologia do *Psammolestes tertius* Lent & Jurberg, 1965 (Hemiptera, Reduviidae), *Rev. Brasileira Biol.* **27**:13–25.
21. Barretto, M.P., and Carvalheiro, J.R., 1968, Estudos sôbre reservatórios e vectores silvestres do *Trypanosoma cruzi*. XXVIII: Sôbre o encontro de *Triatoma sordida* Stal, 1859 e de *Rhodnius neglectus*, Lent, 1954 em ninhos de pássaros da família Furnariidae (Hemiptera, Reduviidae), *Rev. Brasileira Biol.* **28**:289–293.
22. Barretto, M.P., and Ribeiro, R.D., 1981, Wild reservoirs and vectors of *Trypanosoma cruzi*. LXXVII: Observations on the ecology of the *Triatoma arthurneivai* Lent & Martins, 1940, *Rev. Brasileira Biol.* **41**:317–320.
23. Barretto, M.P., Siqueira, A.F., Ferriolli Filho, F., and Carvalho, J.R., 1968, Estudos sôbre reservatórios e vectores silvestres de *Trypanosoma cruzi*. XXIII. Observações sôbre criadouros do *Rhodnius neglectus* Lent, 1954 em biótopos artificiais (Hemiptera, Reduviidae), *Rev. Inst. Med. Trop. S. Paulo* **10**:163–170.
24. Barretto, M.P., Siqueira, A.F., and Freitas, J.L.P., 1964, Estudos sôbre reservatórios e vetores silvestres do *Trypanosoma cruzi*. II. Encontro do *Panstrongylus megistus* em ecótopos silvestres no Estado de São Paulo. (Hemiptera, Reduviidae), *Rev. Inst. Med. Trop. S. Paulo* **6**:56–63.
25. Barros, G.C., Mayrink, W., Salgado, A.A., Barros, R.G.C., and Sessa, P.A., 1975, Contribuição para o conhecimento da doença de Chagas autóctone no Estado do Espirito Santo, *Rev. Inst. Med. Trop. S. Paulo* **17**: 313–329.
26. Bento, D.N.C., Branco, A.Z.C.L., Freitas, M.R., and Pinto, A.S., 1984, Epidemiologic studies of Chagas' disease in the urban zone of Teresina, State of Piauí, Northeastern Brazil, *Rev. Soc. Brasileira Med. Trop.* **17**:199–203.
27. Bondar, G., 1964, *Palmeiras do Brasil*. São Paulo, Secretaria de Agricultura do Estado de São Paulo. Instituto de Botânica, Boletim 2, pp. 1–159.
28. Brazil, R.P., 1986, Observations on the feeding habits of *Triatoma rubrofasciata* (Hemiptera: Reduviidae), *Trans. R. Soc. Trop. Med. Hyg.* **80**: 349–350.
29. Carcavallo, R.U., Barreto, P., Martinez, A., and Tonn, R.J., 1976, El género *Microtriatoma* Prosen e Martínez, 1952 (Hemiptera: Reduviidae), *Bol. Dir. Malariol. Saneamiento Ambiental* **16**:231–240.
30. Carcavallo, R.U., Otero, M.A., Tonn, R.J., and Ortega, R., 1975, Notas sobre a biologia, ecologa y distribución geográfica de *Psammolestes arthuri* (Pinto) 1926 (Hemiptera, Reduviidae). Descripción de los estadios preimaginales, *Bol. Dir. Malariol. Saneamiento Ambiental* **15**:231–239.
31. Carcavallo, R.U., Rabinovich, J.E., and Tonn, R.J., eds, 1985, Factores Biologicos y Ecologicos en la Enfermedad de Chagas, OPAS y Ministério de Salud y Acción Social, Vol. 1: Buenos Aires, 250 p, Vol. 2: 251–472. Vol. 3: bibliography, not seen, fide vol. I. [If not found, search under *Chagas* (número especial)].
32. Carcavallo, R.U., Tonn, R.J., and Carrasquero, B., 1977, Distribución de triatominos en Venezuela, (Hemiptera, Reduviidae). Actualización por entidades y zonas biogeográficas, *Bol. Dir. Malariol. Saneamiento Ambiental* **17**:53–65.

33. Carcavallo, R.U., Tonn, R.J., González, J., and Otero, M.A., 1976, Notas sobre la biología, ecología y distribución geográfica de *Cavernicola pilosa* Barber, 1937 (Hemiptera, Reduviidae), *Bol. Dir. Malariol. Saneamiento Ambiental* **16**:172–175.
34. Carcavallo, R.U., Tonn, R.J., and Jiménez, J.C., 1976, Notas sobre la biología, ecología y distribución geográfica de *Rhodnius neivai* Lent, 1953 (Hemiptera, Reduviidae), *Bol. Dir. Malariol. Saneamiento Ambiental* **16**: 169–171.
35. Carcavallo, R.U., Tonn, R.J., Ortega, R., Betancourt, P., and Carrasqueiro, B., 1978, Notas sobre la biología, ecología y distribución geográfica de *Rhodnius prolixus* Stal, 1859 (Hemiptera, Reduviidae), *Bol. Dir. Malariol. Saneamiento Ambiental* **18**:175–198.
36. Christensen, H.A., and Vasquez, A.M., 1981, Host feeding profiles of *Rhodnius pallescens* (Hemiptera: Reduviidae) in rural villages of central Panama, *Am. J. Trop. Med. Hyg.* **30**:278–283.
37. D'Alessandro, A., 1976, Biology of *Trypanosoma (Herpetosoma) Rangeli* Tejera, 1920, Lumsden, W.H.R., and Evans, D.A. (eds): in Biology of the Kinetoplastida Vol. 1, Academic Press, London, pp. 327–403.
38. D'Alessandro, A., Barreto, P., and Duarte, C.A.R., 1971, Distribution of triatomine-transmitted trypanosomiasis in Colombia and new records of the bugs and infections, *J. Med. Entomol.* **8**:159–172.
39. D'Alessandro, A., Barreto, P., Saravia, N., and Barreto, M., 1984, Epidemiology of *Trypanosoma cruzi* in the Oriental Plains of Colombia, *Am. J. Trop. Med. Hyg.* **33**:1084–1095.
40. D'Alessandro, A., Barreto, P., and Thomas, M., 1981, Nuevos registros de Triatominos domiciliarios y extradomiciliarios en Colombia, *Colombia Méd.* **12**:75–85.
41. Deane, M.P., and Damasceno, R.M.G., 1949, Encontro do *Panstrongylus lignarius* naturalmente infectado por *Trypanosoma* do tipo *cruzi* e algumas notas sobre sua biologia, *Rev. Serv. Esp. Saúde Púb.* **2**:809–814.
42. Deneris, J., and Marshall, N.A., 1989, Biological characterization of a strain of *Trypanosoma cruzi* Chagas isolated from a human case of trypanosomiasis in California, *Am. J. Trop. Med. Hyg.* **41**:422–428.
43. De Santis, L., Silva, M.S.L., and Larramendy, M.C.C., 1981, Lucha biologica contra las vinchucas (Hem. Reduvioidea). El empleo de insectos entomofagos, *Rev. Museo de la Plata*, Nueva serie **12** Zoologia (123):239–260.
44. Dias, E., and Dias, J.C.P., 1968, Variações mensais da incidência das formas evolutivas do *Triatoma infestans* e do *Panstrongylus megistus* no municipio de Bambui, Estado de Minas Gerais. (IIa nota: 1951–1964), *Mem. Inst. Oswaldo Cruz* **66**:209–226.
45. Dias, E., Mello, G.B., Costa, O., Damasceno, R., and Azevedo, M., 1942, Investigações sôbre esquisotripanose de morcegos no Estado do Pará. Encontro do barbeiro *Cavernicola pilosa* como transmissor, *Rev. Brasileira Biol.* **2**:103–110.
46. Dias, J.C.P., 1985, Aspectos socio-culturales y economicos relativos al vector de la enfermedad de Chagas, Carcavallo, R.U., Rabinovitch, J.E., and Tonn, R.J. (eds): in Factores Biologicos y Ecologicos en la Enfermedad de Chagas, Opas y Ministerio de Salud y Accion Social, 472 p.

47. Dias, J.C.P., 1985, Aspectos socio-culturais e economicos na expansão e no contrôle da doença de Chagas humana, *Ann. Soc. Belge Med. Trop.*, **65** (Suppl. 1):119–126.

48. Dias, J.C.P., Gadelha, M.C.A., and Garcia, M.H.M., 1985, Doença de Chagas, Marques, A.C. (ed): in Síntese dos Programas da SUCAM 1985, Ministério da Saúde, Brasilia, pp. 21–25.

49. Dujardin, J.P., and Tibayrenc, M., 1985, Étude de 11 enzymes données de génétique formelle pour 19 loci enzymatiques chez *Triatoma infestans* (Hemiptera: Reduviidae), *Ann. Soc. Belge Med. Trop.* **65**:271–280.

50. Dujardin, J.P., and Tibayrenc, M., 1985, Études isoenzymatiques du vecteur principal de la maladie de Chagas: *Triatoma infestans* (Hemiptera: Reduviidae), *Ann. Soc. Belge Med. Trop.* **65**(Suppl. 1):165–169.

51. Dujardin, J.P., Tibayrenc, M., Venegas, E., Maldonado, L., Desjeux, P., and Ayala, F.J., 1987, Isozyme evidence of lack of speciation between wild and domestic *Triatoma infestans* (Heteroptera: Reduviidae) in Bolivia, *J. Med. Entomol.* **24**:40–45.

52. Else, J.G., Cheong, W.H., Mahadevan, S., and Zárate, L.G., 1977, A new species of cave-inhabiting *Triatoma* (Hemiptera: Reduviidae) from Malaysia, *J. Med. Entomol.* **14**:367–369.

53. Espínola, H.N., 1971, Reproductive isolation between *Triatoma brasiliensis* Neiva, 1911 and *Triatoma petrochii* Pinto & Barreto, 1925 (Hemiptera, Reduviidae), *Rev. Brasileira Biol.* **31**:277–282.

54. Espinoza, L., 1955, Epidemiología de la enfermedad de Chagas en la República del Ecuador, *Rev. Ecuatoriana Hig. Med. Trop.* **12**:25–105.

54a. Fernández-Loayza, R., 1988 (publ. 1989), *Triatoma matsunoi* nueva especie del notre peruano (Hemiptera, Reduviidae: Triatominae), *Rev. Per. Ent.* **31**: 21–24.

55. Ferraroni, J.J., Nunes de Mello, J.A., and Camargo, M.E., 1977, Molestia de Chagas na Amazonia. Ocorrência de seis casos suspeitos, autoctones, sorologicamente positivos. *Acta Amazonica* **7**:438–440.

56. Forattini, O.P., 1980, Biogeografia, origem e distribuição da domicilição de triatomíneos no Brasil, *Rev. Saúde Públ.* **14**:265–299.

57. Forattini, O.P., Barata, J.M.S., Santos, J.L.F., and Silveira, A.C., 1981, Hábitos alimentares, infecção natural e distribuição de triatomíneos domiciliados na região nordeste do Brasil, *Rev. Saúde Públ.* **15**:113–164.

58. Forattini, O.P., Barata, J.M., Santos, J.L., and Silveira, A.C., 1982, Hábitos alimentares, infecção natural e distribuição de triatomíneos domiciliados na região central do Brasil, *Rev. Saúde Públ.* **16**:171–204.

59. Forattini, O.P., Ferreira, O.A., Rocha e Silva, E.O., and Rabello, E.X., 1978, Aspectos ecológicos da tripanossomíase americana. XII—Variação regional da tendência de *Panstrongylus megistus* à domiciliação, *Rev. Saúde Públ.* **12**:209–233.

60. Forattini, O.P., Santos, J.L.F., Ferreira, O.A., Rocha e Silva, E.O., and Rabello, E.X., 1979, Aspectos Ecológicos da Tripanossomiase Americana. XVI—Dispersão e ciclos anuais de colônias de *Triatoma sordida* e de *Panstrongylus megistus* espontaneamente desenvolvidas em ecótopos artificiais, *Rev. Saúde Públ.* **13**:299–313.

61. Forattini, O.P., Rabello, E.X., Ferreira, O.A., Rocha e Silva, E.O., and Santos, J.L.F., 1984, Aspectos ecológicos da tripanosomiase americana. XXI.

Comportamento de espécies de triatomíneos silvestres na reinfestação do intra e peri-domicilio, *Rev. Saúde Públ.* **18**:185–206.

62. Forattini, O.P., Rocha e Silva, E.O., Ferreira, O.A., Rabello, E.X., and Patoli, D.G.B., 1971, Aspectos ecológicos da tripanossomiase americana. III-Dispersão local de triatomíneos, com especial referência a *Triatoma sordida*, *Rev. Saúde Públ.* **5**:193–205.
63. Frías, L.D., and Kattan, F., 1989, Estudios de taxonomia molecular en poblaciones de *Triatoma infestans* (Klug, 1934) y *Triatoma spinolai* Porter, 1933 (Hemiptera: Triatominae), *Acta Entomol. Chilena* **15**:205–210.
64. Galindo, P., and Fairchild, G.B., 1962, Notes on habits of two bloodsucking bugs, *Triatoma dispar* Lent, 1950, and *Eratyrus cuspidatus* Stal, 1859 (Hemiptera: Reduviidae), *Proc. Entomol. Soc. Washington* **64**:229–230.
65. Galloway, C.B., 1971, Forty-second annual report of the work and operations of the Gorgas Memorial Laboratory, Fiscal Year 1970, U.S. Government Printing Office, Washington, 40 p.
66. Galloway, C.B., 1973, Forty-fourth annual report of the work and operations of the Gorgas Memorial Laboratory, Fiscal year 1972, U.S. Government Printing Office, Washington, 37 p.
67. Gamboa, C.J., 1963, Comprobación de *Rhodnius prolixus* extradomiciliario en Venezuela, *Bol. Of. Sanit. Panamericana* **54**:18–25.
68. Gamboa, C.J., 1974, Ecologia de la tripanosomiasis americana (enfermedad de Chagas) en Venezuela, *Bol. Inf. Dir. Malariol. Saneamiento Ambiental* **13**: 158–163.
69. García-Zapata, M.T., Virgens, D., and Marsden, P.D., 1985, Comparison of vigilance methods in three houses with different *Triatoma infestans* densities, *Rev. Soc. Brasileira Med. Trop.* **18**:183–186.
70. García-Zapata, M.T., Virgens, D., Soares, V.A., Bosworth, A., and Marsden, P.D., 1985, House invasion by secondary triatomine species in Mambaí, Goiás-Brazil, *Rev. Soc. Brasileira Med. Trop.* **18**:199–201.
71. Ghauri, M.S.K., 1976, The Indian Triatomine genus *Linshcosteus* (Reduviidae), *Systematic Entomology* **1**:183–187.
72. Glassman, S.F., 1972, A Revision of B.E. Dahlgren's Index of American Palms. Phanerogramarum Monographiae 6, J. Cramer, Lehre, Germany, 294 p.
73. Gómez-Núñez, J.C., 1963, Notas sobre la ecologia del *Rhodnius prolixus*, *Bol. Inf. Dir. Malariol. Saneamiento Ambiental* **3**:330–335.
74. Gonzalez-Angulo, W., and Ryckman, R.E., 1967, Epizootiology of *Trypanosoma cruzi* in Southwestern North America. Part IX: An investigation to determine the incidence of *Trypanosoma cruzi* infections in Triatominae and man on the Yucatan Peninsula of Mexico, *J. Med. Entomol.* **4**:44–47.
75. Gorla, D.E., and Schofield, C.J., 1985, Analysis of egg mortality in experimental populations of *Triatoma infestans* under natural climatic conditions in Argentina, *Bull. Soc. Vector Ecologists* **10**:107–117.
76. Gorla, D.E., and Schofield, C.J., 1989, Population dynamics of *Triatoma infestans* under natural climatic conditions in the Argentine Chaco, *Med. Vet. Entomol.* **3**:179–194.
77. Guimarães, F.N., and Jansen, G., 1943, Novo transmissor silvestre do *Trypanosoma (Schizotrypanum) cruzi* (Chagas, 1909), *Mem. Inst. Oswaldo Cruz* **38**:437–441.

78. Herrer, A., 1955, Trypanosomiasis americana en el Peru. II Repercusión del uso de DDT en la incidencia de la enfermedad de Chagas en algunos valles de la región sudoccidental, *Rev. Med. Exp.* **9**:38–43.
79. Herrer, A., 1955, Trypanosomiasis Americana en el Peru. IV Ingresso del *Triatoma infestans* al territorio peruano, su dispersión en éste y posibilidades de ser erradicado, *Rev. Med. Exp.* **9**:57–67.
80. Herrer, A., 1955, Trypanosomiasis Americana en el Peru. V. Triatominos del Valle interandino del Marañon, *Rev. Med. Exp.* **9**:69–81.
81. Herrer, A., 1960, Distribución geográfica de la enfermedad de Chagas y de sus vectores en el Peru, *Bol. Of. Sanit. Panamericana* **49**:572–581.
82. Herrer, A., Wygodzinsky, P., and Napan, M., 1972, Presencia de *Trypanosoma rangeli* Tejera, 1920 en el Peru. I. El insecto vector, *Rhodnius ecuadoriensis* Lent and León, 1958, *Rev. Biol. Trop.* **20**:141–149.
83. Hoare, C.A., 1972, The Trypanosomes of Mammals. A Zoological Monograph, Blackwell, Oxford, 749 p.
84. Lainson, R., Shaw, J.J., Naiff, R.D., 1980, Chagas' disease in the Amazon Basin: Speculations on transmission per os, *Rev. Inst. Med. Trop. S. Paulo* **22**:294–297.
85. Leal, H., Ferreira Neto, J.A., and Martins, C.M., 1961, Dados ecológicos sobre os triatomíneos silvestres da Ilha de Santa Catarina (Brasil), *Rev. Inst. Med. Trop. S. Paulo* **3**:213–220.
86. Lehane, M.J., and Schofield, C.J., 1981, Field experiments of dispersive flight by *Triatoma infestans*, *Trans. R. Soc. Trop. Med. Hyg.* **75**:399–400.
87. Lent, H., and Jurberg, J., 1981, As espécies insulares de Cuba do gênero *Triatoma* Laporte (Hemiptera, Reduviidae), *Rev. Brasileira Biol.* **41**:431–439.
88. Lent, H., and Valderrama, A., 1973, Hallazgo en Venezuela del triatomino *Rhodnius robustus* Larrouse, 1927 en la palma *Attalea maracaibensis* Martius (Hemiptera, Reduviidae), *Bol. Inf. Dir. Malariol. Saneamiento Ambiental* **13**:175–179.
89. Lent, H., and Wygodzinsky, P., 1979, Revision of the Triatominae (Hemiptera, Reduviidae) and their significance as vectors of Chagas' disease, *Bull. Am. Museum Natl. Hist.* **163**:123–520.
90. Maekelt, G.A., 1983, La epidemiologia de la enfermedad de Chagas en relacion al ecosistema domiciliario, *Interciencia* **8**:353–366.
91. Maguire, J.H., Hoff, R., Sleigh, A.C., Mott, K.E., Ramos, N.B., and Sherlock, I.A., 1986, An outbreak of Chagas' disease in southwestern Bahia, Brazil, *Am. J. Trop. Med. Hyg.* **35**:931–936.
92. Marin, R.E., and Vargas, M.V., 1986, *Rhodnius pallescens* (Hemiptera: Reduviidae) in Costa Rica, *J. Med. Entomol.* **23**:333.
93. Marsden, P.D., Cuba Cuba, C., Alvarenga, N.J., and Barreto, A.C., 1979, Report on a field collection of *Dipetalogaster maximus* (Hemiptera, Triatominae) (Uhler, 1894), *Rev. Inst. Med. Trop. S. Paulo* **21**:202–206.
94. Marshall, N.A., Liebhaber, M., Dyer, Z., and Saxon, R., 1986, The prevalence of allergic sensitization to *Triatoma protracta* (Heteroptera: Reduviidae) in a Southern California, U.S.A., community, *J. Med. Entomol.* **23**:117–124.
95. Martinez, A., Carcavallo, R.U., and Peláez, D., 1984, *Triatoma brailovskyi*, nueva especie de Triatominae de México, *Chagas* **1**(2):39–42. [Not seen, fide ref. 129].

96. Matta, A., 1919, Notas para o estudo da biologia do *Rhodnius brethesi* n. sp., *Amazonas Médico* **2**:104–107.
97. May, P.H., Anderson, A.B., Balick, M.J., and Frazão, J.M.F., 1985, Subsistence benefits from the babassu palm (*Orbignya martiana*), *Econ. Bot.* **39**: 113–129.
98. May, P.H., Anderson, A.B., Frazão, J.F.M., and Balick, M.J., 1985, Babassu palm in the agroforestry systems in Brazil's Mid-North region, *Agroforest. Syst.* **3**:275–295.
99. Mendez, E., and Souza, O.E., 1979, Identificación y distribución de los triatominos de Panamá (Hemiptera: Reduviidae: Triatominae), *Rev. Med. Panamá* **4**:258–280.
100. Miles, M.A., Apt, W.B., Widmer, G., Póvoa, M.M., and Schofield, C.J., 1984, Isozyme heterogeneity and numerical taxonomy of *Trypanosoma cruzi* stocks from Chile, *Trans. R. Soc. Trop. Med. Hyg.* **78**:526–535.
101. Miles, M.A., Arias, J.R., and Souza, A.A., 1983, Chagas' disease in the Amazon Basin. V. Periurban palms as habitats of *Rhodnius robustus* and *Rhodnius pictipes*—triatomine vectors of Chagas' disease, *Mem. Inst. Oswaldo Cruz* **78**:526–535.
102. Miles, M.A., Póvoa, M.M., Souza, A.A., Lainson, R., Shaw, J.J., and Ketteridge, D.S., 1981, Chagas' disease in the Amazon Basin: II. The distribution of *Trypanosoma cruzi* zymodemes 1 and 3 in Pará State, north Brazil, *Trans. R. Soc. Trop. Med. Hyg.* **75**:667–674.
103. Miles, M.A., Souza, A.A., and Póvoa, M., 1981, Chagas' disease in the Amazon Basin. III. Ecotopes of ten triatomine bug species (Hemiptera: Reduviidae) from the vicinity of Belém, Pará State, Brazil, *J. Med. Entomol.* **18**:266–278.
104. Miles, M.A., Souza, A.A., and Póvoa, M.M., 1981, Mammal tracking and nest location in Brazilian forest with an improved spool-and-line device, *J. Zool.* **195**:331–347.
105. Miles, M.A., Souza, A.A., and Póvoa, M.M., 1982, O ecótopo de *Panstrongylus megistus* (Hemiptera: Reduviidae) na floresta do Horto (Rio de Janeiro), *Rev. Brasileira Biol.* **42**:31–35.
106. Monteith, G.B., 1974, Confirmation of the presence of Triatominae (Hemiptera: Reduviidae) in Australia, with notes on Indo-Pacific species, *J. Austral. Entomol. Soc.* **13**:89–94.
107. Nocerino, F., 1972, Selección de una cepa de *Rhodnius prolixus* resistente al Dieldrín, *Bol. Inf. Dir. Malariol. Saneamiento Ambiental* **12**:210–216.
108. Otero, M.A., Carcavallo, R.U., and Tonn, R.J., 1976, Notas sobre la biologia, ecologia y distribución geográfica de *Rhodnius pictipes* Stal, 1872 (Hemiptera: Reduviidae), *Bol. Dir. Malariol. Saneamiento Ambiental* **16**: 163–168.
109. Ozete, H.J., 1981, Observaciones sobre la biologia de *Triatoma flavida* neiva, 1911 en Cuba, *Rev. Cubana Med. Trop.* **33**:42–50.
110. Picado, C., 1913, Les broméliacées épiphytes considérées comme milieu biologique, *Bull. Scientifique France Belgique* Tom. 47, série 7, Vol. **5**: 215–360 and plates 6–24 (plates not included in pagination).
111. Piesman, J., Sherlock, I.A., and Christensen, H.A., 1983, Host availability limits population density of *Panstrongylus megistus*, *Am. J. Trop. Med. Hyg.* **32**:1445–1450.

112. Piesman, J., Sherlock, I.A., Mota, E., Todd, C.W., Hoff, R., and Weller, T.H., 1985, Association between household triatomine density and incidence of *Trypanosoma cruzi* infection during a nine-year study in Castro Alves, Bahia, Brazil, *Am. J. Trop. Med. Hyg.* **34**:866–869.
113. Pinto, A.S., and Bento, D.N.C., 1986, The palm tree *Copernicia cerifera* (carnaúba) as an ecotope of *Rhodnius nasutus* in rural areas of the State of Piauí northeastern Brazil, *Rev. Soc. Brasileira Med. Trop.* **19**:243–245.
114. Rabinovich, J.E., 1985, Ecologia Poblacional de los Triatominos, Carcavallo, R.U., Rabinovitch, J.E., and Tonn, R.J. (eds): in Factores Biologicos y Ecologicos en la Enfermedad de Chaga, OPAS y Ministerio de Salud y Accion Social, Buenos Aires, pp. 121–147.
115. Rambajan, I., 1984, The first autochthonous case of Chagas' disease with notes on possible vectors in Guyana, *Trop. Geogr. Med.* **36**:73–76.
116. Rocha e Silva, E.O., 1975, Ciclo evolutivo do *Hepatozoon triatomae* (Sporozoa, Haemogregarinidae) parasita de triatomineos, *Rev. Saúde Públ.* **9**:383–391.
117. Rodriguez, J.D., 1959, Epidemiologia de la enfermedad de Chagas en la Republica del Ecuador, *Rev. Goiana Med.* **5**:411–438.
118. Rojas, J.C., Malo, E.A., and Espinoza-Medinilla, E., 1989, Sylvatic focus of Chagas disease in Oaxaca, Mexico, *Ann. Trop. Med. Parasitol.* **83**:115–120.
119. Ryckman, R.E., 1962, Biosystematics and hosts of the *Triatoma protracta* complex in North America, *Univ. Calif. Publ. Entomol.* **27**(2):93–240.
120. Ryckman, R.E., 1971, The genus *Paratriatoma* in western North America (Hemiptera: Reduviidae). *J. Med. Entomol.* **8**:87–97.
121. Ryckman, R.E., 1984, The Triatominae of North and Central America and West Indies: A checklist with synonomy (Hemiptera: Reduviidae: Triatominae), *Bull. Soc. Vector Ecologists* **9**:71–83.
122. Ryckman, R.E., 1984, The Triatominae of South America: A checklist with synonomy (Hemiptera: Reduviidae: Triatominae), *Bull. Soc. Vector Ecologists* **11**:199–208.
123. Ryckman, R.E., 1986, The Vertebrate host of the Triatominae of North and Central America and the West Indies (Hemiptera: Reduviidae: Triatominae), *Bull. Soc. Vector Ecologists* **11**:221–241.
124. Ryckman, R.E., and Archbold, E.F., 1981, The Triatominae and Triatominae-borne trypanosomes of Asia, Africa, Australia, and The East Indies, *Bull. Soc. Vector Ecologists* **6**:143–166.
125. Ryckman, R.E., Archbold, E.F., and Bentley, D.G., 1981, The *Neotoma* group in North and Central America: A checklist, literature review and comprehensive bibliography (Rodentia: Cricetidae: Cricetinae), *Bull. Soc. Vector Ecologists* **6**:1–92.
126. Ryckman, R.E., and Blankenship, C.M., 1984, The parasites, predadors and symbionts of the Triatominae (Hemiptera: Reduviidae: Triatominae), *Bull. Soc. Vector Ecologists* **9**:84–111. [Not seen, fide ref. 129].
127. Ryckman, R.E., and Ryckman, A.E., 1967, Epizootiology of *Trypanosoma cruzi* in Southwestern North America Part X: The Biosystematics of *Dipetalogaster maximus* in Mexico (Hemiptera: Reduviidae) (Kinetoplastida: Trypanosomatidae), *J. Med. Entomol.* **4**:180–188.
128. Ryckman, R.E., and Ryckman, J.V., 1967, Epizootiology of *Trypanosoma cruzi* in Southwestern North America. Part XII: Does Gause's rule apply to

the ectoparasitic Triatominae? (Hemiptera: Reduviidae) (Kinetoplastida: Trypanosomatidae) (Rodentia: Cricetidae), *J. Med. Entomol.* **4**:379–386.

129. Ryckman, R.E., and Zackrison, J.L., 1987, A bibliography to Chagas' disease, the Triatominae and Triatominae-borne trypanosomes of South America (Hemiptera: Reduviidae: Triatominae), *Bull. Soc. Vector Ecologists* **12**:1–464.
130. Schaub, G.A., 1989, Does *Trypanosoma cruzi* stress its vectors? *Parasitol. Today* **5**:185–188.
131. Schaub, G.A., Böker, C.A., Jensen, C., and Reduth, D., 1989, Cannibalism and coprophagy are modes of transmission of *Blastocrithidia triatomae* (Trypanosomatidae) between Triatomines, *J. Protozool.* **36**:171–175.
132. Scheone, H., Carrasco, J., Dedios, F., Oyrazun, E., Gazani, A., Madariaga, L., and Ercilla, A., 1961, Determinación del limite austral de dispersión del triatomismo domiciliario e infección trypanosómica en Chile, *Bol. Chileno Parasitol.* **16**:59–62.
133. Schofield, C.J., 1979, The Behaviour of Triatominae (Hemiptera, Reduviidae): A review, *Bull. Entomol. Res.* **69**:363–379.
134. Schofield, C.J., 1980, Density regulation of domestic populations of *Triatoma infestans* in Brazil, *Trans. R. Soc. Trop. Med. Hyg.* **74**:761–769.
135. Schofield, C.J., 1982, The role of blood intake in density regulation of populations of *Triatoma infestans* (Klug) (Hemiptera: Reduviidae), *Bull. Entomol. Res.* **72**:617–629.
136. Schofield, C.J., 1985, Population Dynamics and Control of *Triatoma infestans*, *Ann. Soc. Belge Med. Trop.* **65**(Suppl. 1):149–164.
137. Schofield, C.J., 1988, Biosystematics of the Triatominae, Service, M.W. (ed): in Biosystematics of Haematophagous Insects, Systematics Association Special Volume No 37, Clarendon, Oxford, pp. 284–312.
138. Schofield, C.J., Apt, W., and Miles, M.A., 1982, The Ecology of Chagas' disease in Chile, *Ecol. Dis.* **1**:117–129.
139. Schofield, C.J., and Marsden, P.D., 1982, The effect of wallplaster on a domestic population of *Triatoma infestans*, *Bull Pan Am. Health Organ.* **16**: 356–360.
140. Schofield, C.J., Marsden, P.D., and Virgens, D., 1980, Notes on the biology of *Triatoma costalimai* Verano & Galvão, 1958, *An. Soc. Entomol. Brasil* **9**:295–301.
141. Schofield, C.J., and Matthews, J.N.S., 1985, Theoretical approach to active dispersal and colonization of houses by *Triatoma infestans*, *J. Trop. Med. Hyg.* **88**:211–222.
142. Schofield, C.J., and White, G.B., 1984, House design and domestic vectors of disease, *Trans. R. Soc. Trop. Med. Hyg.* **78**:285–292.
143. Schofield, C.J., Williams, N.G., and Kirk, M.L., 1985, Dispersal of *Triatoma spinolai*, *Trans. R. Soc. Trop. Med. Hyg.* **79**:280–281.
144. Schofield, C.J., Williams, N.G., and Marshall, T.F., 1986, Density-dependent perception of triatomine bug bites, *Ann. Trop. Med. Parasitol.* **80**:351–358.
145. Sherlock, I.A., 1979, Vetores, Brener, Z., and Andrade, Z.A. (eds): in Trypanosoma cruzi e Doença de Chagas, Guanabara Koogan, Rio de Janeiro, pp. 42–88.

146. Sherlock, I.A., and Serafim, E.M., 1967, *Triatoma lenti* sp. n., *Triatoma pessoai* sp. n. e *Triatoma bahiensis* sp. n. do Estado do Bahia, Brasil (Hemiptera, Reduviidae), *Gaz. Méd. Bahia* **67**:75–92.
147. Silva, L.J., 1985, A Doença de Chagas no Brasil. Indicios de sua ocorrência e distribuição até 1909. *Rev. Inst. Med. Trop. S. Paulo* **27**:219–223.
148. Silva, L.J., 1986, Desbravamento, agricultura e a doença de Chagas no Estado de São Paulo, *Cadernos de Saúde Pública* **2**:124–140.
149. Silveira, A.C., Feitosa, V.R., and Borges, R., 1984, Distribuição de Triatomíneos capturados no ambiente domiciliar, no periodo 1975/83, Brasil, *Rev. Brasileira Malariol. Doenças Trop.* **36**:15–312.
150. Soler, C.A., Sheone, H., and Reyes, M., 1969, Problemas derivados de la reaparición de *Triatoma infestans* en viviendas desinsectadas y el concepto de reinfestación, *Bol. Chileno Parasitol.* **24**:83–87.
151. Sousa, O.E., and Adames, A.J., 1977, Geographical extension in a new ecological association of *Panstrongylus humeralis* (Hemiptera: Reduviidae), natural host of *Trypanosoma cruzi* in Panama, *J. Med. Entomol.* **6**:748–749.
152. Sousa, O.E., Wolda, H., and Batista, L.F., 1983, Triatominos encontrados en el ambiente silvestre de la isla de Barro Colorado, *Rev. Méd. Panamá* **8**:50–55.
153. Spinola, M., 1852, Hemípteros, VII. Reduviteos, Gay, C. (ed): in Historia Física y Política de Chile, Fauna Chilena, *Zoologia* 7, Museo de Historia Natural, Santiago, pp. 210–226.
154. Superintendência de Campanhas de Saúde Públiса, 1986, *Síntese dos programas da SUCAM-1986*, Ministerio da Saúde, Brasília, 59 p.
155. Tibayrenc, M., Hoffmann, A., Poch, O., Echalar, L., Le Pont, F., Lemesre, J.L., Desjeux, P., and Ayala, F.J., 1986, Additional data on *Trypanosoma cruzi* isoenzyme strains encountered in Bolivian domestic transmission cycles, *Trans. R. Soc. Trop. Med. Hyg.* **80**:442–447.
156. Tonn, R.J., Carcavallo, R.U., and Ortega, R., 1976, Notas sobre la biologia, ecologia y distribución geográfica de *Rhodnius robustus* Larrousse, 1927 (Hemiptera: Reduviidae), *Bol. Dir. Malariol. Saneamiento Ambiental* **16**: 158–162.
157. Tonn, R.J., Otero, M.A., More, R., Espinola, H., and Carcavallo, R.U., 1978, Aspectos biológicos, ecológicos y distribución geográfica de *Triatoma maculata* (Erichson, 1848) (Hemiptera, Reduviidae) en Venezuela, *Bol. Dir. Malariol. Saneamiento Ambiental* **18**:16–24.
158. Travassos, L.P., 1972, *Triatoma williami* Galvão, Souza and Lima, 1965, capturado em Mato Grosso, Brasil, novo vector da moléstia de Chagas, *Mem. Inst. Butantan* **36**:263–266.
159. Usinger, R.L., Wygodzinsky, P., and Ryckman, R.E., 1966, The Biosystematics of Triatominae, *Annu. Rev. Entomol.* **7**:309–330.
160. Vargas, V.M., and Montero-Gei, F., 1971, *Triatoma dispar* Lent, 1950 in Costa Rica (Hemiptera: Reduviidae), *J. Med. Entomol.* **8**:454–455.
161. Weinmann, D., Wallis, R.C., Cheong, W.H., and Mahadevan, S., 1978, Triatomines as experimental vectors of trypanosomes of Asian monkeys, *Am. J. Trop. Med. Hyg.* **27**:232–237.
162. Wessels Boer, J.G., 1988, Palmas Indigenas de Venezuela, *Pittieria* **17**:1–332.
163. Whitlaw, J.T., and Chaniotis, B.N., 1978, Palm trees and Chagas' disease in Panama, *Am. J. Trop. Med. Hyg.* **27**:873–881.

164. Yaeger, R.G., 1988, The prevalence of *Trypanosoma cruzi* infection in armadillos collected at a site near New Orleans, Louisiana, *Am. J. Trop. Med. Hyg.* **38**:323–326.
165. Zapata, M.T.G., Schofield, C.J., and Marsden, P.D., 1985, A simple method to detect the presence of live triatomine bugs in houses sprayed with residual insecticides, *Trans. R. Soc. Trop. Med. Hyg.* **79**:558–559.
166. Zárate, L.G., 1984, Comportamiento de los triatomíneos en relación a su potencial transmisor de la enfermedad de Chagas (Hemiptera: Reduviidae), *Fol. Entomol. Mexicana* **61**:257–271.
167. Zeledón, R., 1974, Epidemiology, modes of transmission and reservoir hosts of Chagas' disease, *Trypanosomiasis and Leishmaniasis*, Ciba Foundation Symposium **20**:51–85.
168. Zeledón, R., 1981, *El Triatoma dimidiata (Latreille, 1811) y su relación con la enfermedad de Chagas*, San José (Costa Rica): Editorial Universidad Estatal a Distancia, 146 p.
169. Zeledón, R., 1983, Vectores de la enfermedad de Chagas y sus características ecofisiológicas, *Interciencia* **8**:384–395.
170. Zeledón, R., 1985, El *Triatoma dimidiata* (Latreille), Carcavallo, R.U., Rabinovitch, J.E., and Tonn, R.J. (eds): in Factores Biologicos y Ecologicos en la Enfermedad de Chagas, OPAS y Ministerio de Salud y Accion Social, Buenos Aires, 250 p.
171. Zeledón, R., and Rabinovich, J.E., 1981, Chagas' disease: An ecological appraisal with special emphasis on its insect vectors, *Annu. Rev. Entomol.* **26**:101–133.
172. Zeledón, R., and Vargas, L.G., 1984, The role of dirt floors and of firewood in rural dwellings in the epidemiology of Chagas' disease in Costa Rica, *Am. J. Trop. Med. Hyg.* **33**:232–235.

7
Tick Paralyses: Pathogenesis and Etiology

Rainer Gothe and Albert W.H. Neitz

Introduction

As has already been reviewed (33, 60), certain tick species or populations and strains of individual species are potentially capable of causing pathological and/or pathophysiological changes in humans and animals by inoculating noninfectious noxious substances during the repletion process. These substances are generally considered to be toxins. On the basis of different clinical manifestations eight forms of toxicosis may be distinguished. The most important of these toxicoses for veterinary as well as for human medicine are the tick paralyses, which basically differ both etiologically and clinically from tick-borne infections and notably from virus-mediated encephalitides.

The capability to induce paralysis, as already documented (33, 60), has been demonstrated, described, or suspected from the family Ixodidae for *Amblyomma americanum*, *A. cajannense*, *A. maculatum*, *A. ovale*, *A. testudinis*, *A. variegatum*, *Dermacentor albipictus*, *D. andersoni*, *D. auratus*, *D. occidentalis*, *D. silvarum*, *D. variabilis*, *Dermacentor* sp. in Italy, *Haemaphysalis inermis*, *H. kutchensis*, *H. parva*, *H. punctata*, *Haemaphysalis* spp. (as *cholodkovskyi* and *cinnabarina*), *Hyalomma scupense*, *H. truncatum*, *Hyalomma* spp. (as *aegypticum* and *savignyi*), *Ixodes brunneus*, *I. cornuatus*, *I. crenulatus*, *I. gibbosus*, *I. hexagonus*, *I. holocyclus*, *I. muris*, *I. pacificus*, *I. pari*, *I. redikorzevi*, *I. ricinus*, *I. rubicundus*, *I. scapularis*, *I. tasmani*, *Ixodes* sp. in Mexico, *Rhipicentor nuttalli*, *R. tricuspis*, *Rhipicephalus bursa*, *R. evertsi evertsi*, *R. evertsi mimeticus*, *R. sanguineus*, and *R. simus*, and from the family Argasidae for *Argas africolumbae*, *A. arboreus*, *A. mimiatus*, *A. persicus*, *A. radiatus*,

Rainer Gothe, Institute for Comparative Tropical Medicine and Parasitology, University of Munich, W-8000 Munich 40, Germany.
Albert W.H. Neitz, Department of Biochemistry, University of Pretoria, Pretoria 0002, Republic of South Africa.

A. reflexus, *A. sanchezi*, *A. walkerae*, *Ornithodoros lahorensis*, *O. savignyi*, and *Otobius megnini*. This enumeration is now to be extended with a *Rhipicephalus* spp. belonging to the *pravus* group and causing paralysis in Angora goat kids in South Africa (19, 91, 92) as well as with *Dermacentor nuttalli* inducing the same syndrome in sheep in the People's Republic of Mongolia (12) and possibly also with *Argas robertsi* with respect to the cattle egret *Ardeola ibis* in Australia (94) and *Ornithodoros capensis* affecting sea gulls of the genus *Larus* in South Africa (15).

Thus, of the approximately 810 tick species so far described (74) at least 60 species belonging to 10 genera have to be considered as potential paralysis inducers. However, for many of these species only a few and often inadequate or dubious records regarding the actual toxicity have appeared in the literature. Moreover, the identity of some tick species associated with paralysis must be accepted with caution. According to case reports documented in the scientific literature as well as from our own experiences, it is evident that of these 60 potentially paralysis-inducing tick species, essentially only *I. holocyclus* in Australia as well as *D. andersoni* and *D. variabilis* in North America are of particular interest in human medicine. In addition to these three tick species, which have the same epidemiological and causative relevance in veterinary medicine, *I. rubicundus*, *R. evertsi evertsi*, *R. evertsi mimeticus*, and *A. walkerae* in Africa south of the Sahara as well as presumably *A. radiatus* in North America are important inducers of paralysis in domestic and wild animals. The pathogenetic basis of this antibiotic relationship between ticks and their vertebrate hosts as well as the causality of the toxicoses has already been discussed comprehensively and in detail with respect to *A. walkerae*, *D. andersoni*, *D. variabilis*, and *I. holocyclus* (33, 60). However, because of new investigations and earlier unconsidered literature, in this review the current state of knowledge regarding the modus operandi of the pathomechanism as well as the toxin etiology of tick paralyses is actualized and presented separately for the hitherto studied tick species.

Argas (Persicargas) walkerae

Investigations to elucidate the pathomechanism of paralyses due to argasid ticks are confined to the disease syndrome caused by *A. walkerae* (40–42). As the paralysis-inducing developmental stage of this tick species, only larvae are responsible, whose clinically effective toxicity must be assigned to the active initial sucking phase around day 5 to day 6 of feeding and later (24). With the use of an in vivo test system it was confirmed that crude extracts of replete larvae only produced paralysis. Extracts of unfed larvae as well as those of all other stages, either fed or unfed, evoked no overt effects when inoculated at high dosage rates into 1-day-old chickens (134, 135).

In this tick paralysis, after a very constant time span of 5 to 6 days post-infestation, a flaccid tetraplegia develops. The incubation period until the appearance of this is entirely independent of the infestation load and the host age and can be shortened experimentally by transferring preinfested larvae to new vertebrate hosts. However, the rate of infestation is of primary importance for the severity of clinical symptoms, which increase in intensity and extent approximately directly proportional to the number of parasitizing larvae (24). A host age disposition has to be excluded but there are marked age-related differences in the number of larvae necessary to produce various degrees of paresis (24, 25). Only after repeated reinfestations does a weak protective mechanism become effective, which is mainly directed against the repletion process and in some animals probably also against the inoculated toxin (25).

As it was stated that paralytic symptoms appearing in chicken hosts during infestation of *Argas* (*Persicargas*) *persicus* are not the result of a toxic effect due to these parasites but rather caused by blood loss (69), pareses and paralyses induced by larvae of *A. walkerae* were hematologically analyzed at first. In these investigations it was clearly demonstrated that, even in fatally ending paralyses of chickens, the blood picture was not or only very slightly altered. The hematological changes were not greater than those in noninfested chickens after experimental withdrawal of an equivalent quantity of blood, which led to neither debility nor paresis nor paralysis (2, 59). Therefore, elucidation of the pathomechanism started with the neurophysiological differentiation of this tetraplegia.

Electromyographic investigations with chickens (26, 34, 45, 47, 51, 59, 65, 83, 84, 88) revealed a generalized affection of the peripheral nervous system especially of fast conducting nerve fibers. During the course of severe paralyses maximal motor conduction velocity slowed down to 55% of the initial value from 38.7 m/s and 37.7 m/s before larval infestation to 20.4 m/s and 20.3 m/s at the peak of the disease for the median-ulnar and sciatic nerves, respectively. Simultaneously motor threshold and supramaximal stimuli to the nerves had to be increased six- and threefold, respectively. The amplitudes of the evoked potentials from the corresponding distal musculature decreased from 3.0 mV to 0.46 mV for the wing muscles and from 2.7 mV to 0.75 mV for the leg muscles. Distal latencies changed only slightly from 1.9 ms to 2.8 ms for the N. median-ulnaris and from 2.5 ms to 3.7 ms for the N. ischiadicus. Upon repetitive distal nerve stimulation at a frequency of 30 stimuli/s, muscle action potential amplitudes fell to ca. 65% of the initial value (84).

From these findings it was concluded (84) that as paralysis advances, there is blockage of a steadily increasing number of nerve fibers, particularly in those of the rapid conduction type with fibers of the distal nerve sector finally also becoming involved. Experimental confirmation of this conclusion was obtained by direct neurophysiological differentiation of exposed sciatic nerves in normal and paralyzed chickens (46, 47). Rapidly conducting fibers were reduced in their impulse propagation from 85 to 86 m/s in normal chickens to 39 to 40 m/s in completely paralyzed animals. A functional impairment of the more slowly conducting fibers was also demonstrated but not statistically confirmed. The conduction velocity of afferent fibers, on the other hand, was not affected to that extent, the decrease totalled only 30% from 50.4 m/s in noninfested chickens to 35.5 m/s during complete paralysis. Thus, this tick paralysis is characterized basically as a motor polyneuropathy with only slight or moderate participation of the afferent paths.

Functional impairment during this paralysis also affects the efferent nerve fibers serving the breathing muscles, resulting in a decrease of compound potential amplitudes of the intercostal musculature from 297 μV in normal chickens to 45 μV in paralyzed, moribund animals. Simultaneously, the respiration rate was reduced from 32/min to 22/min, the duration of respiration, however, remained with 0.8 to 1.0 s constant. After stimulation of the Plexus brachialis the amplitudes of evoked potentials from the breathing musculature slowed down to only 15% of the initial value during the course of paralysis. There was no direct effect on the myocardium or on the stimulus-conducting system of the heart. The heart rate, however, was depressed from 392 beats per minute (bpm) to 227 bpm in completely paralyzed, moribund chickens. From these experiments it was concluded that as the paralysis progresses an increasing number of nerve fibers are blocked until innervation of the intercostal musculature and of the auxillary breathing muscles finally ceases (61).

Due to the resulting hypoventilation the P_{CO_2} increased from 38.8 mmHg in normal chickens to 81.3 mmHg after development of a complete paralysis. Simultaneously, partial oxygen pressure decreased from 37.4 mmHg to 16.3 mmHg and blood pH from 7.46 to 7.12. As a pathophysiological consequence, a respiratory acidosis develops, which may result in an impairment of the organs bearing on the hemodynamic functions (66). Further experiments revealed a significant elevation of serum glucose and nonesterified fatty acid concentrations during paralysis, indicating a direct toxic effect on the adrenal cortex. Serum electrolytes remained unchanged, but activity of the pseudocholine esterases in serum was reduced, which may be due to a direct action of the toxin (43, 44).

In order to investigate whether acetylcholine is causally responsible for the functional impairment of the peripheral nerves appearing during paralysis, the sciatic nerve was supramaximally stimulated distally at a frequency of up to 30 impulses/s, the response potential was derived from the foot muscles, and the pharmacological effect of the application of acetylcholine, prostigmine, and edrophonium chloride was determined quantitatively (48, 49). The results of these investigations clearly demonstrated that application of acetylcholine, as well as of blockers of its specific splitting enzyme, markedly improved neuromuscular impulse propagation in diseased animals, particularly in severe and extreme stages of paralysis.

Administration of acetylcholine to healthy animals caused an initial depression of excitation responses, which fell to 20% of their initial value. This depression weakened after 1 to 2 min and was again reinforced after 4 to 5 min. At the same time, there was a dissociation between the amplitudes of the first and the 30th potential of each excitatory series. In most pronounced cases of this tick paralysis, with an initial muscle potential of only 0.027 mV and a maximal motor nerve conduction velocity of 20 m/s, there was an immediate marked increase in the amplitudes of both potentials, in contrast to healthy and to untreated paralytic animals. At the fourth pulse the first and 30th potential increased to 160%, and at the fifth pulse to approximately 200% of the initial values.

Under the influence of edrophonium chloride, a short-duration cholinesterase inhibitor, depression of the first potential was much less marked in healthy animals than it was with acetylcholine; after 3 min it faded out. The 30th potential showed a steady depression at 60% of the initial value. In paralytic animals, both the first and the 30th potential increased, as with acetylcholine; this effect was maintained evenly in each of the excitatory series for several minutes but the amplitude reduction for the 30th potential simultaneously lessened.

Application of prostigmine to normal chickens resulted in slowly developing and progressive depression of amplitudes of the first and 30th potential, which after 10 min attained a minimum of approximately 20% of the initial values. In paralyzed animals, the amplitudes of both potentials first increased but after 1 to 2 min they fell to initial values.

From these experiments it was concluded that the toxin affects motor and sensory nerves and also influences neuromuscular transmission. Its action on efferent nerves results in a diminished acetylcholine liberation and in an alteration of the receptor sensitivity at the myoneural synapse.

To characterize the vulnerability of peripheral nerves, we investigated isolated sciatic nerves of normal and paralyzed chickens under standardized oxygen-saturated and anoxic conditions (50, 52, 53, 85–87). The nerves were first kept in Tyrode's solution, perfused by a carbogenic gas, and constantly maintained at 41°C, they were then transferred to a nerve chamber and incubated with a carbogenic or an anoxic gas. It was demonstrated that, independently from the duration of storage in a carbogenically perfused Tyrode's solution, the maximum nerve conduction velocities determined on the isolated sciatic nerve of normal and paralyzed animals were characterized by a rise after the first anoxic incubation, a clear-cut reduction of normal nerves and an increase of impaired nerves during the second carbogenic phase, and by almost equivalent values in the second anoxic phase. After completing the entire experimental in vitro series, the nerve conduction velocities measured on the isolated sciatic nerves of paretic and paralyzed animals were found to be higher or at least corresponding to that of normal nerves. Thus, under this experimental design, a more pronounced vulnerability of impaired nerves was not observed. The survival times of isolated sciatic nerves after anoxic exposure, which were determined by the temporal persistence of the potentials, revealed that this neurophysiological parameter always resulted in a higher value for the toxically damaged nerves after every two anoxic phases. After the first anoxic phase, the survival times of normal nerves amounted to 7.3 to 7.9 min and those of toxically impaired nerves up to 14.2 min. The survival times were reduced after the second anoxic phase, reaching only 5.6 to 6.4 min for normal nerves but 8.5 to 9.2 min for nerves from paralyzed animals. This means that toxically impaired nerves tolerate anoxia longer and better than do nerves of normal chickens with respect to excitability and function of impulse propagation. These in vitro investigations led to the conclusion that the noxious substance responsible for the paresis or paralysis is not located in the cell, but circulates humorally. The toxin must possess membranophilic properties, with a possible primary point of attack in the region of the nodes of Ranvier and/or in the totality of the membrane, but the somatic toxin linkage is very labile. This assumption is also supported by experiments in which chickens, whose entirely neurectomized wings only were infested, developed a degree of paresis corresponding to the intensity of infestation (R. Gothe and K. Kunze, unpublished data).

The functional changes in the cable properties of the peripheral nerves are not manifest morphologically, as even animals that were paralyzed for a prolonged period due to repeated larval infestation showed no ultrastructural lesions or reactions in the function-carrying parenchyma (26, 39). Structural modifications are not to be expected in tick paralysis on the basis of its clinical course, which is characterized as a generalized peripheral nervous system affection reaching a peak in a few hours, as paretic or paralytic symptoms only exist up to full engorgement of larvae and the extensive flaccid tetraplegia quickly regresses, if the ticks are removed in time (24).

In an attempt to isolate and define the toxin responsible for the paralysis gel permeation chromatography, chromatofocusing and DEAE-Sephacryl ion-exchange chromatography of crude extracts of replete larvae were employed. A fraction was obtained that induced paralysis in 1-day-old chickens when inoculated subcutaneously. SDS-PAGE revealed two bands with molecular weight of 32 kDa and 60 kDa. This result indicates that the toxin may exist as an oligomer, as gel permeation chromatography revealed a molecular weight in the region of 80–100 kDa. Analytical isoelectrical focusing showed one band with a pI of 4.5 (108, 135).

The paralysis caused by *A. walkerae* in chickens provides a suitable research model for detailed elucidation of all factors of these particular host–parasite interactions, especially of the structure–function relationship of the toxin owing to the ease of breeding of this tick species and to the economic value of the chicken host (89) and because of the availability of a relatively simple, but effective toxicity bioassay (134, 135). Similar models could be established with *Argas (P.) arboreus*, a parasite of the cattle egret

(67) and *Argas* (*P.*) *radiatus* (37), because each parasitic stage of these tick species is also well adapted to chickens, but their larvae have a greater paralysis-inducing capacity than do those of *A. walkerae*. The larval toxicity of *Argas* (*P.*) *persicus* (35, 37, 67), *Argas* (*P.*) *sanchezi* (37), and *Argas* (*A.*) *africolumbae* (54) is less pronounced.

Dermacentor spp.

The pathomechanism of paralyses due to *Dermacentor* has been studied probably in the disease syndromes caused by *D. andersoni* and *D. variabilis* only and was first hypothetically discussed as a severe impairment of the motor neurons as well as a mild irritative lesion of the posterior sensory roots in the spinal cord (3, 4) or it was thought that the toxin is neurotrophic and acts on the spinal cord and nuclear bulbar regions (1). Because of the typical clinical picture as an ascending flaccid tetraplegia it became reasonable and necessary to differentiate and characterize the neurophysiological status of affected hosts.

In a first respective investigation it was demonstrated that after electrical stimulation of the thigh muscles of a child, who was totally paralyzed probably by *D. andersoni*, a reaction was obtained leading to the conclusion that the point of attack of the "toxin" was located proximal to these muscles (114). Subsequent studies revealed indubitably and for the first time that the peripheral nerves are functionally damaged in tick paralysis (97). Using completely or partially paralyzed dogs, each probably affected by *D. andersoni*, the anterior tibial muscle responded to direct but not to indirect or reflex stimulation through the peroneal and posterior tibial nerve, respectively. When acetylcholine was injected rapidly into the femoral artery the muscle contracted. In contrast to healthy animals the potentials measured on the peroneal nerve after exciting the posterior tibial nerve were completely lacking in paralyzed dogs and differed distinctly in the pattern of the amplitude in partial paralysis. The modus operandi of pathogenesis was interpreted as an impairment of impulse propagation in the region of the myoneural and spinal cord synapses, due either to failure to liberate acetylcholine or to the action of an anticholinesterase.

In further experiments (115) considering only the muscle reaction and not, additionally, the compound nerve action potentials, the pathogenic principle of *D. andersoni* paralysis was also explained as a block in myoneural synapses. After electrically stimulating a peripheral nerve in a severely paralyzed dog no corresponding muscular reaction was observed; the animal merely expressed the sensation of pain. From this response it was deduced that the afferent paths are not impaired, that is, the impulse propagation is interrupted in the motor fibers only. In a severely paralyzed sheep, the voltage necessary for an impulse propagation had to be increased to 150 V and higher to trigger even a weak muscular reaction. However, after recovery from the paralysis, a voltage as low as 10 V sufficed to transmit a stimulus to a muscle with a stronger reaction. In a severely paralyzed dog, stimulation with potentials of up to 250 V had no effect on the corresponding muscle, but after clinical recovery a voltage of only 10 V induced a strong muscle response. Because of the speedy clinical restitution after removing the responsible ticks it was supposed that paralysis is caused by a mechanism similar to that of curare. The tick toxin, however, is not identical with curare, as curare antagonists such as prostigmine did not influence this disease (115).

A mechanism resembling the action of a competitive neuromuscular blocking agent was, however, then excluded, because of a normal sensitivity to acetylcholine in the motor end plates (98). This finding was also confirmed by results of a repetitive series of stimulations that corresponded in paralyzed and healthy dogs after both indirect and direct stimulation. A depolarizing-type block was ruled out, because intraarterial application of prostigmine reinforced, and pentamethonium, an antagonist to depolarizing blocking agents, failed to improve muscle contraction in paralyzed animals. Furthermore, a neuromuscular block due to cholinesterase inhibitors was not assumed, as the response to intraarterially applied acetylcholine was normal; prostigmine did not decrease the muscle contractions and the muscle maintained a tetanus upon indirect stimulation. The pathomechanism at the myoneural synapse was thought to involve a conduction block in the fine terminal nonmyelinated fibers, an inhibition in acetylcholine synthesis and the inability to release acetylcholine from the depots. Because motor as well as sensory conduction was said to be functionally maintained it was continued to suggest that the cause of paralysis due to *D. andersoni* was an impairment in neuromuscular transmission. The change in the flexing reflex reaction was interpreted as an additional impairment of transmission in the spinal cord (98).

In an attempt to localize the exact site of the neuromuscular block, the anterior tibial muscle of a dog completely paralyzed by *D. andersoni* was directly stimulated before and after administration of curare (99). As no differences were observed, it was concluded that the impairment of impulse propagation must occur in the region of the terminal motor nerve fibers. Further experimentation revealed that the fully paralyzed anterior tibial muscle contracted after intraarterial infusion of acetylcholine and that neither cathodal nor anodal current facilated stimulus transmission. The paralysis was intensified by curare, but was uninfluenced by pentamethonium. The maintenance of functional activity of the end plates during paralysis was indicated by the capacity of the muscle to contract after intraarterial injection of acetylcholine and by depolarization through succinylcholine. From these results it was deduced that the probable mechanism of tick paralysis is due to a failure in the liberation or the biosynthesis of acetylcholine at the nerve terminals. The tick toxin thereby acts specifically on the neuromuscular junctions, because cholinergic fibers of the vegetative system were not affected (99). Using two marmots (*Marmota flaviventris avara*), one guinea pig, and two hamsters, suffering from *D. andersoni* paralysis, reactions described as generalized body twitches were observed after stimulation of the lateral popliteal nerves by 250 V at 0.5 and 1 impulse/s as compared with normal responses before paralysis or after recovery. In contrast, muscles reacted normally to direct stimulation. These results were taken as further evidence of a neuromuscular block on the assumption that the conduction in the motor nerves had not changed during paralysis (68). These findings were confirmed in marmots, as electrical stimuli applied through motor nerves failed to induce contractions, whereas direct stimulation of the muscles was effective. Additionally, it was proven that nerve impulses do not increase the proportion of acetylcholine in a perfusion fluid following cannulation of the iliac artery and vein of fully paralyzed marmots due to *D. andersoni*. The sciatic nerve of the marmots was maximally stimulated at a frequency of 10 impulses/s and the acetylcholine content was determined by bioassay according to the lowering effect on blood pressure of the outflowing perfusion medium in an eviscerated cat. However, the question was left open of whether this acetylcholine release impairment occurred because of inhibited synthesis or suppressed liberation of acetylcholine. The probable involvement of yet unknown factors acting on the central nervous system was also discussed (16). It was further demonstrated that a deficit of choline and acetyl-Co A, which are essential for acetylcholine biosynthesis, is not a causative factor, as their application did not alter the disease course in dogs. Therefore, the failure of the nerve impulses to liberate acetylcholine was considered due to a defect in the release mechanism rather than an inability to synthesize it (100). In further complementary investigations on *D. andersoni* paralysis, the acetylcholine output of the perfused anterior tibial muscle in normal and paralyzed dogs were compared during nerve stimulation and also by perfusion with high-potassium Locke solution. The cholineacetylase activity as well as the acetylcholine content of the ventral lumbar root and of the peroneal nerve were also measured to determine whether the inability of the nerve impulse to liberate acetylcholine in the paralyzed muscle was due to an impairment in synthesis of the transmitter substance. Acetylcholine was shown to be liberated in normal and in paralyzed dogs, but the output was greater in the normal animals. No significant differences were found in cholineacetylase activity and in the acetylcholine content of the ventral lumbar root and of the peroneal nerve, leading to the explanation of the pathomechanism that nerve impulses are incapable of traversing the terminal presynaptic fibers of the somatic motor axons to activate the necessary release of acetylcholine (101).

Further experiments finally demonstrated that in the *D. andersoni* paralysis of marmots acetylcholine synthesis is not impaired in peripheral nerves or in the spinal cord and the cerebral cortex, and that the absence of this transmitter substance in perfusates of the peripheral and central nerve tissue following stimulation may be due to its depressed release or to an inhibition of the motor nerve conduction. For, in the paralyzed marmots, after stimulation of the exposed sciatic nerve, the amplitudes of the nerve action potentials were much lower than those in normal animals. Concomitantly, the amplitude of the electromyographic response in the gastrocnemius muscle was also reduced. Additionally, the impulse propagation in centripetally conducting nerve fibers as well as the monosynaptic reflex actions were clearly impaired. Changes in the electrocardiogram were suggestive of a slowed rate of auricular and ventricular depolarization and repolarization (17). In experiments with dogs and marmots, paralyzed by *D. andersoni*, attention was drawn to the loss in function of the stretch reflexes, which failed even in animals with only slightly impaired neuromuscular impulse transmission. In the results, however, the neurophysiological findings and the degree of neuromuscular impairment are only tabulated in the form of a percentage proportion, but now this percentage was defined is not stated. The disturbances in coordination appearing early in the disease course and the ascending character of the paralysis were considered to be due to a loss of the stretch reflexes. It was also conjectured that the toxin blocks fine terminal fibers in the central and peripheral nervous system (18).

Comparing the conduction capacity of the motor fibers in the peroneal nerve of normal and *D. andersoni* paralyzed dogs it was shown that, after stimulation of the ventral root of the sixth lumbar nerve in cases of paresis of medium severity, the potential of the α fibers was reduced threefold and that of β and γ fibers decreased 30 times. The amplitudes of the δ fibers seemed to be even smaller. The speed of conduction was also clearly reduced, particularly in the β, γ, and δ fibers. In cases of severe paralysis, only a very low potential could be obtained, presumably originating from the α fibers. From these measurements it was concluded that this tick paralysis is due to a conduction block in the motor nerve fibers and that the toxin attacks especially motor nerve fibers of small diameter (102).

In further experiments to determine the action potential and conduction velocity, the ventral root of the sixth lumbar nerve was stimulated in six normal and eight *D. andersoni* paralyzed dogs, and the derived potentials were measured at two sites on the sciatic and peroneal nerves in the upper thigh, as well as on the peroneal nerve at the neck of the fibula. Paralysis was defined as severe when voluntary muscle contraction was no longer possible and when no visible contraction of the anterior tibial muscle occurred upon indirect stimulation. In medium-grade paralysis, the dogs still showed weak muscle movements and the muscular response after nerve stimulation was distinctly less than in normal animals. In the normal animals and in four moderately paralyzed dogs, the potentials derived from three measurement sites were characterized by a biphasic initial component of small amplitude and short latency apparently due to the thick, rapidly conducting fibers, and a subsequent multiple complex of large amplitude and longer latency, probably caused by the fibers of smaller diameter and slower conductance. The amplitude of the action potentials in fastest conducting fibers was diminished three times than that of normal animals, and in fibers of slower conduction was more pronouncedly reduced to 1/14 of the normal value. In four animals with severe paralysis, however, only a single potential of small amplitude could be recorded, presumably originating from thick fibers. Conductance capacity was also lessened in the sensory nerve fibers (103, 104). From these experiments the pathogenic principle of this tick paralysis was explained as a progressive block in impulse propagation of the efferent and afferent fibers, probably caused by suppression of an increasing number of Ranvier's nodes. Smaller-diameter, slower-conducting fibers were considered to be involved to a greater degree than fibers with larger diameter and faster conduction (104, 106). However, the original records (104) contain only one potential complex, so that a typification of the fibers is impossible. In addition, Aα fibers usually have a markedly higher potential than do the Aβ, Aγ, or Aδ fibers, which, moreover, have almost exclusively afferent or vegetative functions. This in turn cannot be correlated with the typical clinical symptom complex of *D. andersoni* paralysis, which essentially is a motor polyneuropathy.

The central nervous system may also be affected in *D. andersoni* paralysis, because the electroencephalogram in a paralyzed child showed a gross abnormality in the right occipital area which, however, was quickly reversible after removing the tick (131). This abnormality was not observed in another human case (6).

In further studies on *D. andersoni* paralysis it was found that in vivo the average action potential of the peroneal nerve of paralyzed dogs was reduced by ca. 50% of that of normal animals, but in vitro there were no differences. To explain these contradictory findings, it was suggested that the toxin might be leached out of the nerve during its incubation in Locke solution or that the high partial oxygen pressure in vitro may have favorably affected the reduced impulse propagation. The impairment of impulse propagation was hypothetically explained to be caused by a sensitivity of the nodes of Ranvier to the toxin and that, with increasing length of the nerve fiber investigated, the probability becoming greater for the impulse to meet an affected node (105). However, the proposed hypothesis (105) is problematic, as no dissected preparations of single nerve fibers were investigated, but only mixed nerves with numerous single fibers. Investigation of a larger or smaller section of peripheral nerve containing internodal distances within a 0.1 to 1.0 mm range is theoretically unimportant, provided that the distances are large enough, the in vitro setup is arranged to protect against formation of artifacts arising from stimulation, and that a clear assay of nerve conduction velocity is possible.

Electrophysiological investigations of a 5-year-old girl with typical signs of paralysis probably caused by *D. andersoni* revealed that the conduction velocity in the right median nerve was decidedly lowered and reached normal values only after clinical restitution. Thus, the impulse propagation rose from 43.3 m/s on the second day after removing the responsible tick to 47.6 m/s on the third day and to 50.0 m/s about 3 weeks later. Corresponding with these increasing values, the amplitudes of the muscle action potentials measured in the right thenar muscle changed from 0.8 mV to 4.0 mV and 12.5 mV, respectively. However, conduction capacity of the afferent fibers and the neuromuscular impulse transfer were not impaired. The electroencephalogram, as well as the creatine kinase level, were normal. As another partial pathogenic aspect, the possibility of a depolarizing block at the myoneural synapse and/or muscle lesion were also discussed (6). In another case report concerning a 5-1/2-year-old girl paralyzed probably by *D. variabilis*, the disease symptoms were interpreted differently with respect to the pathomechanism. Without clarifying the neurophysiological parameters of the peripheral nerves, the symptoms were considered to be of a characteristically cerebellar type, because they consisted of severe ataxia with incoordination, dysmetria, intention tremor, and absent stretch reflexes. The possible cause of these signs was explained to be due to an impairment of the cerebellar-vestibular-spinal pathways (90).

In a 4-year-old girl paralyzed probably by *D. variabilis* a diminished conductance velocity in the ulnar and median nerves with a simultaneously retarded latency was again demonstrated (70). Investigations on the ulnar nerve of a 4-year-old boy paralyzed by the same tick species also showed a reduced conduction velocity and an abnormally small compound muscle action potential (13).

These neurophysiological values became normal within 3 and 2 weeks, respectively, after removing the responsible ticks (13, 70). A similar neurophysiological pattern, but including the afferent nerve fibers, was also observed in a 5-year-old girl paralyzed by *D. variabilis*. The amplitudes of muscle action potentials evoked by stimulation of motor nerves were reduced initially, returning to normal after tick removal. Distal motor and sensory latencies also shortened after removing of the tick. There was no obvious evidence of a defect in neuromuscular transmission, because muscle action potentials did not change significantly in amplitude on repetitive stimulation even up to 50 Hz (130). On the other hand, the pathogenic principle of the *D. variabilis* paralysis was again interpreted as a neuromuscular junction blockade. This assumption was deduced from electromyographic results in a diseased dog, which, however, were not presented and from the unresponsiveness of peripheral nerves to direct electrical stimulation (7).

Acetylcholine liberation interference was regarded as a partial aspect of the pathomechanism of *D. andersoni* paralysis, but the exact site of impairment in the area of the neuromuscular junction could not be located clearly. In vitro, the frequency of the miniature end-plate potentials in phrenic nerve-diaphragma preparations obtained from normal and paralyzed hamsters did not differ when the bathing solution contained the usual potassium concentration. The frequency at paralyzed junctions lessened only with increased potassium concentrations. The mean quantum content of evoked end-plate potentials in a magnesium-containing solution was normal but their amplitudes and that of the miniature end-plate potentials were heightened. Thus, the assumption of additional damage in the neuromuscular end-plate area was not excluded or proven in this particular tick paralysis (95). During the most severe clinical manifestation of *D. andersoni*-induced paralysis, the creatine kinase activity in the serum increases significantly. In an 8-year-old paralyzed girl the level rose namely to 108 IU/l as compared to 60 and 56 IU/l during clinical convalescence 10 and 24 days, respectively, after removing the responsible tick. The increased creatine kinase activity was considered to result from the direct effect of the paralysis-inducing toxin on either muscle or nerve tissue, with the explanation that the enzyme was released by the damaged muscle cell membrane owing to interference by the tick toxin with the cellular energy metabolism. The impairment of pyruvate production from the muscle tissue of paralytic marmots was interpreted as supporting this hypothesis (5). Electrophysiologic measurements in a 9-year-old girl with tick paralysis, probably caused by *D. variabilis* demonstrated a prolonged distal latency and a decremental response to repetitive stimulation. The amplitudes of the extensor digitalis muscles remained decreased by 20.8% after stimulation at 30 impulses/s even as long as 27 h after removing the tick, showing a relatively persistent defect in myoneural transmission (96).

The mechanism of pathogenicity in *Dermacentor*-caused paralysis, investigated almost exclusively in the syndrome induced by *D. andersoni*, has been interpreted differently in various investigations, despite frequently clear evident findings. This mechanism was first thought to be due to impaired impulse propagation in the myoneural synapse area (97, 115), either by failure to liberate acetylcholine or by the action of an anticholinesterase (97), or to an impairment caused by a mechanism similar to that operating in curare (115). Other possibilities suggested subsequently were a conduction block in the fine terminal, nonmyelinated nerve fibers, impairment in acetylcholine synthesis, and incapacity of the impulses to release acetylcholine from the depots (68, 98, 99). The nerve impulses were also thought to be incapable of passing the terminal presynaptic fibers of the somatic motor axons in order to activate the necessary acetylcholine release (18, 101). The total function of the peripheral nerves was considered pathogenetically only in later investigations. Thus, *Dermacentor*-induced paralyses are now defined essentially as motor polyneuropathies with only limited participation of the afferent pathways. The following pathogenetic factors have been demonstrated experimentally: (1) diminution of the maximal motor nerve conduction velocities (6, 13, 70, 102–104, 130); (2) clear decrease in nerve compound action potentials (17, 97, 102–105) as well as in the compound potentials from the corresponding muscles (6, 13, 17, 68, 97, 115, 130); (3) impairment of impulse propagation of afferent fibers (17, 103, 104, 130); and (4) the simultaneously required heightening of the stimulating current potentials necessary to elicit a response (115).

A causal pathogenic role of inhibited acetylcholine biosynthesis can be excluded (17, 95). Whether, or to what extent, a central defect also exists cannot be decided from the few contradictory available findings (6, 90, 131).

With respect to the toxin etiology of *Dermacentor*-induced paralyses, no studies additional to the already documented and reviewed investigations (33) have been reported in the scientific literature. As has been stated there (33), from the hitherto published, often inadequate investigations certain aspects convincingly explain the cause of these paralyses also to be a toxin. Its chemical nature, however, has not yet been studied.

Rhipicephalus evertsi evertsi

Experimental in vivo investigations with sheep (27–32, 34, 55–58) revealed that the pathomechanism of the induced paralysis due to female *R. evertsi evertsi* is primarily also characterized as a generalized affection of the peripheral nervous system and essentially as a motor polyneuropathy with strong functional but simultaneous fast reversible impairment of impulse propagation. Thereby, these functional disturbances were directly correlated with the degree of this flaccid tetraplegia and thus with the infestation rate. Neuropathophysiologically, most obvious was the marked decrease of the amplitudes of evoked compound muscle action potentials after proximal and distal stimulation of the sciatic nerve in the corresponding distal leg musculature, which, in temporal parallelism and quantitatively analogous convergency with the severity as well as in comparison with normal animals, amounted to 28% in animals with moderate paresis and 44% in completely paralyzed sheep. The maximal motor conduction velocities, however, were only slightly reduced by 13.5% and 17.5%, respectively. The minimal slow conducting fibers were according to the double stimulus technique used in the investigation (57) not affected. Likewise neither quantitative nor qualitative differences were noted with respect to the electroencephalogram and the amplitude pattern by repetitive stimulation of the sciatic nerve with high frequencies between sheep before tick-infestation and during maximum intensity of tetraplegia. Correspondingly, a pathogenetic causal participation of the myoneural synapses or the central nervous system was considered not to be involved. From these investigations, it was concluded that with increasing intensity of the tetraplegia a steadily larger number of nerve fibers, particularly the slow conducting axons but also those of the rapid conduction type are blocked with respect to their excitability and impulse propagation (28, 30–32, 34, 56, 57). In further complementary neurophysiological investigations of exposed tibial nerves in normal and paralyzed sheep, it was confirmed that primarily not the fast but the slower conducting nerve fibers are functionally inhibited or blocked. The amplitudes of nerve action potentials and evoked compound muscle action potentials namely slowed down by 46% and 88.3%, respectively, when the paralysis became clinically manifest, whereas the conduction velocity of the Nervus tibialis and the maximum motor conduction velocity were only slightly reduced by 21.6% and 20%, respectively (32, 34, 58).

As a pathophysiological consequence of this motor polyneuropathy, as elucidated by parallel analysis of serum enzymes, blood glucose levels as well as blood gas and blood pH (31, 32, 34, 117) a secondary toxin action also becomes operative in sheep. During the course of this paralysis the activities of creatine kinase (CK), aspartate aminotransferase (AST), and alanine aminotransferase (ALT) always increased markedly and maximally with 735%, 200%, and 373%, respectively, whereas the values of alkaline phosphatase (AP) and cholinesterase were reduced up to 48% and 24%, respectively. Simultaneously, the blood glucose concentrations was elevated by 14%, whereas the total leukocyte count as a result of a mononuclear leucopenia and eosinopenia was diminished. The hemoglobin content and hematocrit as well as the plasma urea concentration remained unchanged. Blood gas analysis of the arterio-venous blood from skin vessels revealed an increase of Pco_2 with a corresponding decrease of Po_2 as well as blood pH. However, all values reached their normal levels still in the clinical restitution phase. The elevation in activity of the almost muscle-specific CK in temporal parallelism with the increase in severity of this toxicosis and its corresponding diminution upon clinical restitution is thereby to be considered as an expression of a functional rather than as a structural myopathy and as a consequence of a heightened but fast reversible permeability of the muscle cell membrane. The simultaneous marked increase and the CK-analogous time curve of the almost ubiquitous and muscle-unspecific AST and ALT also indicate a muscle cell damage. The increase in the AST and ALT activities even imply an impairment of the liver parenchyma probably resulting from injury to cellular obturation. In addition, the increased AST values can be evaluated as an expression of a necrosis of liver cells. Damage of the liver, however, is clearly confirmed by the parallel decrease of the liver-specific secretion enzyme, cholinesterase. Whether this decrease of cholinesterase is based on a direct damage of the liver cells or is due to malnutrition with simultaneous hypoproteinemia as a clinical consequence of the ascending, also muscles for chewing and swallowing affecting tetraplegia cannot be deduced. Because of the parallel decrease of the AP, the decline of the cholinesterase has rather to be explained with the long hunger period as the result of a considerably reduced or for days completely inhibited food uptake (71). This extended nutritional abstinence possibly also induces the mild to moderate hypoglycemia, whereby the basal insulin secretion is probable insufficient to handle the total metabolism, thus a hunger diabetes develops.

The neurotoxin also affects, as is indicated by the increase of Pco_2 with a corresponding decrease of Po_2 as well as blood pH (31, 34, 117), the efferent fibers serving the breathing muscles. Thus, as the paralysis advances in severity, a respiratory acidosis is established, which can initially still be compensated by an increase in the breathing frequencies from 15/ to 76/min (36, 71). With further progress of the paralysis, continuing larger numbers of nerve fibers become impaired, concomitantly the breathing frequency now diminishes also as the result of the steadily increasing damage to the muscle cells. Thus, the still remaining alveolar ventilation is inadequate for the required oxygen demand of the internal breathing. With the lowered alveolar oxygen pressure a continual portion of the hemoglobin remains unsaturated with the consequence that a hypoxemia develops and, because of the increasing arterial carbonic acid concentration, retention of CO_2 in the blood results leading ultimately to a hypercapnia and a decrease in blood pH. If compensating possibilities no longer exist, a respiratory acidosis with impairment of the regulatory circuit of breathing is established, which, as a life-threatening situation, eventually causes irreversible damage particularly to the central nervous system as well as to all vital organs and thereby leads to the death of the sheep (34, 117).

In temporal parallelism with the clinical manifestation of a paresis or paralysis, the plasma lysozyme activity also increased in sheep. As the result of the toxin action on neurons and possibly even on glia cells, it is to be considered that the cell-bound lysozyme is liberated in a reactive form as a mechanism of the natural defence against microorganisms in or near the function-carrying parenchyma of the peripheral nerves and is subsequently passaged into the blood plasma (31, 32, 34, 111).

In order to isolate the neurotoxin, the changes in the protein pattern of female *R. evertsi evertsi* during infestation on sheep were investigated first (107, 109). Results showed that the total protein content increased from 4.2 µg/gland before feeding to 33 µg/gland on the fourth day of repletion. This amount remained relatively constant during the entire repletion process. SDS-gradient gel electrophoresis of salivary gland extracts revealed the presence of 35 distinct protein bands at positions corresponding to the molecular mass of 15.5 kDa to 145 kDa. Twenty proteins were present in unfed as well as in fed female ticks and 13 additional proteins appeared from the fourth day of infestation and persisted up to complete engorgement. Two proteins with a molecular mass of 65 kDa and 37 kDa were only observed after mating from the fifth feeding day, at which time ticks reach their in vivo identified toxic phase of the extremely narrow individual body mass range of 15 to 21 mg (28, 30, 31, 34, 35, 38, 63, 65).

Because mice, rats, hamsters, *Meriones unguiculatus*, *Mastomys natalensis*, guinea pigs, and rabbits are not or only slightly sensitive to the neurotoxin (64) a very sensitive in vitro assay employing a nerve muscle preparation of *Xenopus laevis* was developed. In this in vitro assay it was eventually shown (82, 110, 132, 133) that only one fraction, obtained through chromatofocusing from salivary glands of female ticks in exclusively the sucking phase of 15 to 21 mg, caused complete inhibition of impulse propagation. The inhibition was reversible since washing of the nerve with Ringer solution restored its conduction capacity completely. Through isoelectric focusing the HPLC gel permeation a pI of 6 and a molecular mass of 68 kDa were demonstrated for the toxic fraction. The toxin was inhibited by pronase and neutralized by immune serum. Therefore, the toxin has to be defined as a protein and corresponds to the noxious substance which is inoculated during the natural repletion process (82, 110, 132, 133) and induces an immunity (62).

Ixodes holocyclus

The pathogenetic principle of the paralysis due to *I. holocyclus*, of which essential aspects have probably not been studied yet, was initially interpreted as an affection of the central nervous system, particularly the medulla (14). The earliest experimental neurophysiological investigations showed no differences between reactions of normal and paralyzed dogs after electrical stimulation of the peroneal, femoral, and median nerves. It was thus concluded that in *I. holocyclus* paralysis only the motor anterior horn neurons as well as the cranial nerve cells were affected; the peripheral nerves and the cerebral cortex appeared to be functionally unimpaired (116). It was also contemplated that the tick toxin has a wide range of action with selective points of attack at the vagus center and at the synapses and also functions as an allergen (93). A toxin complex with components acting either specifically on the spinal cord or on the vagus center in the medulla oblongata was also postulated (73) and the causal participation of several toxins in this disease syndrome was emphasized (81). As a biochemical abnormality in paralytic mice, an extra- and intramitochondrial inhibition of enzyme reactions dependent on nicotinamide adenine dinucleotide coenzyme and a suppression of oxidative phosphorylation in tissue homogenates and subcellular particle preparations of the gastrocnemius muscle, central nervous system, and liver were indicated. In contrast, the functions of acetylcholine esterase as well as those of the acetylcholine synthesizing enzyme in the central nervous system were normal (81). In further investigations into the pathomechanism, no morphological manifest ultrastructural changes were demonstrated in the motor end plate of rats and mice dead or dying from *I. holocyclus* paralysis (72). The possibility was also discussed that the toxin intervenes presynaptically (8, 9). Furthermore, the toxin seems to act extremely slowly in vivo and in vitro, because the normal functioning of a nerve muscle preparation was unaffected by a 4-h exposure to the toxin (129).

Neuropathophysiologically, the paralysis due to *I. holocyclus* is still evaluated differently. Thus, a reduction of the nerve conduction velocity from 60 to 30 m/s in a paralyzed human was documented (112), but it was also reported that the amplitudes of the nerve compound action potentials in paralyzed mice remained unchanged (10, 11). In vitro investigations on nerve muscle preparations from paralyzed mice showed temperature-dependent differences in the muscle reaction after nerve stimulation as well as in end-plate potentials, also under the action of *d*-tubocurarine and increased concentrations of $MgCl_2$. End-plate potentials with amplitudes up to 10 mV could be recorded in the range of 15° to 30°C but not upon incubation at higher temperatures. Accordingly it was deduced that the toxin of *I. holocyclus* has a direct temperature-sensitive action on the excitation-secretion mechanism at the myoneural synapse, and thereby prevents the liberation of acetylcholine above 30°C. Because the spontaneous diffusion of the transmitter substance was unaffected by blockage of the induced liberation, it was considered that the toxin does not interfere with the direct liberation of the transmitter but rather with some steps between depolarization of the terminal membrane and the release. In addition a possible impairment in the influx of Ca^{2+} ions, essential for induced liberation was discussed (10, 11). The clinical practice in Australia of keeping patients with paralysis cool may thus have some scientific basis. Because of a temperature-dependent inhibition of transmitter release at the myoneural synapse, it was suspected that even a very small drop in body temperature could have a favorable influence on the course of the disease (118).

Further investigations do not relate to the actual modus operandi of the pathogenesis, but to the secondary actions of the toxin only, revealing at first that the toxicosis induced by female adult ticks in dogs is clinically manifested as a rapid, ascending, flaccid paralysis within 5.5 to 7 days post-infestation and leads to death after 18.4 to 31.2 h of disease duration. The reflex excitability was diminished and totally suppressed in the final stages, the breathing became continuously difficult during the course of the disease, whereas the reaction to painful stimuli was progressively reduced (80). With advancing paralysis the arterial Po_2 dropped from 97.45 to 55.64 mmHg, simultaneously the Pco_2 rose from 25.4 to 51.36 mmHg and pH changed from 7.395 to 7.203. The plasma values of standard bicarbonate fell from 19.20 to 17.74 mmol/l and that of potassium, urea, and bilirubin declined significantly, whereas those for glucose, cholesterol, and creatine kinase were increased. The hemoglobin concentration changed significantly from 147.1 to 166.8 g/l (76). An assessment of the respiratory functions revealed a progressive fall in the respiratory rate from 29.9 to 13.3 breaths/min, in the expiratory minute volume from 5.686 to 2.556 l with simultaneous increase in the expiratory time from 1.29 to 2.68 s. Furthermore, the Pco_2 and the pH value of the arterial blood increased, whereas the Po_2 decreased (77). Electrocardiographic changes varied considerably. Dysrhythmias tended to be a sinus or ventricular tachycardia or sinus arrest in the initial phases of the disease. In moribund dogs, sinus bradycardia predominated. Cardiovascular measurements indicated an increase in peripheral vascular resistance with significant elevation of the arterial pressure including the pulmonary arterial pressure (75, 79). Arterial hypertentions were attenuated by therapeutic intervention with phenoxybenzamine hydrochloride, an α-adrenergic blocker and through combined administration of hyperimmune serum, the survival rate of dogs with advanced degree of paralysis could be considerably enhanced (78). The hypertension and peripheral vasoconstriction possibly impair the perfusion at the neuromuscular junction and thus prolong the paralysis (113).

In continuation of the already documented findings and conclusions concerning the noxious substance responsible for the paralysis (33), it was further demonstrated that the toxin is most probably a protein, the paralyzing activity being reduced by 50% through papain. This enzyme hydrolyzed 88% of the protein present in a crude extract of salivary glands. However, pronase, which is a mixture of proteolytic enzymes, caused no loss of paralyzing activity but digested 78% of the total protein in these extracts (119). The molecular mass was determined to be between 40 and 80 kDa (118). The toxin was supposedly been isolated in a highly purified from (120). Details of its chemical characteristics are, however, not reported yet. Female ticks also secrete potent allergens (20, 22, 23).

In addition to the already reviewed results (33), it was further established that rabbits were successfully immunized against the toxin by intramuscular injection of a crude extract or by a partially purified toxic fraction of salivary glands obtained from female *I. holocyclus* ticks on the fifth to sixth day of infestation; 33.4 μg and 19.5 μg IgG obtained from the serum totally or approximately by 50%, respectively, neutralized 1 μg of crude toxin (125, 126). A long lasting, effective immunity was also observed in dogs after subcutaneous application of salivary gland crude extracts (21, 127, 128, 136) with pronounced toxin neutralizing potency in their serum (21, 127). Glutaraldehyde treatment resulted in a detoxication for rabbits (123) and dogs (124) with simultaneous enhancement of the immunogenicity of the toxoid.

The toxin is present in the saliva of the ticks as shown by in vitro feeding using silicone membranes (121, 122) and was isolated and enriched by means of ultrafiltration and gelpermeation chromatography. One of two main fractions separated through gel chromatography contained most of the toxin as assayed by inoculation into 4- to 5-g mice. In addition, the elution behavior on Ultragel AC44 of the toxic fraction obtained from the feeding medium was similar to that of the toxic component extracted from salivary glands (122).

Ultrastructural investigations of salivary glands first suggested that the paralysis toxin probably originates in the "b" cells of acinus II because of the coincidence of maximal toxicity of female ticks on the fourth to the sixth repletion day and the highest level of synthesizing activity and the peak of granular accumulation (118, 119). In contrast, transmission electron microscopic investigations of salivary glands, treated with IgG antibodies against a highly purified component from a paralyzing fraction and labelled by means of a protein-A-colloidal gold conjugate, rather indicated "e" cells of acinus III as source of the toxin (120).

Conclusions

In further investigations, it should be aspired to isolate the toxins and to pursue the dynamics of toxin production by means of in vitro cultivation of the responsible tick species as well as to develop an in vitro test system for the demonstration of the toxin and for detailed elucidation of the pathomechanism. In vitro systems are essential premises for standardizable and thus reproducible experimental investigations, which should be conducted with pure toxins. Sufficient quantities of toxin ought to become available for this purpose through use of recombinant DNA technology.

References

1. Alexander, R.M., 1952, Tick paralysis. Report of a case in Florida, *J.A.M.A.* **149**:931–932.
2. Alt, H., 1971, Die Zeckenparalysen bei Mensch und Tier sowie ein Beitrag zur Pathogenese der durch *Argas (Persicargas) persicus* (Oken, 1818)—Larven bedingten Lähme der Hühner, *Inaug. Diss.* Justus-Liebig-Universität Giessen.
3. Amese, J.W., and Lyday, J.H., 1939, Tick paralysis in Colorado, *Rocky Mount. Med. J.* **36**:640–641.
4. Barnett, E.J., 1937, Wood tick paralysis in children, *J.A.M.A.* **109**:846–848.
5. Boffey, G.C., and Paterson, D.C., 1973, Creatine phosphokinase elevation in a case of tick paralysis, *Can. Med. Assoc. J.* **108**:866–868.
6. Cherington, M., and Snyder, R.D., 1968, Tick paralysis: neurophysiological studies, *N. Engl. J. Med.* **278**;95–97.
7. Chrisman, C.L., 1975, Differentiation of tick paralysis and acute idiopathic polyradiculoneuritis in the dog using electromyography, *J. Am. Anim. Hosp. Asosc.* **11**:455–458.
8. Cooper, B.J., 1974, (Personal communication quoted in: Sutherland, S.K., 1974, Venomous Australian creatures: The action of their toxins and the care of the envenomated patient, *Anaesth. Intensive Care* **4**:316–328.

9. Cooper, B.J., 1975, (Discussion on the mechanism of action of the toxin. Bagnall, B.C., and Doube, B.M. (eds): in The Australian paralysis tick *Ixodes holocyclus*, *Aust. Vet. J.* **51**:159–160.
10. Cooper, B.J., Cooper, B.L., Ilkiw, J.E., and Kelly, J.D., 1976, Tick paralysis, *Sydney Univ. Postgrad. Comm. Vet. Sci. Proc.* **30**:57–61.
11. Cooper, B.J., and Spence, I., 1976, Temperature-dependent inhibition of evoked acetylcholine release in tick paralysis, *Nature, London* **263**:693–695.
12. Dash, M., and Byambaa, B., 1989, Ixodid ticks as parasites, *Proc. 13. Conf. World Assoc. Adv. Vet. Parasitol.* p. 42, Berlin.
13. De Busk, F.L., and O'Connor, S., 1972, Tick toxicosis, *Pediatrics* **50**:328–329.
14. Dodd, S., 1921, Tick paralysis, *J. Comp. Pathol. Ther.* **34**:309–323.
15. Duffy, D.C., 1985, (Personal communication quoted in Hoogstraal, H., Argasid and Nuttalliellid ticks as parasites and vectors. *Adv. Parasitol.*, **24**:135–238.
16. Emmons, P., and McLennan, H., 1959, Failure of acetylcholine release in tick paralysis, *Nature, London* **183**:474–475.
17. Emmons, P., and McLennan, H., 1980, Some observations on tick paralysis in marmots, *J. Exp. Biol.* **37**:355–362.
18. Esplin, D.W., Philip, C.B., and Hughes, L.E., 1960, Impairment of muscle stretch reflexes in tick paralysis, *Science* **132**:958–959.
19. Fourie, L.J., Horak, I.G., and Marais, L., 1988, An undescribed *Rhipicephalus* species associated with field paralysis of Angora goats, *J. South Afr. Vet. Assoc.* **59**:47–49.
20. Gauci, M., Loh, R.K.S., Stone, B.F., and Thong, Y.H., 1989, Allergic reactions to the Australian paralysis tick, *Ixodes holocyclus*: Diagnostic evaluation by skin test and radioimmunoassay, *Clin. Exp. Allergy* **19**:279–283.
21. Gauci, M., Morrison, J.J., and Stone, B.F., 1986, Determination of serum antibody titres to salivary gland antigens of the Australian paralysis tick *Ixodes holocyclus*, Howell, M.J., (ed): in *Handb. 6th Int. Congr. Parasitol. Brisbane*, Aust. Acad. Sci., Canberra, p. 135.
22. Gauci, M., Stone, B.F., and Thong, Y.H., 1988, Detection in allergic individuals of IgE specific for the Australian paralysis tick, *Ixodes holocyclus*, *Int. Arch. Allergy Appl. Immunol.* **85**:190–193.
23. Gauci, M., Stone, B.F., and Thong, Y.H., 1988, Isolation and immunological characterisation of allergens from salivary glands of the Australian paralysis tick *Ixodes holocyclus*, *Int. Arch. Allergy Appl. Immunol.* **87**:208–212.
24. Gothe, R., 1971, Die durch *Argas (Persicargas) persicus*-Larven bedingte Paralyse der Hühner. I. Über den Einfluss des Saugzustandes und der Infestationsrate auf die klinische Manifestation, *Z. Parasitenkd.* **35**:298–307.
25. Gothe, R., 1971, Die durch *Argas (Persicargas) persicus*-Larven bedingte Paralyse der Hühner. II. Untersuchungen zur Immunität, *Z. Parasitenkd.* **35**: 308–317.
26. Gothe, R., 1972, Pathogenitätsmechanismen bei Zeckenparalysen, *Proc. 6th Tag. Dtsch. Tropenmed. Ges. Montreux*, pp. 21–22.
27. Gothe, R., 1981, Biological and pathogenic aspects of the *Rhipicephalus evertsi evertsi*—paralysis, *Proc. 9th Int. Conf. World Assoc. Adv. Vet. Parasitol. Budapest*, p. 185.
28. Gothe, R., 1981, The toxic phase of paralysis inducing female *Rhipicephalus evertsi evertsi* Neumann, 1897, during repletion and aspects on the patho-

mechanism of this toxicosis. Whitehead, G.B., and Gibson, J.D. (eds): in *Proc. Int. Conf. Tick Biol. Control*, Grahamstown, South Africa, p. 13.

29. Gothe, R., 1982, Pathophysiology of *Rhipicephalus evertsi evertsi* infestations implicating a tick paralysis, *Toxicon* **20**(Suppl. 1)22.
30. Gothe, R., 1982, Parasite–host interactions, pathogenic mechanisms and immunity of *Rhipicephalus evertsi*-paralysis, *Proc. 5th Int. Congr. Parasitol. Toronto, Canada*, Vol. 1:422.
31. Gothe, R., 1983, The *Rhipicephalus evertsi evertsi*-paralysis: On the causal genesis in the repletion and the pathogenic effect, *Zentralbl. Bakteriol. Hyg.* [*A*]**256**:262.
32. Gothe, R., 1984, Pathophysiological consequences of a tick infestation: *Rhipicephalus evertsi evertsi* in sheep, *Proc. 4th Eur. Multicolloq. Parasitol. Izmir, Turkey*, p. 246.
33. Gothe, R., 1984, Tick paralyses: Reasons for appearing during ixodid and argasid feeding. *Curr. Top. Vector Res.* **2**:199–223.
34. Gothe, R., 1985, Pathogenese bei Befall mit Arthropoden, *Berl. Muench. Tieraerztl. Wochenschr.* **98**:274–279.
35. Gothe, R., and Bezuidenhout, J.D., 1986, Studies on the ability of different strains or populations of female *Rhipicephalus evertsi evertsi* (Acarina: Ixodidae) to produce paralysis in sheep, *Onderstepoort J. Vet. Res.* **53**:19–24.
36. Gothe, R., and Budelmann, K., 1980, Zur toxischen Phase Paralyse—induzierender weiblicher *Rhipicephalus evertsi evertsi* Neumann, 1897, während der Repletion, *Zentralbl. Veterinaermed. B* **27**:524–543.
37. Gothe, R., and Englert, R., 1978, Quantitative Untersuchungen zur Toxinwirkung von Larven neoarktischer *Persicargas* spp. bei Hühnern, *Zentralbl. Veterinaermed. B* **25**:122–133.
38. Gothe, R., Gold, Y., and Bezuidenhout, J.D., 1986, Investigations into the paralysis-inducing ability of *Rhipicephalus evertsi mimeticus* and that of hybrids between this subspecies and *Rhipicephalus evertsi evertsi*, *Onderstepoort J. Vet. Res.* **53**:25–29.
39. Gothe, R., Hager, H., Jehn, E., Kunze, K., and Thoenes, W., 1971, Pathologisch—anatomische Untersuchungen an peripheren Nerven bei der durch *Argas (Persicargas) persicus*-Larven bedingten Zeckenparalyse der Hühner, *Z. Tropenmed. Parasitol.* **22**:285–291.
40. Gothe, R., and Koop, E., 1974, Zur biologischen Bewertung der Validität von *Argas (Persicargas) persicus* (Oken, 1818), *Argas (Persicargas) arboreus* Kaiser, Hoogstraal und Kohls, 1964 und *Argas (Persicargas) walkerae* Kaiser und Hoogstraal, 1969. I. Untersuchungen zur Entwicklungsbiologie. *Z. Parasitenkd.* **44**:299–317.
41. Gothe, R., and Koop, E., 1974, Zur biologischen Bewertung der Validität von *Argas (Persicargas) persicus* (Oken, 1818), *Argas (Persicargas) arboreus* Kaiser, Hoogstraal und Kohls, 1964 und *Argas (Persicargas) walkerae* Kaiser und Hoogstraal, 1969. II. Kreuzungsversuche, *Z. Parasitenkd.* **44**:319–328.
42. Gothe, R., and Koop, E., 1974, Biological evaluation on the validity of *Argas (Persicargas) persicus*, *Argas (Persicargas) arboreus* and *Argas (Persicargas) walkerae*, *Proc. 3th Int. Congr. Parasitol. (Munich)* **2**:957–958.
43. Gothe, R., and Kraft, W., 1972, Untersuchungen von Serum-Elektrolyten, Pseudocholinesterasen, Glukose und unveresterten Fettsäuren bei der durch *Argas (Persicargas) persicus*-Larven induzierten Zeckenparalyse der Hühner, *Zentralbl. Veterinaermed. B* **19**:213–216.

44. Gothe, R., and Kraft, W., 1972, Zur Pathophysiologie der durch *Persicargas* induzierten Zeckenparalyse. *Z. Parasitenkd.* **39**:73.
45. Gothe, R., and Kunze, K., 1970, Untersuchungen zur Pathogenese und Klinik der durch *Argas (Persicargas) persicus*—Larven bedingten Paralyse der Hühner, *J. Parasitol.* **56**:123.
46. Gothe, R., and Kunze, K., 1971, Zur Erregungsleitung von efferenten und afferenten peripheren Nervenfasern bei der durch *Argas (Persicargas) persicus*—Larven bedingten Zeckenparalyse der Hühner. *Z. Tropenmed. Parasitol.* **22**:292–296.
47. Gothe, R., and Kunze, K., 1971, Untersuchungen der afferenten und efferenten Anteile peripherer Nerven im Verlauf der durch *Argas (Persicargas) persicus*—Larven bedingten Paralyse der Hühner, *Proc. 5th Tag. Dtsch. Tropenmed. Ges. (Tübingen)* p. 38.
48. Gothe, R., and Kunze, K., 1973, Zur Neuropharmakologie der Zeckenparalyse, *Proc. 6th Int. Conf. World Assoc. Adv. Vet. Parasitol. (Vienna)* (Abstract).
49. Gothe, R., and Kunze, K., 1974, Neuropharmacological investigations on tick paralysis of chickens induced by larvae of *Argas (Persicargas) walkerae*, Soulsby, E.J.L. (ed): in Parasitic zoonoses. *Clinical and experimental studies*, Acad. Press, Inc., New York, San Francisco, London, pp. 369–382.
50. Gothe, R., and Kunze, K., 1976, Zur Vulnerabilität des Nervus ischiadicus bei der durch *Argas (Persicargas) walkerae* induzierten Zeckenparalyse, *Z. Parasitenkd.* **50**:188.
51. Gothe, R., and Kunze, K., 1977, New aspects in pathogenicity of tick paralysis, *Proc. 8th Int. Conf. World Assoc. Adv. Vet. Parasitol. (Sydney)*, (Abstract No. 70).
52. Gothe, R., and Kunze, K., 1978, The in vitro vulnerability of peripheral nerves in tick paralysis, *Proc. 4th Int. Conf. Parasitol. (Warsaw)* Sect. C, p. 213.
53. Gothe, R., and Kunze, K., 1978, Neurophysiologische Differenzierung der Zeckenparalyse in vitro, *Zentralbl. Bakteriol. Parasitenkd. Infektionskr. Hyg. Abt. I: Ref.* **257**:34–35.
54. Gothe, R., Buchheim, C., and Schrecke, W., 1981, Zur Paralyse-induzierenden Kapazität wildstämmiger *Argas (Persicargas) persicus*- und *Argas (Argas) africolumbae*-Populationen aus Obervolta. *Berl. Muench. Tieraerztl. Wochenschr.* **94**:299–302.
55. Gothe, R., and Kunze, K., 1979, Die durch *Rhipicephalus evertsi evertsi* induzierte Zeckenparalyse der Schafe, *Proc. 21st World Vet. Congr. (Moskwa)* **2**:62–63.
56. Gothe, R., and Kunze, K., 1980, The *Rhipicephalus evertsi evertsi* paralysis, biological aspects and pathogenesis, *Proc. 3rd Eur. Multicolloq. Parasitol. (Cambridge)*, p. 73.
57. Gothe, R., and Kunze, K., 1981, Zur Neuropathophysiologie der *Rhipicephalus evertsi evertsi*—Paralyse, *Zentralbl. Veterinaermed. B* **28**:241–248.
58. Gothe, R., and Kunze, K., 1982, Aktionspotentiale und Leitungsgeschwindigkeiten des Nervus tibialis bei der *Rhipicephalus evertsi evertsi*—Paralyse der Schafe, *Zentralbl. Veterinaermed. B* **29**:186–192.
59. Gothe, R., Kunze, K., and Alt, H., 1970, Zur Zeckenparalyse der Hühner, *Z. Parasitenkd.* **34**:31.

60. Gothe, R., Kunze, K., and Hoogstraal, H., 1979, The mechanisms of pathogenicity in the tick paralyses. *J. Med. Entomol.* **16**:357–369.
61. Gothe, R., Kunze, K., and Mechow, O., 1971, Untersuchungen über die Todesursache bei der durch *Argas (Persicargas) persicus*—Larven bedingten Zeckenparalyse der Hühner, *Z. Tropenmed. Parasitol.* **22**:430–435.
62. Gothe, R., and Lämmler, M., 1981, Zur antitoxischen Immunität bei der *Rhipicephalus evertsi evertsi*—Paralyse der Schafe, *Zentralbl. Veterinaermed. B* **29**:107–118.
63. Gothe, R., and Lämmler, M., 1982, Zur sektoralen Einordnung der Toxizität im Repletionsprozeß Paralyse—induzierender weiblicher *Rhipicephalus evertsi evertsi* Neumann, 1897, *Zentralbl. Veterinaermed. B* **29**:37–50.
64. Gothe, R., and Lämmler, M., 1982, Zur Sensitivität von Laboratoriumstieren gegenüber der *Rhipicephalus evertsi evertsi*—Paralyse, *Zentralbl. Veterinaermed. B* **29**:249–252.
65. Gothe, R., Neitz, A.W.H., and Bezuidenhout, J.D., 1987, *Argas walkerae* and *Rhipicephalus evertsi* paralysis: Etiology and mechanisms of pathogenesis, *Proc. 6th Entomol. Congr. Entomol. Soc. South. Afr. (Stellenosch)*, pp. 113–114.
66. Gothe, R., and Riethmüller, H., 1972, Untersuchungen über den Partialdruck von Kohlendioxyd und Sauerstoff sowie den pH-Wert des Blutes bei der durch *Argas (Persicargas) persicus*—Larven induzierten Zeckenparalyse der Hühner, *Zentralbl. Veterinaermed. B* **19**:217–220.
67. Gothe, R., and Verhalen, K.H., 1975, Zur Paralyse-induzierenden Kapazität verschiedener *Persicargas*-Arten und -Populationen bei Hühnern. *Zentralbl. Veterinaermed. B* **22**:98–112.
68. Gregson, J.D., 1959, Tick paralysis in groundhogs, guinea pigs and hamsters, *Can. J. Comp. Med.* **23**:266–268.
69. Gulyásh, M., 1952, Untersuchungen über die Ursache der Lähmungserscheinungen von mit Hühnerzecken (*Argas persicus*) befallenen Hühnern. *Acta. Vet. Hung.* **2**:41–67 (In Russian, German summary).
70. Haller, J.S., and Fabara, J.A., 1972, Tick paralysis. Case report with emphasis on neurological toxicity, *Am. J. Dis. Child.* **124**:915–917.
71. Hamel, H.D., and Gothe, R., 1978, Influence of infestation rate on tick-paralysis in sheep induced by *Rhipicephalus evertsi evertsi* Neumann, 1897, *Vet. Parasitol.* **4**:183–191.
72. Hamilton, R.C., and Cooper, B.J., 1974, (Personal communication quoted in Sutherland S.K., 1974, Venomous Australian creatures: The action of their toxins and the care of the envenomated patient, *Anaesth. Intensive Care* **4**: 316–328.
73. Hindmarsh, W.L., and Pursell, R.T., 1935, Tick paralysis of dogs. Mortality after serum treatment, *Aust. Vet. J.* **11**:229–243.
74. Hoogstraal, H., 1985, Argasid and nutalliellid ticks as parasites and vectors. *Adv. Parasitol.* **24**:135–238.
75. Ilkiw, J.E., 1980, Tick paralysis in Australia, Kirk, R.W., (ed): in *Curr. Vet. Ther. VII Small Anim. Pract.*, Philadelphia, London, Toronto, W.B. Saunders Comp., pp. 777–779.
76. Ilkiw, J.E., and Turner, D.M., 1987, Infestation in the dog by the paralysis tick *Ixodes holocyclus*. 2. Blood-gas and pH, haematological and biochemical findings, *Aust. Vet. J.* **64**:139–142.

77. Ilkiw, J.E., and Turner, D.M., 1987, Infestation in the dog by the paralysis tick *Ixodes holocyclus*. 3. Respiratory effects, *Aust. Vet. J.* **64**:142–144.
78. Ilkiw, J.E., and Turner, D.M., 1988, Infestation in the dog by the paralysis tick, *Ixodes holocyclus*. 5. Treatment, *Aust. Vet. J.* **65**:236–238.
79. Ilkiw, J.E., Turner, D.M., and Goodman, A.H., 1988, Infestation in the dog by the paralysis tick, *Ixodes holocyclus*. 4. Cardiovascular effects, *Aust. Vet. J.* **65**:232–235.
80. Ilkiw, J.E., Turner, D.M., and Howlett, C.R., 1987, Infestation in the dog by the paralysis tick *Ixodes holocyclus*. 1. Clinical and histological findings, *Aust. Vet. J.* **64**:137–139.
81. Koch, J.H., 1967, Some aspects of tick paralysis in dogs, *Proc. Aust. Vet. Assoc. N.S.W. Div.* **3**:34–35.
82. Kraiss, A., Gothe, R., Gold, Y., and Neitz, A.W.H., 1987, *Rhipicephalus evertsi mimeticus*: Developmental biology and pathogenicity for sheep, *Int. J. Microbiol. Hyg. Ser. A* **265**:519.
83. Kunze, K., and Gothe, R., 1971, Neurophysiological investigations in tick paralysis, *Proc. 4th Int. Congr. Electromyography (Brussels)*, pp. 86–87.
84. Kunze, K., and Gothe, R., 1971, Die durch *Argas (Persicargas) persicus*—Larven bedingte Paralyse der Hühner. III. Neurophysiologische Untersuchungen. *Z. Parasitenkd.* **36**:251–264.
85. Kunze, K., and Gothe, R., 1978, Zur Vulnerabilität peripherer Nerven und Toxinbindung bei der durch *Argas (Persicargas) walkerae* induzierten Zeckenparalyse der Hühner, *Z. Parasitenkd.* **56**:275–285.
86. Kunze, K., and Gothe, R., 1979, Neurophysiologische Untersuchungen bei Zeckenparalyse, *Z. Electroencephalgr. Electromyogr. verw. Geb.* **10**:48.
87. Kunze, K., and Gothe, R., 1979, Nerve function and anoxia in tick paralysis, *Acta Neurol. Scand.* **73**:184.
88. Kunze, K., Gothe, R., and Muskat, E., 1970, Neurophysiologische Untersuchungen bei experimentellen Polyneuropathien, *Pfluegers Arch.* **319**:125.
89. Lämmler, G., Gothe, R., Zahner, H., and Schütze, H.-R., 1977, Parasitäre Modellinfektionen und -Infestationen als Grundlage angewandter Forschung, *Tieraerztl. Umsch.* **32**:354–358.
90. Lagos, J.C., and Thies, R.E., 1969, Tick paralysis without muscle weakness, *Arch. Neurol., Chicago* **21**:471–474.
91. Marais, L.C., 1987, A new paralysis tick, *Proc. 6th Entomol. Congr. Entomol. Soc. South. Afr. (Stellenbosch)*, p. 99.
92. Marais, L., Fourie, L.J., and Horak, I.G., 1987, An addition to the list of paralysis inducing ticks of veterinary importance, *Proc. 6th Entomol. Congr. Entomol. Soc. South. Afr. (Stellenbosch)*, p. 100.
93. McKay, W.J.S., 1933, Facial paralysis following tick-bite, *Med. J. Aust.* **1**:204–205.
94. McKilligan, N., 1987, Causes of nesting losses in the cattle egret *Ardeola ibis* in eastern Australia with special reference to the pathogenicity of the tick *Argas (Persicargas) robertsi* to nestlings, *Aust. J. Ecol.* **12**:9–16.
95. McLennan, H., and Oikawa, I., 1972, Changes in function of the neuromuscular junction occurring in tick paralysis, *Can. J. Physiol. Pharmacol.* **50**: 53–58.
96. Morris, H.H., 1977, Tick paralysis: Electrophysiologic measurements, *South. Med. J.* **70**:121–122.

97. Murnaghan, M.F., 1955, Tick paralysis, *Rev. Can. Biol.* **14**:273–274.
98. Murnaghan, M.F., 1958, Tick paralysis in the dog: a neurophysiological study, *Proc. 10th Int. Congr. Entomol. (Montreal)* **3**:841–847.
99. Murnaghan, M.F., 1958, Neuro-anatomical site in tick paralysis. *Nature London* **181**:131.
100. Murnaghan, M.F., 1959, A defect in the release mechanism of acetylcholine caused by tick paralysis, *Proc. Can. Fed. Biol. Soc.* **2**:48–49.
101. Murnaghan, M.F., 1960, Conduction block of terminal somatic motor fibers in tick paralysis, *Can. J. Biochem. Physiol.* **38**:287–295.
102. Murnaghan, M.F., 1960, Motor nerve fibre conduction in tick paralysis, *Fed. Proc. Fed. Am. Soc. Exp. Biol.* **19**:298.
103. Murnaghan, M.F., 1960, Site and mechanism of tick paralysis, *Science* **131**: 418–419.
104. Murnaghan, M.F., 1961, Nerve fiber conduction block in tick paralysis, *Rev. Can. Biol.* **20**:19–24.
105. Murnaghan, M.F., and McConnaill, M., 1967, Peroneal nerve conduction in tick paralysis, *Ir. J. Med. Sci.* **502**:473–477.
106. Murnaghan, M.F., and O'Rourke, F.J., 1978, Tick paralysis, Bettini, S. (ed): in *Arthropod venoms*, Springer-Verlag, Berlin, Heidelberg, New York, pp. 419–464.
107. Neitz, A.W.H., and Gothe, R., 1986, Changes in the protein pattern in the salivary glands of paralysis inducing female *Rhipicephalus evertsi evertsi* during infestation, *Zentralbl. Veterinaermed. B* **33**:213–220.
108. Neitz, A.W.H., Viljoen, G.J., Bezuidenhout, J.D., Gothe, R., Oberem, P.T., and Vermeulen, N.M.J., 1987, Partial purification of toxic component present in *Argas (Persicargas) walkerae* larvae, *Proc. 6th Entomol. Congr. Entomol. Soc. South Afr. (Stellenbosch)*, pp. 103–104.
109. Neitz, A.W.H., Viljoen, G.J., Gothe, R., Bezuidenhout, J.D., Oberem, P.T., and Vermeulen, N.M.J., 1987, Quantitative changes in the protein pattern in the salivary glands of paralysis—inducing female *Rhipicephalus evertsi evertsi* during infestation, *Proc. 6th Entomol. Congr. Entomol. Soc. South Afr. (Stellenbosch)*, pp. 114–115.
110. Neitz, A.W.H., Viljoen, G.J., Gothe, R., Visser, L., and Vermeulen, N.M.J., 1986, Isolation of a neurotoxin from the salivary glands of female *Rhipicephalus evertsi evertsi* causing spring lamb paralysis, *Proc. 1st Jt. Congr. South Afr. Biochem. Soc., South Afr. Genet. Soc., South Afr. Soc. Microbiol. (Witwatersrand)*, p. 161.
111. Nolte, I., and Gothe, R., 1982, Zur Plasmalysozymaktivität bei der durch *Rhipicephalus evertsi evertsi* induzierten Zeckenparalyse der Schafe, *Berl. Muench. Tieraerztl. Wochenschr.* **95**:143–145.
112. Pearn, J., 1982, Clinical aspects of tick envenomation of humans. International seminar on the nature of the problem of tick envenomation for man and animals, the extent of the problem and its treatment, *Working paper*, 7 pp. *7th World Congr. Anim. Plant Microb. Toxins (Brisbane)*.
113. Prescott, C.W., 1984, Ticks, spiders, insects, cane toads, platypus venom intoxications, *Aust. Vet. Pract.* **14**:111–116.
114. Rose, I., 1954, (Unpublished data quoted in: Rose I., Gregson, J.D., 1956, Evidence of a neuromuscular block in tick paralysis, *Nature London* **178**: 95–96.)

115. Rose, I., and Gregson, J.D., 1956, Evidence of a neuromuscular block in tick paralysis, *Nature London* **178**:95–96.
116. Ross, I.C., 1926, An experimental study of tick paralysis in Australia, *Parasitology* **18**:410–429.
117. Schniewind, A., Gothe, R., and Neu, H., 1983, Zur Pathophysiologie der durch *Rhipicephalus evertsi evertsi* Neumann, 1897, induzierten Zeckenparalyse der Schafe, *Berl. Muench. Tieraerztl. Wochenschr.* **96**:81–85.
118. Stone, B.F., 1988, Tick paralysis, particularly involving *Ixodes holocyclus* and other *Ixodes* species, *Adv. Dis. Vector Res.* **5**:61–85. Heidelberg, London, Paris, Tokyo.
119. Stone, B.F. and Binnington, K.C., 1986, The paralyzing toxin and other immunogens of the tick *Ixodes holocyclus* and the role of the salivary gland in their biosynthesis, Saven, J.R., and Hair, J.A. (eds): in Morphology, physiology, and behavioral biology of ticks, Ellis Horwood Limited Publishers, Chichester, pp. 75–99.
120. Stone, B.F., Binnington, K.C., Gauci, M., and Aylward, J.H., 1989, Tick/host interactions for *Ixodes holocyclus*: Role, effects, biosynthesis and nature of its toxic and allergenic oral secretions, *Exp. appl. Acarol.* **7**:59–69.
121. Stone, B.F., Commins, M.A., and Kemp, D.H., 1982, Membrane feeding of the Australian paralysis tick *Ixodes holocyclus* and secretion of toxin, *Toxicon* **20**(Suppl. 1):55.
122. Stone, B.F., Commins, M.A., and Kemp, D.H., 1983, Artificial feeding of the Australian paralysis tick, *Ixodes holocyclus* and collection of paralysing toxin, *Int. J. Parasitol.* **13**:447–454.
123. Stone, B.F., and Neish, A.L., 1984, Tick-paralysis toxoid: An effective immunizing agent against the toxin of *Ixodes holocyclus*, *Aust. J. Exp. Biol. Med. Sci.* **62**:189–191.
124. Stone, B.F., Neish, A.L., Morrison, J.J., and Uren, M.F., 1986, Toxoid stimulation in dogs of high titres of neutralising antibodies against holocyclotoxin, the paralysing toxin of the Australian paralysis tick *Ixodes holocyclus*, *Aust. Vet. J.* **63**:125–127.
125. Stone, B.F., Neish, A.L., and Wright, I.G., 1982, Vaccination of rabbits against the toxin of the Australian paralysis tick *Ixodes holocyclus* and production of high serum titres of neutralizing antibodies, *Toxicon* **20**(Suppl. 1): 56.
126. Stone, B.F., Neish, A.L., and Wright, I.G., 1982, Immunization of rabbits to produce high serum titres of neutralizing antibodies and immunity to the paralyzing toxin of *Ixodes holocyclus*, *Aust. J. Exp. Biol. Med. Sci.* **60**: 351–358.
127. Stone, B.F., Neish, A.L., and Wright, I.G., 1983, Tick (*Ixodes holocyclus*) paralysis in the dog—quantitative studies on immunity following artificial infestation with the tick, *Aust. Vet. J.* **60**:65–68.
128. Stone, B.F., Wright, J.G., and Neish, A.L., 1982, Natural and artificial immunisation of dogs against tick paralysis induced by the Australian paralysis tick *Ixodes holocyclus*, *Toxicon* **20**(Suppl. 1):56.
129. Sutherland, S.K., 1974, Venomous Australian creatures: The action of their toxins and the care of the envenomated patient, *Anaesth. Intensive Care* **4**:316–318.

130. Swift, T.R., and Ignacio, O.J., 1975, Tick paralysis: Electrophysiologic studies, *Neurology* **25**:1130–1133.
131. Taylor, C.W., 1966, Tick paralysis, *Can. Med. Assoc. J.* **95**:125.
132. Viljoen, G.J., Bezuidenhout, J.D., Oberem, P.T., Gothe, R., Vermeulen, N.M.J., and Neitz, A.W.H., 1987, Toxity of salivary gland extracts from paralysis-inducing female *Rhipicephalus evertsi evertsi*, *Proc. 6th Entomol. Congr. Entomol. Soc. South. Afr. (Stellenbosch)*, p. 118.
133. Viljoen, G.J., Bezuidenhout, J.D., Oberem, P.T., Vermeulen, N.M.J., Visser, L., Gothe, R., and Neitz, A.W.H., 1986, Isolation of a neutrotoxin from the salivary glands of female *Rhipicephalus evertsi evertsi*, *J. Parasitol.* **72**:865–874.
134. Viljoen, G.J., Neitz, A.W.H., Bezuidenhout, J.D., Oberem, P.T., Gothe, R., and Vermeulen, N.M.J., 1987, Paralysis-inducing capability of larval and postlarval stages of *Argas (Persicargas) walkerae*, *Proc. 6th Entomol. Congr. Entomol. Soc. South. Afr. (Stellenbosch)*, pp. 109–110.
135. Viljoen, G.J., Van Wyngaardt, S., Gothe, R., Visser, L., Bezuidenhout, J.D., and Neitz, A.W.H., 1990, The detection and isolation of a paralysis toxin present in *Argas (Persicargas) walkerae*, *Onderstepoort J. Vet. Res.* **57**: 163–168.
136. Wright, I.G., Stone, B.F., and Neish, A.L., 1983, Tick (*Ixodes holocyclus*) paralysis in the dog—induction of immunity by injection of toxin, *Aust. Vet. J.* **60**:69–70.

Index